Mechanisms and Treatment of Cardiac Arrhythmias; Relevance of Basic Studies to Clinical Management

Proceedings of the A. N. Richards Symposium sponsored by the Physiological Society of Philadelphia—May 5–6, 1983.

Mechanisms and Treatment of Cardiac Arrhythmias; Relevance of Basic Studies to Clinical Management

Edited by

H. Joseph Reiser, Ph. D.
Berlex Laboratories, Inc.
Cedar Knolls, New Jersey

Leonard N. Horowitz, M.D.
Likoff Cardiovascular Institute
Philadelphia, Pennsylvania

Urban & Schwarzenberg
Baltimore-Munich • 1985

Urban & Schwarzenberg, Inc.
7 E. Redwood Street
Baltimore, Maryland 21202
USA

Urban & Schwarzenberg
Pettenkoferstrasse 18
D-800 München 2
West Germany

Printed in the United States of America

NOTICES

The Editors (or Author(s)) and the Publisher of this work have made every effort to ensure that the drug dosage schedules herein are accurate and in accord with the standards accepted at the time of publication. The reader is strongly advised, however, to check the product information sheet included in the package of each drug he or she plans to administer to be certain that changes have not been made in the recommended dose or in the contraindications for administration.

The Publishers have made an extensive effort to trace original copyright holders for permission to use borrowed material. If any has been overlooked, it will be corrected at the first reprint.

Library of Congress Cataloging in Publication Data

Mechanisms and treatment of cardiac arrhythmias.

Includes index.
1. Arrhythmia. 2. Myocardial depressants. I. Reiser, H. Joseph. II. Horowitz, Leonard. [DNLM: 1. Anti-Arrhythmia Agents—therapeutic use. 2. Anti-Arrhythmia Agents—pharmacodynamics. 3. Arrhythmia—drug therapy.
QV 150 M486]
RC685.A65M418 1984 616.1'28 84-10363
ISBN 0-8067-1621-5

Compositor: Douglas-Innes & Co.
Printer: Port City Press
Manuscript editor: Nancy Wachter
Indexer: Susan Lohmeyer
Production and design: Norman Och and Karen Babcock

ISBN 0-8067-1621-5 Baltimore

ISBN 3-541-71621-5 Munich

To my family for their enduring support; they make it all worthwhile.

Joe

To my wife, Dona, and Adam, Joshua, and Aimee for their patience and support.

Len

Contents

Part I
Mechanisms of Arrhythmias and Antiarrhythmic Drug Action

Part II
Basic and Clinical Effects of Antiarrhythmic Drugs: Classification of Drug Effects

Part III
Therapeutic Applications of Antiarrhythmic Drugs: Cutting Across Drug Classifications

Contributors

Gary J. Anderson, M.D.
Professor of Medicine and Physiology
Likoff Cardiovascular Institute
Hahnemann University School of Medicine
Broad and Vine Streets
Philadelphia, PA 19102

John C. Bailey, M.D.
Professor of Medicine
Krannert Institute of Cardiology
1001 West 10th Street
Indianapolis, Indiana 46202

J.T. Bigger, Jr., M.D.
Professor of Medicine and Pharmacology
Columbia University
Director, Arrhythmia Control Unit
Columbia Presbyterian Medical Center
622 West 168th Street
New York, NY 10032

Paul F. Cranefield, M.D., Ph.D.
Professor, Rockefeller University
1230 York Avenue
New York, NY 10021

Peter Danilo, Jr., Ph.D.
Assistant Professor, Pharmacology and Pediatrics
Department of Pharmacology
Columbia University
College of Physicians and Surgeons
630 West 168th Street
New York, NY 10032

N.A. Mark Estes, III, M.D.
Director, Cardiac Electrophysiology Laboratory
Massachusetts General Hospital
171 Harrison Avenue
Boston, MA 02111

William H. Frishman, M.D.
Chief of Medicine
Hospital of the Albert Einstein College of Medicine
1825 Eastchester Road
Bronx, NY 10461

Hassan Garan, M.D.
Co-Director, Cardiac Electrophysiology Laboratory
Massachusetts General Hospital
171 Harrison Avenue
Boston, MA 02114

Frank J. Green, M.D.
Instructor in Medicine
Krannert Institute of Cardiology
1001 West 10th Street
Indianapolis, Indiana 46202

Charles I. Haffajee, M.D.
Associate Professor of Medicine
Director, Cardiac Electrophysiology and Pacing
University of Massachusetts Medical School
Department of Medicine
Worchester, MA 01605

Eric L. Hagestad
Graduate Student
Department of Physiology and Biophysics
Harvard School of Public Health
665 Huntington Avenue
Boston, MA 02115

Jeffrey L. Hill, Ph.D.
Section Head, Cardiac Pharmacology
Berlex Laboratories, Inc.
110 E. Hanover Avenue
Cedar Knolls, New Jersey 07927
(Current address:
Biosensors, Inc.
PO Box 640
Chester, NY 07930)

Leonard N. Horowitz, M.D.
Director, Clinical Cardiac Electrophysiology Laboratory
Likoff Cardiovascular Institute
Hahnemann University Hospital
Broad and Vine Streets
Philadelphia, PA 19102

Richard J. Kovacs, M.D.
Fellow in Cardiology
Krannert Institute of Cardiology
1001 West 10th Street
Indianapolis, Indiana 46202

Lawrence I. Laifer, M.D.
Cardiology Fellow
Division of Cardiology
Department of Medicine
Albert Einstein College of Medicine
1300 Morris Park Avenue
Bronx, NY 10461

Brian McGovern, M.D.
Cardiac Unit
Massachusetts General Hospital
171 Harrison Avenue
Boston, MA 02114

Eric L. Michelson, M.D.
Chief, Clinical Research
Lankenau Medical Research Center
Lancaster and City Line Avenues
Philadelphia, PA 19151

E. Neil Moore, Ph.D., D.V.M.
Professor of Physiology
University of Pennsylvania
School of Veterinary Medicine
3800 Spruce Street
Philadelphia, PA 19104

Joel Morganroth, M.D.
Professor of Medicine & Pharmacology
Hahnemann University Hospital
Likoff Cardiovascular Institute
230 North Broad Street
Philadelphia, PA 19102

Philip J. Podrid, M.D.
Research Associate in Cardiology,
Cardiovascular Laboratories
Associate Physician in Medicine,
Brigham and Women's Hospital
Lown Cardiovascular Laboratories
Richardson Fuller Building
221 Longwood Avenue
Boston, MA 02115

David P. Rardon, M.D.
Fellow in Cardiology
Krannert Institute of Cardiology
1001 West 10th Street
Indianapolis, Indiana 46202

H. Joseph Reiser, Ph.D.
Director, Pharmacology and
Pre-Clinical Development
Berlex Laboratories, Inc.
110 E. Hanover Avenue
Cedar Knolls, New Jersey 07927

Linda Rolnitzky
Biostatistician
Arrhythmia Control Unit
Columbia Presbyterian Medical Center
622 West 168th Street
New York, NY 10032

Michael R. Rosen, M.D., Ph.D.
Professor, Department of Pharmacology & Pediatrics
Department of Pharmacology
Columbia University
College of Physicians and Surgeons
630 West 168th Street
New York, NY 10032

Jeremy Ruskin, M.D.
Director, Cardiac Electrophysiology
Laboratory
Massachusetts General Hospital
171 Harrison Avenue
Boston, MA 02114

Joseph F. Spear, Ph.D.
Professor of Physiology
Department of Animal Biology
University of Pennsylvania
School of Veterinary Medicine
3800 Spruce Street
Philadelphia, PA 19104

Mitchell I. Steinberg, Ph.D.
Cardiovascular Pharmacology
Research Administration
Lilly Research Laboratories
307 East McCarty Street
Indianapolis, Indiana 46285

Richard L. Verrier, Ph.D.
Associate Professor of Physiology
Director of Experimental Studies,
Cardiovascular Laboratories
Department of Nutrition
Harvard School of Public Health
665 Huntington Avenue
Boston, MA 02115

August M. Watanabe, M.D.
Professor of Medicine and
Pharmacology
Chairman, Department of Medicine
Indiana University Medical Center
Emerson Hall, Room 317
545 Barnhill Drive
Indianapolis, Indiana 46223

E. M. Vaughan Williams, D.M., D.Sc., F.R.C.P.
Hertford College, Oxford University
University Department of
Pharmacology
South Parks Road
Oxford, United Kingdom OX1 3QT

Andrew L. Wit, Ph.D.
Professor of Pharmacology
Department of Pharmacology
College of Physicians and Surgeons
Columbia University
630 West 168th Street
New York, NY 10032

Preface

The content of this monograph is based upon the presentations given at the A. N. Richards Symposium of the Philadelphia Physiological Society. The purpose of the symposium was to review our current understanding of the mechanisms of arrhythmias and antiarrhythmic therapy, with particular emphasis on the relevance of basic studies to clinical management. Based upon our present knowledge, we hope to project future areas of basic and clinical research and identify new conceptual frameworks in the evaluation and treatment of arrhythmias. In each area covered in the monograph, we have attempted to present both basic concepts and their clinical counterparts in diagnosis and treatment to bridge the transition from basic principles to applied concepts.

The understanding of the mechanisms of arrhythmias has evolved in concert with our understanding of antiarrhythmic drug action over the past 20 years. This evolution has triggered the development of animal models for investigating antiarrhythmic agents and clinical technologies for investigating antiarrhythmic actions in man. The development of many new antiarrhythmic compounds has provided a vast amount of information on basic and clinical effects of these agents and has had a significant impact on our clinical management of arrhythmias. This evolution and development forms the basis of the presentations in this monograph.

The format of the monograph includes both basic and clinical studies in each area. There are seven major sections of the book in which we have summarized information on the mechanisms of arrhythmias, the mechanisms of antiarrhythmic drug action, indices of antiarrhythmic drug efficacy, the antiarrhythmic effects of conduction-slowing agents, adrenergic blocking agents, agents that selectively prolong the action potential, and calcium channel-blocking agents. In addition, there are three related chapters: one introduces our review of the concepts of arrhythmias and antiarrhythmic drugs; another introduces the classification of antiarrhythmic drugs; and a final chapter provides a synthesis of our concepts of arrhythmogenesis and antiarrhythmic drug action—the clinical application of antiarrhythmic drugs in the prevention of sudden cardiac death. Each section is followed by editorial notes that have been prepared by us to highlight areas of concensus and controversy, with the intent of advancing emerging concepts and suggesting areas for further investigation.

In this monograph we have stressed that the clinical application of our understanding of the mechanisms of arrhythmias and antiarrhythmic drug action begins with the relative simplicity of isolated models and extends to the complexity of the clinical situation. Evolution in both areas is necessary to advance further our overall understanding. For example, animal models for testing antiarrhythmic agents have become more complex and simulate more closely the clinical condition. This evolution of clinically relevant animal models has in turn allowed the application of clinical investigational techniques such as programmed electrical stimulation, which has been extensively employed in the clinical realm both as a research tool and as a basis of drug selection. Thus the use of common techniques in both basic and clinical studies has advanced our understanding of such techniques and allowed an extension of information from the basic to the clinical arena. Similarly, the classification system of Vaughan Williams, originally developed from in vitro data, has been modified and evolved to its current status in which it is now useful for clinical applications, particularly in the investigation of antiarrhythmic agents. In this regard, the concept of a class III antiarrhythmic drug action has evolved by reviewing the effects of older drugs that were originally introduced for other indications thus providing the impetus to develop specific drugs that express a class III activity. Lastly, the interpretation of clinical effects of currently available agents, in view of existing basic research data for such agents, allows drugs to be used as tools in the interpretation of the arrhythmia, which in turn can lead to the development of more potent and useful antiarrhythmic agents.

Finally, we would like to thank the various individuals who helped to complete this monograph. We are especially indebted to our secretaries, Helaine Corr, Janie Tanilli, and Carol Pollette, for their expert assistance in the preparation of this monograph. In addition, we feel indebted to Dr. Thomas Tulenko for his assistance in organizing the symposium. We wish to extend to our publisher, Urban & Schwarzenberg, and its staff our sincere appreciation for their diligent efforts in the preparation of this book. Lastly, we would like to thank the Board of the Philadelphia Physiological Society for making this symposium and publication possible.

H. Joseph Reiser, Ph.D.
Cedar Knolls, NJ

Leonard N. Horowitz, M.D.
Philadelphia, PA

Acknowledgments

The A.N. Richards Symposium was supported by the Philadelphia Physiological Society and by the generous contributions from the following companies:

American Critical Care
Hoechst-Roussel Pharmaceuticals, Inc.
Berlex Laboratories, Inc.
Boehringer Ingelheim Ltd.
Bristol-Myers Company
Merck, Sharp & Dohme Research Laboratories
Miles Laboratories, Inc.
Norwich-Eaton Pharmaceuticals
Ortho Pharmaceutical Corporation
Schering Corporation
Revlon Health Care Group
E. R. Squibb and Sons, Inc.
Stuart Pharmaceuticals, Division of ICI Americas, Inc.
Wallace Laboratories, Division of Carter-Wallace
Wyeth Laboratories
American Cyanamid
USV Pharmaceutical Corporation
Sandoz, Inc.
Ciba-Geigy Corporation, Pharmaceuticals Division
Burroughs Wellcome
Hoffmann-LaRoche, Inc.
McNeil Pharmaceutical
Winthrop Laboratories, Division of Sterling Group
E. I. DuPont de Nemours & Company
Searle Pharmaceuticals
Ives Laboratories
Cordis Corporation

Part I

Mechanisms of Arrhythmias and Antiarrhythmic Drug Action

On Thinking about Arrhythmias

Paul F. Cranefield

There are many models that we use for thinking about arrhythmias and it seems worthwhile to sort them out and see how they relate to one another. For many of us, the most familiar model is the electrical activity detected by an intracellular microelectrode, activity that we used to think of as the activity of a single cell. We always knew, of course, that the microelectrode records changes in potential that arise at points both near to and rather remote from the cell that it impales, if that cell is part of a syncytium. Now that we can record from actual single cells, we have to be a little more careful about terminology!

What kinds of events can arise in a single cell and cause arrhythmias? Obviously, phase 4 depolarization is such an event. So are oscillatory prepotentials that reach threshold to yield an action potential. Delayed afterdepolarizations capable of giving rise to triggered activity can also appear in a single cell. An early afterdepolarization, i.e., an interruption of repolarization leading to a "second upstroke," can occur in a single cell. In short, most and perhaps all of the events ordinarily classified as abnormalities of impulse generation can occur in the isolated single cell, whereas the kinds of abnormalities associated with conduction disturbances obviously cannot.

We have barely begun and it is already time for a caveat. It is true that most abnormal forms of impulse generation, perhaps all such forms, can be seen in isolated single cells. Yet the occurrence of such phenomena in a cell does not mean that if that cell were "plugged into" a syncytium, these arrhythmogenic events would continue to occur and continue to give rise to arrhythmias. The moment the cell is connected to neighboring cells, the possibility arises that a flow of current, resulting from the higher or lower resting potential of those neighboring cells, will suppress the membrane potential changes that were arrhythmogenic in the isolated cell. So our earlier model may well be more representative of the heart in situ. The events that we see with the intracellular microelectrode used to impale a single cell that is part of a syncytium, may be a perfectly sound model because it is possible that no single cell is ever an arrhythmogenic focus. Only a group of cells, sharing more or less similar properties, may be able to sustain, in the whole heart, such behavior as phase 4 depolarization capable of reaching threshold and propagating throughout the heart. And even then the arrhythmogenic focus may need some degree of shielding from the stabilizing effects of its surroundings. The cells of the S-A node, for example, show a wide range of rates of phase 4 depolarization, a wide range of diastolic potentials, and a diverse range of action potential types, from those of the purest ''true'' pacemaker to those of the virtually full-blown atrial cell. The pacemaker could not function as a pacemaker if it were connected directly to contractile cells of the atrium, because the atrial cells would tend to hyperpolarize and suppress the pacemaker cell. The gradual increase of diastolic potential, the gradual change in the type of action potential, the gradual increase in the density of intercellular connections, seen as one moves from the ''true pacemaker'' to the true atrial fiber is essential to the ability of the ''single cell'' that is the ''pacemaker'' actually to initiate the excitation of the entire heart.

Thus, although the electrical activity of the single cell is attractive as a model for thinking about arrhythmias, and it is a very useful, informative, and indispensable model, it must be used with caution. In the heart, the cell is always part of a syncytium and its behavior is always influenced by that fact. Thus, if we begin with the single cell as model, we must always use another model, a group of cells in which that single cell is surrounded by cells of rather similar properties. We must add yet another model in which that group of cells is surrounded by ''transitional'' cells with properties intermediate between those of the single cell with which we started and the cells of the bulk of the heart.

The resting potential and the action potential are determined by the flow of currents across the membrane. A useful model of the resting potential and of the action potential is obtained by thinking in terms of ionic gradients and permeabilities, without special reference to the fact that the membrane is, in fact, wrapped around a cell. In this model, we think of a membrane that has certain properties and that divides two solutions that have certain properties; those of the intracellular and extracellular milieus. Indeed, it is possible and useful to think even of mechanisms such as active sodium/potassium exchange in this way, since the necessary enzymes can be envisioned as being in the necessary places in one side or the other of the membrane, or in it.

This biophysical, circuit diagram model is an essential part of our thinking about the action potential and thus is essential to any kind of thinking about abnormal impulse generation or abnormal conduction. The factors that determine the transmembrane potential and the factors that are determined by the transmembrane potential make up between them the bulk of the electrical properties of the cell. At any stable, constant membrane potential, in the absence of applied current, there is, by definition, zero net flow of current across the membrane. This most certainly does not mean that no current is flowing across the membrane. Many currents are flowing, in different channels with different conductances, carried by different ions and arising from various causes. Currents arising from diffusion potentials and carried by small inorganic ions (Na^+, K^+, Cl^-) dominated our model of the membrane potential for a long time, but we are now aware of the importance of currents generated by active (and electrogenic) ion exchange mechanisms such as the Na^+/K^+ exchange system, and, possibly, currents generated by Na^+/Ca^+ exchange. In thinking about the membrane potential, it is important to think not only about the currents, but about the source impedance of each current, and to bear in mind that the total membrane resistance is an important determinant of some features of electrophysiological importance. A resting potential of a given value that results from the balance of large currents gives a membrane characteristics very different from one that shows the same membrane potential as the result of the balance of small currents. Not only is there a difference in total membrane resistance, there is also the fact that small currents cause less change in the ionic "battery" from which they are drawn than do large currents, and hence, less demand for restoration of the ionic gradients that their flow perturbs. Even at zero current potentials there is another important asymmetry in the behavior of a membrane in that a perturbation of the membrane potential caused by blocking one of the currents (either through blocking the channel or removing the ion that carries the current), or caused by applying a current from an external source, will have a different effect according to whether the change is in the depolarizing or the hyperpolarizing direction. This is because at least some of the channels that carry current across the membrane have voltage-dependent resistances. In other words, all perturbations of membrane potential, however small, and at whatever level of membrane potential they occur, may well be nonlinear (nonohmic). The membrane potential is the result of the transmembrane currents (it is equally the cause of some of them). But the membrane potential also determines how certain channels will behave in response to a perturbation of the membrane potential. An example of this is found in the phenomena of inactivation and the removal of inactivation.

The models of the membrane and of the membrane potential that incorporate the properties outlined above have become increasingly complex; thus, the advent of methods for studying single channels holds out hope for simpler models. The idea of an ohmic channel seems gratifyingly straightforward, yet a channel might rectify, i.e., ions might flow through it more readily in one direction than in the other. Such a channel could be either inwardly or outwardly rectifying. It appears, in fact, that at least some of the important channels are purely ohmic, i.e., they carry current with equal ease in either direction and at any membrane potential, if they are open. It is the probability that a channel will be open that is sensitive to membrane potential. Yet the fact that a single channel is open or closed does not determine the potential across the membrane: that potential is determined by the entire ensemble of channels capable of carrying either inward or outward current. Thus, a second caveat: the contribution of the single channel is dependent on the characteristics of the other channels in its neighborhood, just as the activity of a single cell is dependent on the properties of the other cells to which it is connected. Indeed, we already know enough about the membrane potential and about channels to know that any dream of interpreting even the resting potential as the net effect of a set of currents flowing through ohmic channels is indeed idle.

Let us go to an opposite extreme: from the single channel to a bundle of fibers, and to the abnormalities of conduction and other types of interactions that may occur in a segment of such a bundle when the excitability of its fibers is diminished. This requires models of the action potential propagating in a three-dimensionally nonuniform syncytium, i.e., models that are orders of magnitude more complicated than those that describe the single channel, a family of channels or even the action potential of a single cell. Simplified models thus become almost essential as a guide to our thinking, although we must be constantly alert to the risk that when a conclusion is drawn from a simple model, that conclusion, however plausible, may be wrong.

For example, it is by now well known and widely accepted that certain cardiac cells can produce two essentially different kinds of action potential, the normal action potential and the slow response. A simple model of the importance of this phenomenon would be an unbranched fiber of uniform diameter with uniform passive electrical properties which, over a distance of several length constants, could produce only a slow response action potential. If, for the sake of argument, we take a fiber 10 cm long, that has a 1-cm segment at either end that conducts the normal action potential and a central segment 8 cm long that conducts a slow response, and assume that the pertinent conduction velocities are 1 m/s and 0.1 m/s, that fiber will conduct an action potential for 1 cm at 1 m/s in 10 ms, will conduct a slow response along 8 cm at 0.1 m/s in 800 ms, and then conduct rapidly for another 1 cm in 10 ms, for a total conduction time of 820 ms. That may be compared to a 10-cm-long fiber conducting an impulse throughout its entire length at 1 m/s, for a total conduction time of 100 ms. But this model is unrealistic in many important ways. For example, the most common "physiologic" way to cause a fiber to lose the ability to conduct a normal action potential and acquire the ability to conduct a slow response action potential is to depolarize the fiber. But in a cable, the depolarization of the central segment will of necessity create a gradient of resting potential between each end of the central segment and each normal segment. And that gradient will affect the characteristics of the action potential in the region in which the gradient occurs. A model incorporating those details is probably a bit nearer to what actually happens in the junction between S-A nodal and atrial fibers or in the junctions between the A-V node and atrium or the A-V node and His bundle. But it is also very much harder to think about that model and harder to analyze it mathematically.

Worse is to come, however. If we want a realistic model of the A-V node, we must take into account not only resting potentials and action potentials that change more or less continuously over a considerable stretch, but we also must certainly take into account the complexities of the syncytial structure of the node. In our earliest studies of the A-V node, Hoffman and I called attention to the possibility of decremental conduction, to the possible role of altered core conductor properties, and to the possibility of impairments of cytoplasmic continuity, remarking that the increased transverse resistance caused by the intercalated discs "might become of greater importance in fibers which otherwise possess a low safety factor of conduction." We also called attention to the probable need to include in the model the effects of impulses converging or diverging at branch points of the syncytium.

The model which incorporates branched fibers and variable degrees of depolarization (with the accompanying differences in the characteristics of the action potential) is almost impossible to analyze in exact quantitative detail, and yet is inadequate to explain all of the complex behavior in segments in which the excitability is depressed. Phenomena such as summation and inhibition, particularly when they are evoked by premature excitation, require for their explanation extraordinarily complex models, at present well beyond the reach of full mathematical analysis.

There are, obviously, many models that we use in thinking about the cardiac action potential. The above list is far from complete. The examples I have given show that, almost no matter what simple model we begin with, things rapidly become more complex. It does seem that a more systematic attempt to sort out the various levels of conceptual analysis that are presently in use would be worthwhile. It is certain that we should occasionally step back from our efforts to understand the electrical activity of the heart and ask ourselves which models we are using. Since a model may be too simple or may not be realistic, it is important to remember that although thinking about the predictions of a particular model may be very productive, it may also be misleading.

Acknowledgment

This work was assisted by United States Public Health Service Grant HL 14899.

A. Mechanisms of Arrhythmias

Chapter 1

Cardiac Arrhythmias: Electrophysiologic Mechanisms

Andrew L. Wit

Introduction

Hoffman and Cranefield (1964) originally proposed that arrhythmias may result from abnormalities of impulse initiation, impulse conduction, or a combination of both. In the 20 years that have intervened since this classification of arrhythmia mechanisms was presented, there have been continuous modifications of this basic classification. It is now apparent that there are a variety of mechanisms which can cause abnormal impulse initiation or abnormal conduction. Table 1-1 provides an outline of these mechanisms. As previously stated by Hoffman and Rosen (1981), "Although the new-found complexity of cellular mechanisms and their clinical implications may be the source of some dismay to students of electrophysiology, this need not be the case. The discovery of such complexity probably has put us on the correct track for learning the mechanisms that actually are responsible for specific clinical arrhythmias."

Table 1-1* Mechanisms for Arrhythmias.

I Abnormal impulse generation	II Abnormal impulse conduction	III Simultaneous abnormalities of impulse generation and conduction
A. Normal automatic mechanism	A. Slowing and block (S-A block, A-V block, etc.)	A. Parasystole
B. Abnormal automatic mechanism	B. Unidirectional block and reentry 1. Random reentry 2. Ordered reentry 3. Summation and inhibition (Cranefield et al., 1973)	B. Slow conduction because of phase 4 depolarization (see Hoffman and Rosen, 1981)
C. Triggered activity 1. Early afterdepolarization 2. Delayed afterdepolarization	C. Conduction block, electrotonic transmission and reflection	

*Modified from Hoffman and Rosen (1981) with permission of the publishers.

Arrhythmias Caused by Abnormal Impulse Generation

Abnormal impulse generation occurs because of localized changes in ionic currents which flow across the membranes of single cells or groups of cells. Such impulse generation may be expressed as automaticity or triggered activity.

Normal Automatic Mechanism

Automaticity, the ability to initiate spontaneous action potentials, is a property of normal cardiac cells in the sinus node, in parts of the atria, in the A-V junction and in the His-Purkinje system (Figs. 1-1, 1-2). The basis for automaticity in all

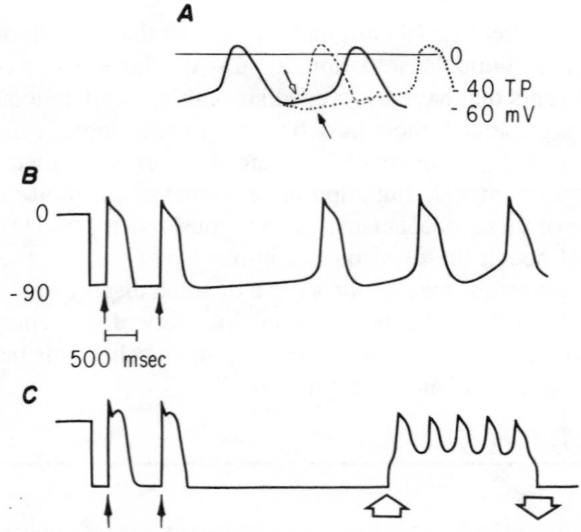

1-1 Normal and abnormal automaticity. The solid trace in panel A shows a schematic depiction of the sinus node transmembrane potential. Spontaneous diastolic depolarization causes automatic firing (normal automaticity). The spontaneous firing rate can be slowed by decreasing the slope of diastolic depolarization (dotted trace and solid arrow). Acetylcholine causes this effect. Spontaneous firing rate is increased by increasing the slope of diastolic depolarization (dashed trace and unfilled arrow). Norepinephrine has this effect. In panel B, a schematic representation of a Purkinje fiber transmembrane potential is shown. The first two action potentials at the left are caused by electrical stimulation at the arrows. Stimulation is then stopped. Spontaneous diastolic depolarization develops causing automatic firing (three action potentials to the right). This is also normal automaticity. In panel C, a schematic representation of a ventricular muscle transmembrane potential is shown. The first two action potentials at the left are caused by stimulation and stimulation is then stopped. Spontaneous diastolic depolarization does not occur. At the unfilled arrow, membrane potential is decreased by depolarizing current passed through a microelectrode. Spontaneous firing (abnormal automaticity) then occurs. (Reproduced from Wit, A.L., and Rosen, M.R. 1981. Cellular electrophysiology of cardiac arrhythmias. I. Arrhythmias caused by abnormal impulse generation. Mod Concepts Cardiovasc Dis 50:1, with permission.)

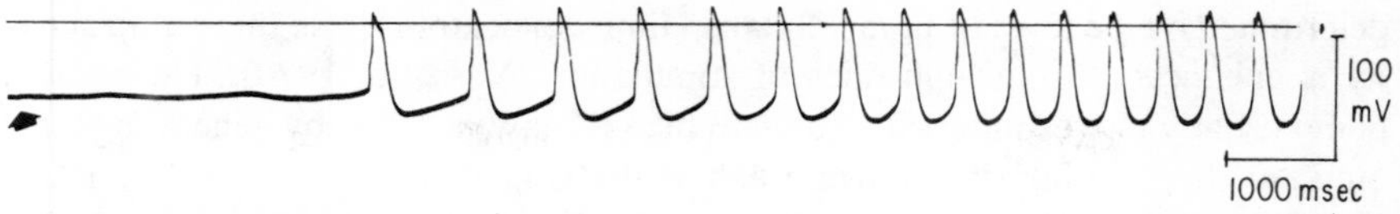

1-2 Normal automaticity in an atrial fiber outside the coronary sinus ostium. The transmembrane potential recording from a fiber which was not being electrically stimulated is shown. Norepinephrine was added to the superfusate at the arrow. Small oscillations in membrane potential then occurred, followed by a spontaneous impulse. The slope of phase 4 depolarization increased with each subsequent spontaneous impulse and cycle length progressively shortened. (Reproduced from Wit, A.L., and Cranefield, P.F. 1977. Triggered and automatic activity in the canine coronary sinus. Circ Res 41:435, with permission of the American Heart Association.)

these cell types is a slow fall in membrane potential during the diastolic interval. This is referred to as phase 4 or diastolic or pacemaker depolarization. When the membrane reaches its threshold potential, an impulse is initiated and the pacemaker conductance is then reactivated. The fall in membrane potential during phase 4 reflects a gradual shift in the balance between inward and outward current components in the direction of net inward (depolarizing) current. Although for many years the pacemaker potential in Purkinje fibers, and perhaps other cardiac fibers as well, was considered to result from an outward pacemaker current carried by K^+ which gradually declines, thereby, allowing the background inward Na^+ current to depolarize the cell membrane (Vassalle, 1965; Trautwein, 1973), recent studies on pacemaker mechanisms have questioned the results of earlier experiments that led to this concept (DiFrancesco, 1981a; DiFrancesco, 1981b). The recently proposed alternative is that an inward Na^+ pacemaker current (called I_f) increases with time, thereby depolarizing the membrane, while the outward K^+ current is constant. This pacemaker current also may be responsible for automaticity in the sinus and A-V nodes (Yanagihara and Irisawa, 1980; Noma et al., 1980). The exact causes of diastolic depolarization is still not settled.

In the normal heart, the rate of impulse initiation due to automaticity of cells in the sinus node is sufficiently rapid that potentially automatic cells (latent pacemakers) elsewhere in the heart are excited by propagated impulses before they can depolarize spontaneously to threshold potential. Not only are ectopic pacemakers prevented from initiating an impulse because they are depolarized before they have a chance to fire, but also the diastolic depolarization of the latent pacemaker cells is actually inhibited by the impulses from the sinus node. This inhibition is called overdrive suppression (Vassalle, 1970; Vassalle, 1977).

Overdrive suppression results from driving a pacemaker cell faster than its intrinsic spontaneous rate and is mediated by enhanced activity of the Na^+/K^+ exchange pump. Since sodium ions enter the cell during each action potential, the higher the rate of stimulation, the greater will be the amount of Na^+ entering the cell over a given period of time. The rate of activity of the sodium pump is largely determined by the level of intracellular sodium concentration, so that pump activity is enhanced during high rates of stimulation (Vassalle, 1970). The sodium pump usually moves more Na^+ outward than K^+ inward, thereby generating a net outward (hyperpolarizing) current across the cell membrane (Vassalle, 1970; Gadsby and Cranefield, 1979). When subsidiary pacemaker cells are driven faster than their intrinsic rate, the enhanced pump current suppresses spontaneous impulse initiation in these cells. When the dominant (overdrive) pacemaker is stopped, this suppression is responsible for the period of quiescence which lasts until the intracellular Na^+ concentration, and hence the pump current, becomes small enough to allow subsidiary pacemaker cells to depolarize spontaneously to threshold. Intracellular Na^+ and pump current continue to decline after the first spontaneous impulse, causing a gradual increase in the discharge rate of the subsidiary pacemaker (Vassalle, 1970).

A shift in the site of impulse initiation to a region other than the sinus node would be expected to occur when the sinus rate falls considerably below the intrinsic rate of the subsidiary pacemakers having the capabilities for normal automaticity, or when impulse initiation in these subsidiary pacemakers is enhanced. Impulse initiation by the sinus node may be slowed or inhibited altogether either by the parasympathetic nervous system or as a result of sinus node disease (Fig. 1-1A). Alternatively, there may be a block of impulse conduction from the sinus node to the atrium. Under any of the above conditions there may be ''escape'' of a subsidiary pacemaker as a result of removal of overdrive suppression by the sinus pacemaker. Several factors can also enhance subsidiary pacemaker activity probably causing impulse initiation to shift to ectopic sites, even when the sinus node function is normal. For example, norepinephrine released locally from sympathetic nerves steepens the slope of diastolic depolarization of most ectopic pacemaker cells (Tsien, 1974) and diminishes the inhibitory effects of overdrive (Vassalle and Carpentier, 1972) (Fig. 1-2).

Another mechanism that may suppress subsidiary pacemakers is the electrotonic interactions between the pacemaker cells and nonpacemaker cells. This suppression was demonstrated by van Capelle and Durrer (1980) using computer simulation studies. Wit and Cranefield (1982) have suggested that this mechanism may be particularly important in normally suppressing A-V nodal automaticity. Although the concept of A-V nodal automaticity and junctional arrhythmias was widely accepted during the first 50 years of this century (Scherf and Cohen, 1964), the occurrence of pacemaker activity in nodal regions was questioned in the 1960's because microelectrode studies often failed to find such pacemaker activity (Hoffman and Cranefield, 1960). More recently it has been observed that small isolated preparations of the rabbit A-V node are highly auto-

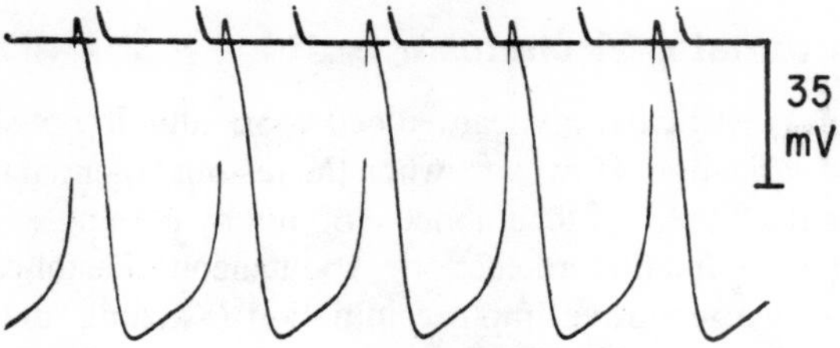

1-3 Automaticity in an A-V nodal fiber. The transmembrane potentials shown were recorded from an isolated 2 × 2 mm preparation dissected from the rabbit A-V node and superfused with Tyrode's solution. Automaticity is commonly found when the connections between the A-V node and surrounding tissue are severed. Time marks are at 250-ms intervals.

matic (Kokubun et al., 1980) (Fig. 1-3). If the atrial connections of the A-V node in the rabbit heart are severed, automatic activity may sometimes arise in the node at rates which are even more rapid than the normal sinus rate (Wit and Cranefield, 1982). Therefore, the automaticity could not have been suppressed by overdrive but rather must have been suppressed through the anatomical connections between the node and atrium. Although the hypothesis still requires more exacting proof, it is proposed that the electrotonic interactions between atrium and node suppress the automaticity (Wit and Cranefield, 1982) through these atrionodal connections. The atrial cells have more negative resting potentials than the nodal cells and are not latent pacemakers. Because of the more negative potentials of the atrial cells, current flow between them and the nodal cells should be in a direction which prevents spontaneous diastolic depolarization of the nodal cells. According to the computer model of van Capelle and Durrer (1980), suppression of automaticity by this mechanism is diminished by increasing the coupling resistance. Any intervention then, which decreases intercellular coupling might increase automaticity. This could result from physical separation of the node from atrium as might occur during fibrosis of the junctional region which causes heart block. Uncoupling might also be caused by factors which increase the intracellular concentration of Ca^{2+} (Dahl and Isenberg, 1980) such as treatment with digitalis (Weingart, 1977).

Abnormal Automatic Mechanism

Working atrial and ventricular myocardial cells normally do not show spontaneous diastolic depolarization. However, when the resting potential of these cells is experimentally reduced to less than about −60 mv by passing depolarizing current through an intracellular microelectrode, spontaneous diastolic depolarization may occur and cause repetitive impulse initiation (Katzung and Morgenstern, 1977; Surawicz and Imanishi, 1976; Brown and Noble, 1969) (Fig. 1-1C). This is called abnormal automaticity. Likewise, cells such as Purkinje fibers which have the property of normal automaticity at normal levels of membrane potential, also show abnormal automaticity when membrane potential is reduced (Cranefield, 1974; Noble and Tsien, 1968). However, if a low level of membrane potential is employed as the only criterion for abnormal automaticity, the automaticity of the S-A node would have to be considered abnormal. Therefore, an important distinction for abnormal automaticity is that the membrane potentials of fibers showing this type of activity are markedly reduced from the normal level (Hoffman and Rosen, 1981).

At the low level of membrane potential at which abnormal automaticity occurs, it is likely that at least some of the ionic currents causing the automatic activity are not the same as those causing normal automatic activity. A likely cause of automaticity at membrane potential of around −50 mv is deactivation of a K^+ current referred to as i_{x_i} (Noble and Tsien, 1968). Under normal conditions, this current functions to help bring about repolarization after the upstroke of an action potential. In addition, because of the low level of membrane potential, the spontaneously occurring action potentials are slow responses (action potentials with upstrokes dependent on slow inward current) (Cranefield, 1975). The decrease in membrane potential of cardiac cells required for abnormal automaticity to occur may be caused by a variety of factors related to cardiac disease which have been described in detail in another review (Gadsby and Wit, 1981). Abnormal automaticity occurs in the Purkinje fibers which survive on the subendocardial surface of canine infarcts and may cause ventricular tachycardia (Friedman et al., 1973; Lazzara et al., 1973). Also, preparations of diseased atrial and ventricular myocardium from human hearts show phase 4 depolarization and automatic firing at membrane potentials in the range of −50 to −60 mv (Fig. 1-4) (Hordof et al., 1976; Singer et al., 1981).

An abnormal automatic focus should manifest itself and cause an arrhythmia when the sinus rate decreases below the intrinsic rate of the focus, as was discussed for latent pacemakers with normal automaticity. However, there may be an important distinction between the effects of the dominant sinus pacemaker on the two kinds of foci. Unlike normal automaticity, abnormal automaticity may not be overdrive suppressed (Carmeliet, 1980; Dangman and Hoffman, In Press).

Therefore, even transient sinus pauses or occassional long sinus cycle lengths may permit the ectopic focus to capture the heart for one or more impulses. On the other hand, an ectopic pacemaker with normal automaticity would probably be quiescent during relatively short, transient sinus pauses because they are overdrive suppressed.

It is also possible that the depolarized level of membrane potential at which abnormal automaticity occurs might cause entrance block into the focus and prevent it from being overdriven by the sinus node (Ferrier and Rosenthal, 1980). This would lead to parasystole, an example of an arrhythmia caused by a combination of an abnormality of impulse conduction and initiation as outlined in Table 1-1. Entrance block may also occur into regions of normal automaticity if they are surrounded by depolarized or inexcitable fibers (Jalife and Moe, 1976; Jalife and Moe, 1979).

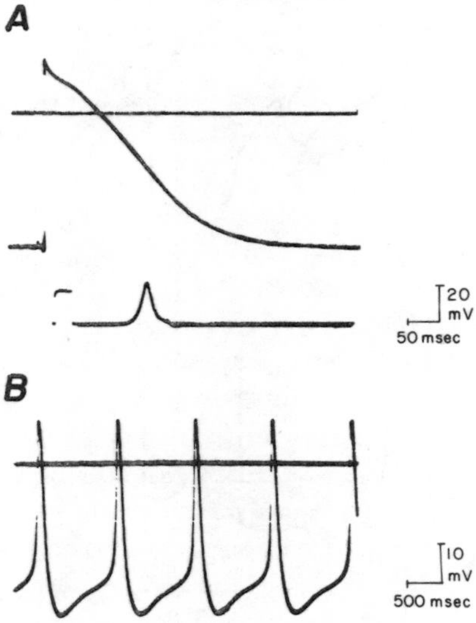

1-4 Abnormal automaticity in an atrial fiber. The top panel shows a transmembrane action potential recorded from a normal human atrial fiber. It has a high resting potential (−80 mv), and rapid upstroke velocity. The bottom panel shows a transmembrane action potential recorded from an isolated sample of diseased human atria. Maximum diastolic potential is low (−40 mv) and there is spontaneous diastolic depolarization and automaticity. Such automaticity does not occur when membrane potential is high. (Modified from Rosen, M.R., Wit, A.L., and Hoffman, B.F. 1975. Electrophysiology and pharmacology of cardiac arrhythmias. VI. Cardiac effects of verapamil. Am Heart J, 89:665, with permission.)

Triggered Activity

Triggered activity is impulse generation caused by afterdepolarizations. An afterdepolarization is a second subthreshold depolarization that occurs either during repolarization (referred to as an early afterdepolarization) (Fig. 1-5A–C) or after repolarization is complete or nearly complete (referred to as a delayed afterdepolarization) (Fig 1-5D, E) (Cranefield, 1977; Wit et al., 1980).

Early Afterdepolarizations and Triggered Activity Early afterdepolarizations usually occur during repolarization of an action potential which has been initiated from a high level of membrane potential, usually between −75 and −90 mv. Early afterdepolarizations appear as a change in membrane potential in a positive direction, relative to the expected membrane potential during normal repolarization (Fig. 1-5A). Under certain conditions, early afterdepolarizations can lead to second upstrokes (Wit et al., 1980); membrane potential during the early

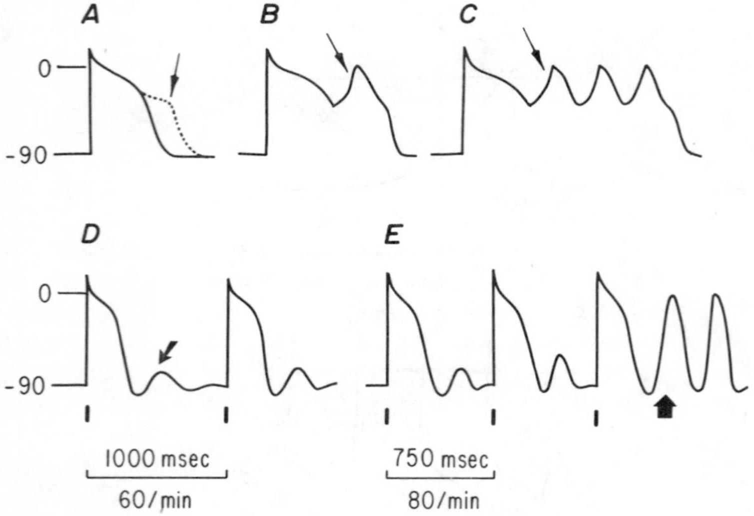

1-5 Early and delayed afterdepolarizations and triggered activity. In panel A, the solid trace represents the normal transmembrane action potential of a Purkinje fiber. The dashed trace shows what happens to repolarization during a subthreshold early afterdepolarization (arrow). In panel B, the early afterdepolarization caused a triggered action potential (arrow), and in panel C, three triggered action potentials occurred prior to repolarization. Delayed afterdepolarizations (arrow) which follow stimulated action potentials are shown in panel D. The stimulus rate is 60/min. In panel E, the stimulus rate was increased causing the amplitude of the delayed afterdepolarization to increase. Triggered activity occurs at the arrow. (Reproduced from Wit, A.L., and Rosen, M.R. 1981. Cellular electrophysiology of cardiac arrhythmias. I. Arrhythmias caused by abnormal impulse generation. Mod Concepts Cardiovasc Dis 50:1, with permission.)

afterdepolarization reaches threshold potential for activation of the slow inward current and a second action potential occurs prior to complete repolarization of the first (Fig. 1-5B). The second upstroke is triggered in the sense that it is evoked by an early afterdepolarization which follows and is caused by the preceding action potential. Without the preceding action potential there would be no second upstroke. The second action potential may also be followed by other action potentials, all occurring at the low level of membrane potential characteristic of the plateau or phase 3 (Fig. 1-5C). These action potentials presumably are slow responses (Cranefield, 1975; Cranefield, 1977; Wit et al., 1980). The sustained rhythmic activity may continue for a variable number of impulses and terminates when the increase in membrane potential associated with repolarization of the initiating action potential returns membrane potential to a high (negative) level. Triggered activity may occur again when the next action potential is initiated from the high level of membrane potential. Sometimes repolarization to the high level of membrane potential may not occur and membrane potential may remain at the plateau level or at a level intermediate between the plateau and the resting potential.

Early afterdepolarizations leading to triggered activity in isolated cardiac preparations may be caused by factors which are present in the heart in situ under some pathologic conditions. Among these factors are hypoxia (Trautwein et al., 1954), high p_{CO_2} (Coraboef and Boistel, 1953), and high concentrations of catecholamines (Brooks et al., 1955). Since catecholamines, hypoxia, and elevated p_{CO_2} may be present in an ischemic or infarcted region of the ventricles, it is possible that early afterdepolarizaions may cause some of the arrhythmias which occur soon after myocardial ischemia. Early afterdepolarizations also can be seen occasionally in Purkinje fibers superfused with a normal Tyrode's solution soon after they have been excised from the heart. These early afterdepolarizations might be caused by relatively nonspecific inward current flowing via incompletely healed cuts made at the ends of the fibers or through other regions injured by stretching or crushing during the dissection (Wit et al., 1980). This suggests the interesting possibility that mechanical injury or stretch of Purkinje fibers in situ might cause triggering. Stretch of Purkinje fibers in the ventricles might occur in heart failure or in ventricular aneurysms. Mechanical injury might occur also in the area of an infarct or aneurysm. Lab (1978) has shown that increased intraventricular pressure may also cause early afterdepolarizations and triggered activity in ventricular muscle possibly by increasing muscle segment length, further reason to believe that triggered activity might be caused by cardiac failure or by ventricular aneurysms.

Some drugs which are used clinically and which markedly prolong the time course for repolarization, such as the β receptor-blocking drug sotolol and the antiarrhythmic drug N-acetylprocainamide (Strauss et al., 1970; Dangman and Hoffman, 1981) cause early afterdepolarizations and triggered activity. These drugs can cause cardiac arrhythmias in patients which may be a result of this triggered activity. Since early afterdepolarizations may occur when action potential duration is markedly prolonged, arrhythmias associated with clinical syndromes characterized by action potentials of long duration such as the prolonged QT syndrome might also be caused by triggered activity (Brachman et al., 1983).

Delayed Afterdepolarizations and Triggered Activity A delayed afterdepolarization is a transient or oscillatory depolarization which occurs after the terminal repolarization of an action potential and which is induced by that action potential. Delayed afterpolarizations may be subthreshold as shown in Figure 1-5D but when they are large enough to bring the membrane potential to threshold a nondriven (triggered) impulse arises which also is followed by an afterdepolarization (Fig. 1-5E). The impulse is said to be triggered since it would not have occurred without the preceding action potential. Delayed afterdepolarizations occur under a number of conditions in which there is a large increase in the intracellular Ca^{2+}. It has been proposed that, under these conditions, an oscillatory uptake and release of Ca^{2+} from the sarcoplasmic reticulum influences the permeability of the sarcolemma to Na^+ and possibly other cations. Intracellular oscillatory release of Ca^{2+} from the sarcoplasmic reticulum following an action potential increases the permeability of an unidentified membrane channel causing a transient inward current which results in the afterdepolarization. The transient inward current is diminished when extracellular Na^+ is decreased, suggesting that Na^+ is a charge carrier (Kass et al., 1978a; Kass et al., 1978b).

One of the most widely recognized causes of afterdepolarizations is toxic amounts of cardiac glycosides. Cardiac glycosides inhibit the Na^+/K^+ pump, thereby leading to an increase in Na_i. The intracellular Na^+ is then probably extruded from the cell in exchange for Ca^{2+} by a Na^+/Ca^{2+} exchange mechanism. Delayed afterdepolarizations caused by digitalis can occur in Purkinje fibers and in working atrial and ventricular muscle fibers, although Purkinje fibers seem to develop them at lower drug concentrations (Ferrier, 1977). Other experimental maneuvers which inhibit the Na^+/K^+ pump also increase Ca_i^{2+} and cause delayed afterdepolarizations similar to those caused by digitalis. A prime example is exposure of cardiac fibers to a K^+-free extracellular environment (Eisner and Lederer, 1979).

Catecholamines can cause delayed afterdepolarizations possibly because they enhance Ca^{2+} entry into cardiac fibers by increasing the slow inward current (Nathan and Beeler, 1975; Wit and Cranefield, 1977; Wit and Cranefield, 1976). Delayed afterdepolarizations and triggered activity caused by catecholamines have been seen in atrial fibers of the mitral valve and coronary sinus, as well as in other regions of the atria. Ventricular muscle fibers and Purkinje fibers can also develop delayed afterdepolarizations in the presence of higher concentrations of catecholamines (Nathan and Beeler, 1975).

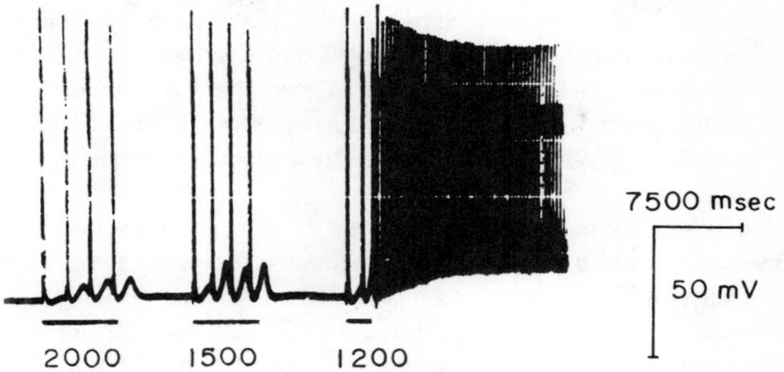

1-6 Effect of stimulus rate on delayed afterdepolarization amplitude. The transmembrane potentials which are shown were recorded from an atrial fiber in the canine coronary sinus superfused with Tyrode's solution containing 0.5 μg/ml norepinephrine. At the left, the fiber was stimulated at a cycle length of 2000 ms for four impulses (underlined). The afterdepolarization following the last driven impulse had an amplitude of 10 mv. In the center, four impulses were stimulated at a cycle length of 1500 ms. The afterdepolarization following the last driven impulse had an amplitude of 17 mv. At the right, after two impulses were stimulated at a cycle length of 1200 ms (underlined), sustained rhythmic activity was triggered. Maximum diastolic potential decreased during the initial period of triggered activity. (Reproduced from Wit, A.L., and Cranefield, P.F. 1977. Triggered and automatic activity in the canine coronary sinus. Circ Res 41:435, with permission.)

Delayed afterdepolarizations may also occur in the absence of drugs or catecholamines. They have been found to occur in fibers in the upper pectinate muscle bordering the crista terminalis in the rabbit heart (Saito et al., 1978), in hypertrophied ventricular myocardium (Aronson, 1981), in human atrial myocardium (Mary-Rabine et al., 1980), and in Purkinje fibers surviving on the subendocardial surface of canine infarcts (El-Sherif et al., 1980).

Delayed afterdepolarizations may not reach threshold, in which case triggered activity does not occur. In fibers showing subthreshold, delayed afterdepolarizations triggering may result if the rate at which the fiber is driven is increased (Fig. 1-6); the amplitude of the afterdepolarizations increases as the drive rate increases. Beyond a certain drive rate the afterdepolarizations reach threshold and triggering occurs. A decrease in the length of even a single drive cycle, i.e., a premature impulse, may increase the amplitude of the afterdepolarization of the action potential that follows the short cycle. The afterdepolarization may reach threshold and initiate triggered activity.

There are some differences in the characteristics of triggered activity, depending upon the cause. In particular, triggered activity caused by digitalis toxicity may have different properties than triggered activity caused by catecholamines. The initial period of triggered activity in coronary sinus atrial fibers caused by catecholamines is often characterized by a gradual decrease in the cycle length after which a constant cycle length occurs (Wit and Cranefield, 1977; Wit et al., 1981). This decrease in cycle length is often accompanied by a decrease in maximum diastolic potential. During triggered activity in Purkinje fibers exposed to toxic amounts of digitalis there is not usually a gradual increase in rate (Ferrier, 1977; Rosen and Reder, 1981).

Triggered activity caused by digitalis or by catecholamines often terminates spontaneously, even in the presence of maintained levels of these agents. When triggered activity in the coronary sinus terminates, the rate usually slows gradually before termination. This gradual slowing is accompanied by a progressive increase in the maximum diastolic potential. A delayed afterdepolarization usually follows the last triggered impulse. Maximum diastolic potential at the time triggered activity ceases may be more negative than when triggering began (Wit et al., 1981). Maximum diastolic potential may continue to increase for some seconds after triggered activity has stopped, but then it returns slowly, over the next few minutes to the control level. The spontaneous termination of triggered activity in canine coronary sinus fibers is caused at least, in part, by an increase in the rate of electrogenic sodium extrusion (Wit et al., 1981). Sodium pump activity is presumably enhanced by the increase in intracellular Na^+ concentration which results from the increase in Na^+ influx during the rapid period of triggered activity. An increase in outward sodium pump current would be expected both to increase the maximum diastolic potential and reduce the rate of triggered activity; a sufficient increase in sodium pump current could thus terminate the triggered activity (Wit et al., 1981). Triggered activity caused by digitalis toxicity probably stops by another mechanism. Termination of a triggered burst is usually not associated with gradual slowing and hyperpolarization but often by speeding of the rate, a decrease in action potential amplitude and a decrease in membrane potential (Rosen and Reder, 1981). Termination is probably not related to activity of the Na^+ pump since the pump is inhibited by the digitalis, but may be caused by Na^+ or Ca^{2+} accumulation in the cell caused by the rapid rate. A decreased transmembrane concentration gradient to either Na^+ or Ca^{2+} might diminish the action potential amplitude and finally lead to cessation of activity.

Since electrical stimulation of the heart is one way in which possible mechanisms of clinical arrhythmias can be ascertained, it is worth reviewing the effects of stimulation on triggered activity. That triggered bursts may be initiated by either overdrive or by programmed premature stimulation has already been discussed. Therefore, triggered arrhythmias might be started by stimulating the heart. Triggered activity can also be terminated by either premature or overdrive stimulation. It is possible to terminate triggered activity in the mitral valve or in the coronary sinus with a single premature stimulus applied late in the cycle (Wit and Cranefield, 1976). The late premature impulse that terminates triggered activity is followed by an increased afterhyperpolarization which, in turn, is fol-

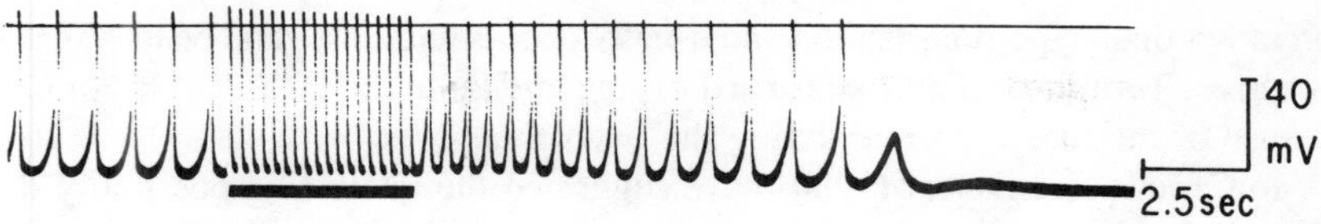

1-7 Overdrive acceleration and termination of triggered activity. The transmembrane potential recorded from an atrial fiber in the canine coronary sinus is shown during a period of triggered activity. Rapid overdrive stimulation is accomplished during the period which is underlined by the black bar. Immediately following this period of overdrive the triggered rate is accelerated. Then, there is a gradual slowing of the rate and a simultaneous increase in maximum diastolic potential until triggered activity stops. (Modified from Wit, A.L., Gadsby, D.C., and Cranefield, P.F. 1981. Electrogenic sodium extrusion can stop triggered activity in the canine coronary sinus. Circ Res 49:1029, with permission.)

lowed by an afterdepolarization that does not reach threshold because it arises from the more negative membrane potential of the preceding afterhyperpolarization. Premature stimulated impulses may terminate digitalis-induced triggered activity in Purkinje fibers, but more frequently, they will simply reset the triggered rhythm. The ability of single prematures to terminate triggered activity is increased if they are preceded by a period of rapid drive.

Triggered activity can also be terminated by overdrive (Fig. 1-7). In the canine coronary sinus fibers, the effects of overdrive are dependent both on the rate and duration of the overdrive (Wit et al., 1981). During a short period of overdrive, at a rate only moderately faster than the triggered rate, there is a decrease in the maximum diastolic potential; following the period of overdrive, the rate of the triggered activity may be faster than it was before overdrive, perhaps because of the decrease in maximum diastolic potential. The postoverdrive accelerated rate then slows, and maximum diastolic potential increases until preoverdrive values are attained. If either the rate of overdrive or the duration of overdrive is increased to a critical degree, the decline in maximum diastolic potential during overdrive is greater as is the postoverdrive acceleration. The maximum diastolic potential then increases and the rate gradually slows until triggered activity stops (Fig. 1-7). The increase in maximum diastolic potential and the slowing and termination of triggered activity following a period of overdrive are caused by enhanced activity of the electrogenic sodium pump. This enhanced activity results from a transient increase in intracellular Na^+ caused by the increased number of action potentials during overdrive (Wit et al., 1981).

Although overdrive stimulation also terminates triggered activity caused by digitalis, the mechanism for the termination probably does not involve enhanced electrogenic Na^+ pump activity since the pump is expected to be inhibited by the digitalis. Termination caused by overdrive usually is associated with depolarization rather than hyperpolarization and usually occurs within several beats after the overdrive. Termination may be caused by an increase in intracellular Na^+ or Ca^{2+} because of the increased rate during the overdrive.

Van Capelle and Durrer (1980) have suggested the interesting possibility that delayed afterdepolarizations might also be caused by the interaction of automatic (pacemaker cells) and nonautomatic cells. As discussed previously, coupling of these two kinds of cells through low resistances suppressed pacemaker activity in their computer simulation studies. When the coupling resistance was increased, delayed afterdepolarizations were shown to follow stimulated action potentials in the cells which were pacemakers before they were coupled to nonautomatic fibers. A further small increase in coupling resistance caused triggered action potentials to follow stimulated (driven) impulses. Further studies are needed to determine whether the characteristics of intercellular coupling can cause afterdepolarizations in cardiac tissue. Whether or not the properties of such triggered activity are similar to the properties of triggered activity caused by increased intracellular Ca^{2+} cannot be predicted at the present time.

Abnormal Impulse Conduction and Reentry

Under special conditions, the propagating impulse may not die out after complete activation of the heart but it may persist to reexcite the atria or ventricles after the end of the refractory period. This is called reentrant excitation (Wit and Cranefield, 1978). Hoffman and Rosen (1981) have further subdivided this mechanism for arrhythmias into two categories, random reentry and ordered reentry. Random reentry is most often associated with atrial or ventricular fibrillation, whereas ordered reentry can cause most other types of arrhythmias. The main distinction between the two is that during random reentry, propagation occurs over reentrant pathways that continuously change their size and location with time, whereas ordered reentry implies a relatively fixed reentrant pathway. However, despite these differences, the basic prerequisite electrophysiologic conditions required for either kind of reentrant excitation are similar. Most mechanisms for reentry require that conduction of the impulse blocks somewhere in part of a reentrant circuit and the block must either be transient or unidirectional (Fig. 1-8). The block enables an excitable pathway to persist through which the reentering impulse can return to reexcite regions it has already excited. Also, the wavelength of the impulse in the reentrant circuit (conduction velocity × refractory period) must be shorter than the length of the circuit so that the tissue into which the impulse is reentering has had time to recover excitability (Mines, 1914). Because of this requirement, it is clear that the relationship between pathlength, conduction velocity and refractory period is crucial (Fig. 1-8). Reentry can be promoted by slowing conduction velocity, shortening the refractory period or a combination of both.

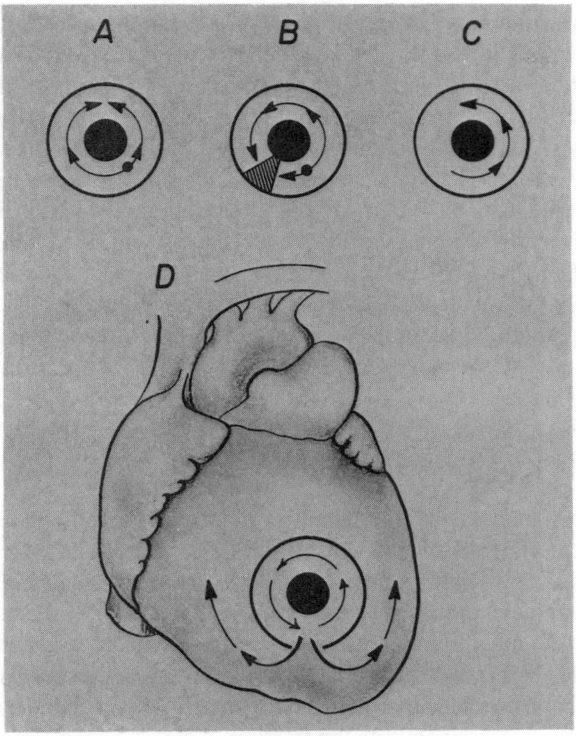

1-8 Schematic representation of reentry in a ring of cardiac tissue as described by Mines in 1914. In A, the ring was stimulated in the area indicated by the small black dot, impulses propagated away from the point of stimulation in both directions and collided; no reentry occurred. In B, the cross-hatched area was compressed while the ring was stimulated again at the black dot. The impulse propagated around the ring in only one direction, having been blocked in the other direction by the area of compression. Then immediately after stimulation, the compression was relieved, and in C, the unidirectionally circulating impulse is shown returning to its point of origin and then continuing around the loop. Identical reentry would occur if the cross-hatched area was a region of unidirectional conduction block, with the conduction block in the right to left direction. D shows how reentry in a loop of the kind described in A–C might cause arrhythmias if located in the heart. In this example, the loop is composed of ventricular muscle which is separated functionally from the rest of the ventricle along most of its border represented by the heavy black line (perhaps caused by fibrosis), but in functional continuity with the ventricles in one place, at its lower end. The arrows show how excitation waves could propagate into the ventricles from the continuously circulating impulse to cause ventricular tachycardia. (Reproduced from Wit, A.L. The genesis of cardiac arrhythmias. In: D.T. Mason, G.G. Neri Seneri, and M.S. Oliver, eds. The Florence International Meeting on Myocardial Infarction. 1979 Excerpta Medica, Amsterdam.)

There can be a number of causes for the slowed conduction and block which are necessary in order for reentrant excitation to occur. The speed at which the impulse conducts in cardiac fibers is dependent on certain features of their transmembrane action potentials, their passive electrical properties, and their microanatomy. Although different groups of investigators who have been studying mechanisms for reentrant excitation have often focused their attention on one or another of these causes and, at one time, have attempted to attribute the cause of all or most reentry to one specific mechanism for slow conduction and block, different mechanisms probably are operative singly or in combination. The cause of slow conduction and block may vary with the type of arrhythmia and the underlying cardiac pathology. Several examples of different mechanisms are discussed below, but this discussion is not all inclusive.

Depressed Resting and Action Potentials Cause Slow Conduction, Block, and Reentry

The influence of transmembrane potential characteristics on conduction is very complex and cannot be discussed here in full. Only some basic principles are presented. An important feature of the transmembrane action potentials of working (atrial and ventricular) myocardial and Purkinje fibers which governs the speed of propagation is the magnitude of the inward Na^+ current flowing through the fast Na^+ channel during the upstroke, and the rapidity with which this current reaches its maximum intensity (the upstroke velocity or V_{max} of phase 0). The intensity of the inward Na^+ current depends on the fraction of Na^+ channels which open when the cell is excited and the size of the Na^+ electrochemical potential gradient (relative concentration of Na^+ outside the cell in the extracellular space to Na^+ concentration inside the cell (Weidmann, 1955; Reuter, 1979)). The fraction of sodium channels available for opening is determined largely by the level of membrane potential at which an action potential is initiated. Immediately after the upstroke, cardiac fibers are inexcitable because of Na^+ channel inactivation at the positive level of membrane potential. During repolarization, progressive removal of inactivation occurs so that, during repolarization from around −60 mv to the diastolic potential, increasingly large Na^+ currents flow through the still partially inactivated Na^+ channels when the cells are excited. The inward Na^+ current and rate of rise of action potentials initiated during this relative refractory period is reduced because the Na^+ channels are only partly reactivated (Weidmann, 1955). Hence, the conduction velocity of these premature action potentials is low.

Premature activation of the heart can induce reentry when premature impulses conduct slowly in regions of the heart where cells are relatively refractory (where Na^+ channels are to some extent inactivated) and, at the same time, block in other regions where cells have not yet repolarized to about −60 mv. Reentry caused by such "inhomogeneous" conduction of premature impulses has been shown to oc-

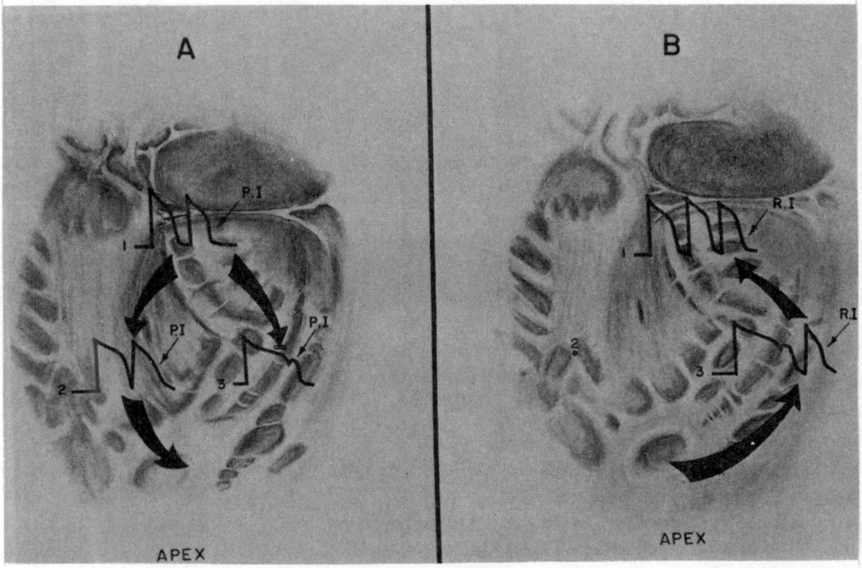

1-9 Mechanism for reentry in the subendocardial Purkinje fiber network surviving over an area of extensive myocardial infarction. Both diagrams show the endocardial surface of the left ventricular anterior papillary muscle (to the left) and the anterior interventricular septum (to the right). The light area on each diagram is the infarcted region which is covered by a blanket of viable Purkinje fibers. Action potential recordings from a subendocardial Purkinje fiber at the border of the infarcted region and normal tissue (site 1), and from subendocardial Purkinje fibers with prolonged repolarization phases (sites 2 and 3) surviving in the infarcted region are shown on the diagrams. In the panel on the left, a premature impulse (PI) occurs at site 1 at the border and conducts into the infarcted regions where action potential duration is prolonged, as indicated by the arrows. The action potential duration at site 3 is longer than at site 2 in the infarct. As a result, the premature impulse can excite cells at site 2 but conduction blocks at site 3. The panel on the right shows a continuation of these events. The premature impulse, after conducting past site 2, returns to activate the cells at site 3 as the reentering impulse (RI) and then conducts back to where it originated at site 1 as the reentrant impulse. (From Wit, A.L., Rosen, M.R., and Hoffman, B.F. 1974. Am Heart J 88: 798, by permission.)

cur in the subendocardial Purkinje system which survives in experimental canine infarcts (Fig. 1-9) (Friedman et al., 1973; Lazzara et al., 1973). Marked differences in the action potential duration (and as a result, the effective refractory period) of cells in adjacent regions exist. Early premature impulses can block in the region with the longest effective refractory period, while conduction continues slowly through regions with a shorter effective refractory period. While the impulse conducts slowly through the excitable tissue, the region of block recovers excitability so that the premature impulse excites this region and then returns to its site of origin as a reentrant impulse. Reentry caused by this mechanism can also be continuous.

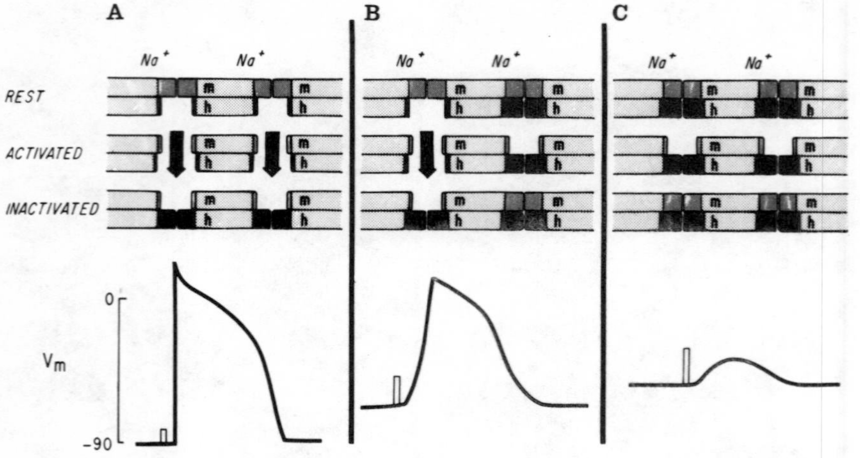

1-10 Effect of reducing membrane potential on function of Na^+ channels. At the top of the figure is a schematic depiction of the sarcolemma of the Na^+ channels at rest, in the activated state, and in the inactivated state. m and h are the "gates" which control channel opening and closing. At the bottom of the figure are representative action potentials. In panel A, at a resting potential of −90 mv, most of the Na^+ channels can be activated causing an action potential with a rapid upstroke. Activation is represented in the diagram by the opened channels and the arrows depicting inward Na^+ current. After the membrane depolarizes, the channels are inactivated; the diagram shows that they are closed. In panel B, resting potential is reduced to −70 mv and about 50% of the Na^+ channels cannot be activated (these channels do not open as shown in the diagram). A depressed fast response action potential with a slow upstroke occurs when the cell is excited. In panel C, at a resting potential less than −60 mv, Na^+channels cannot be activated and an action potential might not be elicited. (Reproduced from Wit, A.L., and Rosen, M.R. 1981. Cellular electrophysiology of cardiac arrhythmias. II. Arrhythmias caused by abnormal impulse conduction. Mod Concepts Cardiovasc Dis 50: 7, with permission.)

Reentry might also occur in cardiac cells with persistently low levels of resting potential (which may be between −60 and −70 mv) caused by disease. At these resting potentials, about 50% of the Na^+ channels are inactivated, and therefore are unavailable for activation by a depolarizing stimulus (Gadsby and Wit, 1981) (Fig. 1-10). The magnitude of the net inward current during phase 0 of the action potential is reduced, and consequently, both the speed and amplitude of the upstroke is diminished, slowing conduction significantly. Such action potentials with upstrokes dependent on inward current flowing via partially inactivated Na^+ channels are sometimes referred to as depressed fast responses. Further depolarization and inactivation of the Na^+ channel may render cardiac fibers inexcitable so that they may become a site of conduction block (Fig. 1-10). Thus, in a diseased region, there may be some areas of slow conduction and some areas of conduction block, possibly depending on the level of resting potential. The

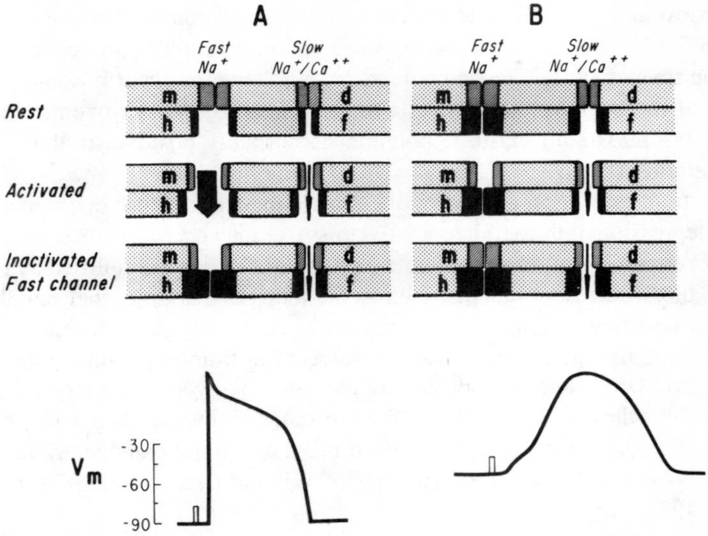

1-11 Slow response action potentials after inactivation of the fast Na^+channel. At the top of the figure is a schematic depiction of the sarcolemma containing the fast Na^+ channels, and the slow Na^+/Ca^{2+} channels. The format of the figure is similar to Figure 2-10. In panel A, the normal action potential, elicited from a resting potential of −90 mv is shown. At rest, both fast and slow channels are closed. After the fiber is stimulated the channels are activated and fast inward current and slow inward current cause the action potential upstroke and plateau. The fast channel inactivates before the slow channel. In panel B, in a cell with resting potential of −50 mv, the fast Na^+ channels are not activated but remain closed when the fiber is stimulated. The slow channels can still be activated and current can pass through them to cause slow response action potentials. (Reproduced from Wit, A.L., and Rosen, M.R. 1981. Cellular electrophysiology of cardiac arrhythmias. II. Arrhythmias caused by abnormal impulse conduction. Mod Concepts Cardiovasc Dis 50: 7, with permission.)

conduction block may be unidirectional (Cranefield et al., 1973). The combination of slow conduction and block may cause reentry.

The slow inward current, under certain conditions, may also underlie the occurrence of reentrant arrhythmias (Cranefield, 1975). Although the fast Na^+ channel may be inactivated largely at membrane potentials near −50 mv, the slow inward channel is not inactivated and still is available for activation (Tsien, 1983) (Fig. 1-11). Under certain conditions, in cells with resting potentials positive to −60 mv (such as when membrane conductance is very low or when catecholamines are present), this normally weak slow inward current may give rise to the regenerative depolarization characteristic of a propagated action potential. This propagated action potential dependent on slow inward current alone is the slow response (Cranefield, 1975). Since this inward current is weak, conduction velocity is slow and both unidirectional and bidirectional conduction block may occur (Cranefield et al., 1973). Slow response action potentials can occur in diseased cardiac fibers with low resting potentials, but they also occur in some normal regions of the heart such as in cells of the sinoatrial and atrioventricular nodes where the maximum diastolic potential is normally positive to about −70 mv (Cranefield, 1975).

Reentrant excitation caused by the slow conduction and block which accompany depression of the action potential upstroke may occur in gross, anatomically distinct circuits (around an anatomical obstacle). This is exemplified by reentry in a loop of cardiac fiber bundles such as the loops of Purkinje fiber bundles in the distal conducting system. Similar anatomical circuits might be formed by bundles of surviving muscle fibers in healed infarcts or in fibrotic regions of the atria and ventricles. Gross anatomical circuits are also involved in reentry utilizing the bundle branches or accessory A-V connecting pathways (Wit and Cranefield, 1978). The basic principles have been discussed quite extensively in other reviews (Vassalle, 1965; Cranefield, 1975; Wit and Cranefield, 1978; Cranefield et al., 1973).

Gross anatomical loops and anatomical obstacles are not absolutely necessary for the occurrence of reentry. Reentry may occur in the sinus or atrioventricular node where no such circuits are obvious. Reentry caused by slow conduction and unidirectional block can also occur in unbranched bundles or "sheets" of muscle fibers. A kind of reentry called reflection occurs in unbranched bundles of Purkinje fibers in which conduction is slow because the resting and action potentials are depressed (Cranefield, 1975; Cranefield et al., 1973). During reflection, excitation occurs slowly in one direction along a bundle of fibers and is followed by excitation occurring in the opposite direction (Fig. 1-12). Wit et al., (1972) proposed that the returning (reflected) impulse is caused by reentry due to longitudinal dissociation of the bundles. This is a type of microreentry.

Recently, Moe and his coinvestigators have described another mechanism which may cause reflection (Antzelevitch et al., 1980; Jalife and Moe, 1981). Slow conduction along the bundles caused by depressed transmembrane potentials as described by Wit et al. (1972) is not necessary, but rather, there is delayed activation of part of the bundle resulting from electrotonic excitation of a region distal to an inexcitable segment. If a segment of a bundle of Purkinje fibers is inexcitable and will not generate action potentials, impulses conducting along the bundle will block at this segment. The blocked action potential, however, can generate axial current flow through the inexcitable segment of the fiber bundle which acts as a passive cable. This electrotonic manifestation of the blocked impulse decays along the cable in the inexcitable segment according to the length constant which is dependent to a large extent on the intra- and extracellular resistances to current flow. If the inexcitable segment is sufficiently short relative to the length constant (2 mm in the experiments of Antzelevitch et al. (1980) and

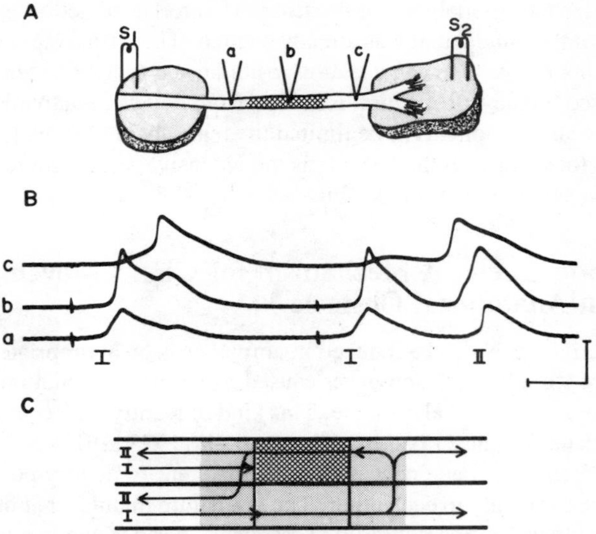

1-12 Reentry (reflection) in a linear bundle of canine Purkinje fibers. A, diagram of preparation showing location of stimulating electrodes (S_1 and S_2) and recording electrodes (a, b, c). The center segment, depressed by high K^+, is indicated by cross-hatched area. The bundle is being stimulated at S_1 only. B, in the first group of action potentials, I shows conduction of impulse originating at S_1 without reentry; conduction from a–c, through the depressed area required 100 ms. In the second group of action potentials, I shows conduction of another impulse from S_1 with a marked increase in the conduction delay between recording sites b and c to 250 ms. A reentrant impulse II returning in the opposite direction is shown at recording sites b and a. C, diagrammatic representation of a possible pathway of impulse propagation during reentry in two parallel fibers. Severely depressed area indicated by cross-hatches, moderately depressed area by stipples. Impulse I is completely blocked in upper fiber at area of unidirectional block but traverses the moderately depressed area in lower fiber, then reenters upper fiber to travel in the reverse direction as impulse II. Calibrations: vertical, 100 mv for traces a and c and 50 mv for trace b; horizontal, 250 ms. (Reproduced from Cranefield, P.F., Wit, A.L., and Hoffman, B.F. 1973. Genesis of cardiac arrhythmias. Circulation 45: 190, with permission.)

Jalife and Moe (1981)), the current flow across the gap can depolarize the excitable fibers distal to the inexcitable region and can excite an action potential. This can occur with a great amount of delay which is dependent to a large extent on the time course and amplitude of the electrotonic current flow. The action potential initiated distal to the point of block not only will conduct distally along the fiber but can itself cause retrograde axial current flow through the inexcitable gap to depolarize the part of the fiber proximal to the gap at the site of the original block. If the sum of excitation times in both directions across the inexcitable gap exceeds the refractory period of the proximal segment, an action potential will be elicited that propagates retrogradely along the fiber. This reflected action potential reenters the part of the bundle that was already excited. Thus, impulse transmission in both directions is over the same pathway unlike the types of reentry that have been discussed already. Reflection resulting from delays in activation caused by electrotonic transmission might be limited to areas where damage to the myocardial fibers is focal since, if the damage is too extensive, electrotonic transmission across the inexcitable area would fail.

The Leading Circle: A Mechanism for Circus Movement without an Anatomical Obstacle

Repetitive activity can also be induced in normal atria by appropriately timed single premature stimuli. Such activity is caused by reentrant excitation occurring in the absence of an anatomical obstacle. This kind of reentry may occur by the leading circle mechanism described by Allessie et al. (1973, 1977) (Fig. 1-13). The initiation of reentry is made possible by the different refractory periods of atrial fibers in close proximity to each other. The premature impulse that initiates repetitive activity blocks in fibers with long refractory periods and conducts in fibers with shorter refractory periods, eventually returning to the initial point of block after excitability recovers there. The impulse may then continue to circulate. Conduction through the reentrant circuit is slowed because impulses are propagating in partially refractory tissue. The circumference of the pathway may be as small as 6–8 mm. Impulses spread centripetally from the circumference of the circulating wave toward the center, and the rates of rise and amplitude of these action potentials gradually decrease as the center is approached. Cells at the center of the circulating wave show only local responses since they are kept in a refractory state by the circulating impulse (Allessie et al., 1977). The length of the circuit is defined completely by the conduction velocity and refractory period of the fibers composing it rather than by some well defined anatomical pathway around an obstacle.

Slow Conduction and Reentrant Excitation Caused by the Anisotropic Structure of Cardiac Muscle

Cardiac muscle is anisotropic; that is, its anatomical and biophysical properties vary according to the direction in the cardiac syncytium in which they are measured (Clerc, 1976). Spach and his co-workers have recently published a series of articles on the effects of anisotropy on conduction properties of normal atrial and ventricular muscle and have shown how anisotropy can cause reentry (Spach et al., 1981; Spach et al., 1982a; Spach et al., 1982b). They have demonstrated that in uniformly anisotropic cardiac tissue (in tissue where the cardiac muscle fibers are closely packed together and arranged parallel to each other in a uniform man-

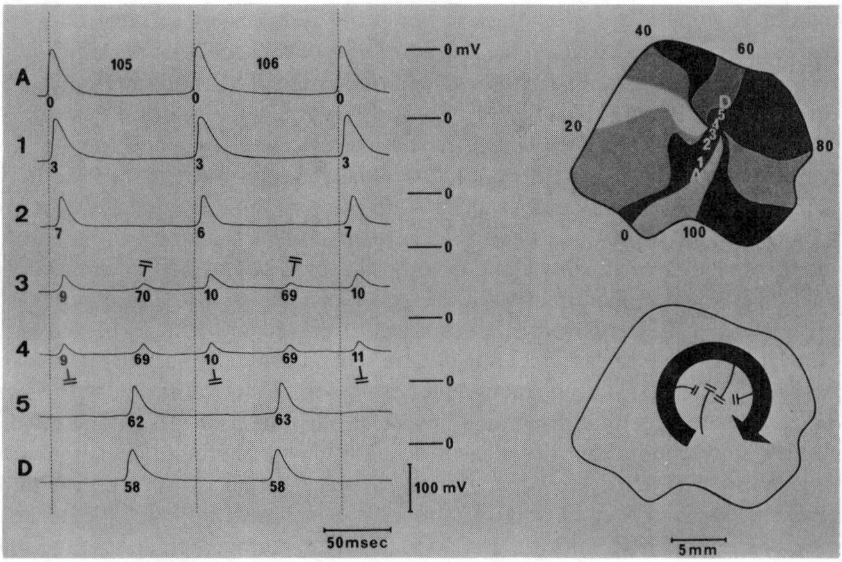

1-13 Reentry in isolated left atrial myocardium by the leading circle mechanism. At the right, above, is the map of the activation pattern of the atrium during circus movement. The impulse was continuously rotating in a clockwise direction; each number and different shading indicates the time in milliseconds during which a given region is activated. Activation proceeds from 0–100 ms and one complete revolution takes 100 ms. At the left, the membrane potentials of seven fibers (marked A, D, and 1–5) located on a straight line through the center of the circus movement are shown (the locations from which these action potentials were recorded are indicated on the map at the upper right). These records show that the fibers in the central point of the circuit (fibers 3 and 4) show double responses of subnormal amplitude during circus movement. These responses result from conduction of the impulse from the circulating wave toward the center. At the lower right, the activation pattern during circus movement is given schematically. It shows the circuit with the converging wavelets in the center. (Reproduced from Allessie, M.A., Bonke, F.I.M., and Schopman, F.J.G. 1977. Circus movement in rabbit atrial muscle as a mechanism of tachycardia. III. The 'leading circle' concept: a new model of circus movement in cardiac tissue without the involvement of an anatomical obstacle. Circ Res 41:9–18, with permission.)

ner), conduction in a direction parallel to the myocardial fiber orientation (along the long axis of the myocardial fibers) is much more rapid than in the direction perpendicular to the long axis. Conduction perpendicular to the long axis of the fibers can be very slow in normal atrial or ventricular muscle (0.1 m/s) even though resting and action potentials of the muscle fibers are normal (Spach et al., 1981). The slow conduction is caused by an effective axial resistivity which is higher in the direction perpendicular to fiber orientation than parallel to fiber orientation. Effective axial resistivity as defined by Spach et al. "is the resistance to current flow in the direction of propagation and is dependent on the intracellular and extracellular resistivities, the size and shape of cells, cellular packing and the resistance, extent and distribution of cell to cell couplings (Spach et al., 1981; Spach et al., 1982a)." The higher axial resistivity perpendicular to fiber orientation results in part from fewer and shorter intercalated discs connecting myocardial fibers in a side-to-side direction than in the end-to-end direction. In addition, although it may seem paradoxical, in spite of more rapid conduction down the long axis of the myocardial fibers than perpendicular to the long axis, premature impulses block more readily along the long axis because the safety factor for conduction is lower in the direction of the lower axial resistivity. The derivation of the principles underlying this concept are discussed in detail by Spach et al. (1981). When myocardial fiber bundles are separated by nonmuscular tissue such as connective tissue, the conduction properties will be altered further by the separation and the structural discontinuities. Such separation of myocardial bundles further slow conduction because of a reduction in intercellular connections (Spach et al., 1982b). The separation of myocardial fibers by connective tissue results in a nonuniform anisotropic structure (Spach et al., 1982b). Spach et al. have shown that both uniform and nonuniform anisotropic structural properties can cause reentry in atrial myocardium with normal transmembrane potentials and uniform refractory periods because anisotropy can cause both slow conduction and conduction block (Spach et al., 1981; Spach et al., 1982b). It has also been proposed that anisotropy of epicardial muscle surviving over healing canine infarcts may cause reentry (Gardner et al., 1983).

Acknowledgment

This work was partly supported by Program Project Grant HL 12738 from the National Institutes of Health.

References

Allessie, M.A., Bonke, F.I.M., and Schopman, F. 1973. Circus movement in rabbit right atrial muscle as a mechanism of tachycardia. Circ Res 33:54–62.

Allessie, M.A., Bonke, F.I.M., and Schopman, F.J.G. 1977. Circus movement in rabbit atrial muscle as a mechanism of tachycardia. III. The "Leading circle" concept: A new model of circus movement in cardiac tissue without the involvement of an anatomical obstacle. Circ Res 41:9–18.

Allessie, M.A., Lammers, W., Smeets, J., Bonke, F., and Hollen, J. 1982. Total mapping of atrial excitation during acetylcholine-induced atrial flutter and fibrillation in the isolated canine heart. In: H.E. Kulbertus, S.B. Olsson, and M. Schlepper, eds. Atrial Fibrillation. Molndal, Sweden: AB Hassle.

Antzelevitch, C., Jalife, J., and Moe, G.K. 1980. Characteristics of reflection as a mechanism of reentrant arrhythmias and its relationship to parasystole. Circulation 61:182–191.

Aronson, R.S. 1981. Afterpotentials and triggered activity in hypertrophied myocardium from rats with renal hypertension. Circ Res 48:720–727.

Brachman, J., Scherlag, B., Rosenstraukh, L.V., and Lazzara, R. 1983. Bradycardia-dependent triggered activity: Relevance to drug-induced multiform ventricular tachycardia. Circulation 68:846–856.

Brooks, C. McC., Hoffman, P.F., Suckling, E.E., and Orias, O. 1955. Excitability of the Heart. New York: Grune and Stratton.

Brown, H.F., and Noble, S.J. 1969. Membrane currents underlying delayed rectification and pacemaker activity in frog atrial muscle. J Physiol (Lond) 204:717–736.

Carmeliet, E. 1980. The slow inward current: non-voltage-clamp studies. In: D.P. Zipes, J.C. Bailey, and V. Elharrar, eds. The Slow Inward Current and Cardiac Arrhythmias. The Hague: Martinus Nijhoff.

Clerc, L., 1976. Directional differences of impulse spread in trabecular muscle from mammalian heart. J Physiol (Lond) 255:335–346.

Coraboef, E., and Boistel, J. 1953. L'action des taux eleves de gaz carbonique sur le tissu cardiaque etudiee a l'aide de microelectrodes intracellulaires. Compt Rend Soc Biol (Paris) 147:654–658.

Cranefield, P.F. 1975. The Slow Response and Cardiac Arrhythmias. Mt. Kisco: Futura Press.

Cranefield, P.F. 1977. Action potentials, afterpotentials and arrhythmias. Circ Res 41:415–423.

Cranefield, P.F., Wit, A.L., and Hoffman, B.F. 1973. Genesis of cardiac arrhythmias. Circulation 47:190–204.

Dahl, G., and Isenberg, G., 1980. Decoupling of heart muscle cells: correlation with increased cytoplasmic calcium activity and with changes in nexus ultrastructure. J Membr Biol 53:63–75.

Dangman, K.H., and Hoffman, B.F. 1981. In vivo and in vitro antiarrhythmic and arrhythmogenic effects of N-acetyl procainamide. J Pharmacol Exp Ther 217:851–862.

Dangman, K.H., and Hoffman, B.F. Studies on overdrive stimulation of canine cardiac Purkinje fibers: Maximum diastolic potential as a determinant of the response. J Am Coll Cardiol In Press.

DiFrancesco, D. 1981a. A new interpretation of the pacemaking current in calf Purkinje fibers. J Physiol 314:359–376.

DiFrancesco, D. 1981b. A study of the ionic nature of the packmaker current in calf Purkinje fibers. J Physiol 314:377–393.

Eisner, D.A., and Lederer, W.J. 1979. Inotropic and arrhythmogenic effects of potassium depleted solutions on mammalian cardiac muscle. J Physiol (Lond) 294:255–277.

El-Sherif, N., Zeiler, R., and Gough, W.B. 1980. Effects of catecholamines, verapamil and tetrodotoxin on triggered automaticity in canine ischemic Purkinje fibers. Circulation 62 Part 2:281.

Ferrier, G.R. 1977. Digitalis arrhythmias: Role of oscillatory afterpotentials. Progr Cardiovasc Dis 19:459–474.

Ferrier, G.R., Rosenthal, J.E. 1980. Automaticity and entrance block induced by focal depolarization of mammalian ventricular tissues. Circ Res 47:238–248.

Friedman, P.L., Stewart, J.R., and Wit, A.L. 1973. Spontaneous and induced cardiac arrhythmias in subendocardial Purkinje fibers surviving extensive myocardial infarction in dogs. Circ Res 33:612–626.

Gadsby, D.C., and Cranefield, P.F. 1979. Direct measurement of changes in sodium pump current in canine cardiac Purkinje fibers. Proc Natl Acad Sci USA 76:1783–1787.

Gadsby, D.C., and Wit, A.L. 1981. Electrophysiologic characteristics of cardiac cells and the genesis of cardiac arrhythmias. In: R.G. Wilkersen, ed. Cardiac Pharmacology. New York: Academic Press.

Gardner, P., Ursell, P.C., Pham, T.D., Fenoglio, J.J., and Wit, A.L. 1983. Experimental chronic ventricular tachycardia: Anatomic and electrophysiologic substrates. In: M.E. Josephson, and H.J.J. Wellens, eds. Tachycardias: Mechanisms and Management. Philadelphia: Lea and Febiger. (In Press)

Hoffman, B.F., and Cranefield, P.F. 1960. Electrophysiology of the Heart. New York: McGraw-Hill.

Hoffman, B.F., and Cranefield, P.F., 1964. The physiological basis of cardiac arrhythmias. Am J Med 37:670–684.

Hoffman, B.F., and Rosen, M.R. 1981. Cellular mechanisms for cardiac arrhythmias. Circ Res 49:1–15.

Hordof, A., Edie, R., Malm, J., Hoffman, B.F., and Rosen, M.R. 1976. Electrophysiological properties and response to pharmacologic agents of fibers from diseased human atria. Circulation 54:774–779.

Jalife, J., and Moe, G.K. 1976. Effects of electrotonic potentials on pacemaker activity of canine Purkinje fibers in relation to parasystole. Circ Res 39:801–808.

Jalife, J., and Moe, G.K. 1979. A biologic model of parasystole. Am J Cardiol 43:761–772.

Jalife, J., and Moe, G.K. 1981. Excitation, conduction and reflection of impulses in isolated bovine and canine cardiac Purkinje fibers. Circ Res 49:233–247.

Kass, R.S., Lederer, W.J., Tsien, R.W., and Weingart, R. 1978a. Role of calcium ions in transient inward currents and aftercontractions induced by strophanthidin in cardiac Purkinje fibers. J Physiol (Lond) 281:187–208.

Kass, R.S., Tsien, R.W., and Weingart, R. 1978b. Ionic basis of transient inward current induced by strophanthidin in cardiac Purkinje fibers. J Physiol (Lond) 281:209–226.

Katzung, B.O., and Morgenstern, J.A. 1977. Effects of extracellular potassium on ventricular automaticity and evidence for a pacemaker current in mammalian ventricular myocardium. Circ Res 40:105–111.

Kokubun, S., Nishimura, M., Noma, A., and Irisawa, A. 1980. The spontaneous action potential of rabbit atrioventricular node cells. Jap J Physiol 30:529–540.

Lab, M.J. 1978. Mechanically dependent changes in action potentials recorded from the intact frog ventricle. Circ Res 42:519–528.

Lazzara, R., El-Sherif, N., and Scherlag, B.J. 1973. Electrophysiological properties of canine Purkinje cells in one-day-old myocardial infarction. Circ Res 33:722–734.

Mary-Rabine, L., Hordof, A.J., Danilo, P., Malm, J.R., and Rosen, M.R. 1980. Mechanisms for impulse initiation in isolated human atrial fibers. Circ Res 47:267–277.

Mines, G.R., 1914. On circulating excitations in heart muscle and their possible relations to tachycardia and fibrillation. Trans Roy Soc Can Ser 3 Sect IV 8:43.

Nathan, D., and Beeler, G.W. 1975. Electrophysiologic correlates of the inotropic effects of isoproterenol in canine myocardium. J Mol Cell Cardiol 7:1–15.

Noble, D., and Tsien, R.W. 1968. The kinetics and rectifier properties of the slow potassium current in cardiac Purkinje fibers. J Physiol (Lond) 195:185–214.

Noma, A., Irisawa, H., Kokubun, S., Kotake, H., Nishimura, M., and Watanabe, Y. 1980. Nature 285:228–229.

Reuter, H. 1979. Properties of two inward membrane currents in heart. Annu Rev Physiol 41:413–424.

Rosen, M.R., and Reder, R.F. 1981. Does triggered activity have a role in the genesis of cardiac arrhythmias. Ann Intern Med 94:794–801.

Saito, T., Otaguro, M., and Matsubara, T. 1978. Electrophysiological studies on the mechanism of electrically induced sustained rhythmic activity in the rabbit right atrium. Circ Res 42:199–206.

Scherf, D., and Cohen, J. 1964. The Atrioventricular Node and Selected Cardiac Arrhythmias. New York: Grune and Stratton.

Singer, D.H., Baumgarten, C.M., and Ten Eck, R.E. 1981. Cellular electrophysiology of ventricular and other dysrhythmias: Studies on diseased and ischemic heart. Progr Cardiovasc Dis 24:97–156.

Spach, M.S., Kootsey, J.M., and Sloan, J.D. 1982a. Active modulation of electrical coupling between cardiac cells of the dog: A mechanism for transient and steady state variations in conduction velocity. Circ Res 51:347–362.

Spach, M.S., Miller, W.T., Dolber, P.C., Kootsey, J.M., Sommer, J.R., and Mosher, C.E. 1982b. The functional role of structural complexities in the propagation of depolarization in the atrium of the dog: Cardiac conduction disturbances due to discontinuities of effective axial resistivity. Circ Res 50:175–191.

Spach M.S., Miller W.T., Jr., Geselowitz, D.B., Barr, R.C., Kootsey, J.M., and Johnson, E.A. 1981. The discontinuous nature of propagation in normal canine cardiac muscle. Evidence for recurrent discontinuities of intracellular resistance that affect the membrane currents. Circ. Res. 48:39–54.

Strauss, H.C., Bigger, J.T., Jr., and Hoffman, B.F. 1970. Electrophysiological and beta-receptor blocking effects of MJ 1999 on dog and rabbit cardiac tissues. Circ Res 26:661–678.

Surawicz, B., and Imanishi, S. 1976. Automatic activity in depolarized guinea pig ventricular myocardium: characteristics and mechanisms. Circ Res 39:751–759.

Trautwein, W. 1973. Membrane currents in cardiac muscle fibers. Physiol Rev 53:793–835.

Trautwein, W., Gottstein, V., and Dudel, J. 1954. Der Aktionsstrom der Myokardfaser im Sauerstoffmangel. Pfluegers Arch Ges Physiol 260:40–60.

Tsien, R.W. 1974. Effects of epinephrine on the pacemaker potassium current of cardiac Purkinje fibers. J Gen Physiol 64:293–319.

Tsien, R.W. 1983. Calcium channels in excitable cell membranes. Annu Rev Physiol 45:341–358.

Van Capelle, F.J.L., and Durrer, D. 1980. Computer simulation of arrhythmias in a network of coupled excitable elements. Circ Res 47:454–466.

Vassalle, M. 1965. Analysis of cardiac pacemaker potential using a "voltage clamp" technique. Am J Physiol 208:770–775.

Vassalle, M. 1970. Electrogenic suppression of automaticity in sheep and dog Purkinje fibers. Circ Res 27:361–377.

Vassalle, M. 1977. The relationship among cardiac pacemakers: Overdrive suppression. Circ Res 41:269–277.

Vassalle, M., and Carpenter, R. 1972. Overdrive excitation: Onset of activity following fast drive in cardiac Purkinje fibers exposed to norepinephrine. Pflueger Arch Ges Physiol 332:198–205.

Weidman, S. 1955. The effect of the cardiac membrane potential on the rapid availability of the sodium carrying system. J Physiol (Lond) 127:213–224.

Weingart, R. 1977. The actions of ouabain on intercellular coupling and conduction velocity in mammalian ventricular muscle. J Physiol (Lond) 264:341–365.

Wit, A.L. and Cranefield, P.F. 1976. Triggered activity in cardiac muscle fibers of the simian mitral valve. Circ Res 38:85–98.

Wit, A.L., and Cranefield, P.F. 1977. Triggered and automatic activity in the canine coronary sinus. Circ Res 41:435–445.

Wit, A.L., and Cranefield, P.E. 1978. Reentrant excitation as a cause of cardiac arrhythmias. Am J Physiol 235:H1–H17.

Wit, A.L., and Cranefield, P.F. 1982. Mechanisms of impulse initiation in the atrioventricular junction and the effects of acetylstrophanthidin (abstr). Am J Cardiol 49:921.

Wit, A.L., Cranefield, P.F., and Gadsby, D.C. 1980. Triggered activity. In: D.P. Zipes, J.C. Bailey, and V. Elharrar, eds. The Slow Inward Current and Cardiac Arrhythmias. The Hague: Martinus Nijhoff.

Wit, A.L., Gadsby, D.C., and Cranfield, P.F. 1981. Electrogenic sodium extrusion can stop triggered activity in the canine coronary sinus. Circ Res 49:1029–1042.

Wit, A.L., Hoffman, B.F., and Cranefield, P.F. 1972. Slow conduction and reentry in the ventricular conducting system. I. Return extrasystole in Canine Purkinje fibers. Circ Res 30:1–22.

Yanagihara, K., and Irisawa, H. 1980. Potassium current during the pacemaker depolarization in rabbit sinoatrial node cell. Pfluegers Arch Ges Physiol 388:255–260.

Chapter 2

Neural Mechanisms in Cardiac Arrhythmias

Richard L. Verrier and Eric L. Hagestad

Introduction

Clinical and experimental studies have provided compelling evidence implicating neural factors in the genesis of cardiac arrhythmias. The contemporary challenge is to define precisely the mechanisms responsible for the arrhythmogenic influence of neural activity. Available evidence indicates the involvement of several interacting factors, including alterations in coronary hemodynamic function and platelet aggregability as well as direct effects of neurotransmitters on myocardial excitable properties.

Central Nervous System Stimulation and Ventricular Arrhythmias

Stimulation of various central nervous system structures by drugs or by means of stereotaxically positioned electrodes can elicit a diversity of ventricular arrhythmias (Lown et al., 1977; Hoff et al., 1963; Korteweg et al., 1957). In normal animals, stimulation of the posterior hypothalamus, for example, rarely provokes ventricular fibrillation (VF) but profoundly lowers the vulnerable period threshold (Verrier et al., 1975). When hypothalamic stimulation was conducted during acute left anterior descending coronary artery occlusion, the occurrence of spontaneous VF increased 10-fold (from 6–63%) as compared to occlusion without neural stimulation (Satinsky et al., 1971). The susceptibility to ventricular arrhythmias associated with stimulation of various cortical and subcortical structures is prevented by cardiac sympathectomy (Manning and Cotten, 1962) or β-adrenergic blockade (Verrier et al., 1975; Hockman et al., 1966). Parasympathetic pathways are probably not involved because bilateral vagotomy leaves unaltered the arrhythmogenic effect of central nervous system stimulation (Verrier et al., 1975; Hockman et al., 1966). The ventricular arrhythmias which immediately follow cessation of diencephalic or hypothalamic stimulation require intact vagi and stellate ganglia (Korteweg et al., 1957; Manning and Cotten, 1962).

Thus, brain stimulation can provoke a variety of ventricular arrhythmias and lower the vulnerable period threshold (Verrier, 1980). In animals with acute myocardial ischemia, such stimuli are sufficient to provoke VF. The sympathetic nervous system appears to be the primary mediator of the arrhythmogenic effect of central nervous system stimulation.

Peripheral Sympathetic Nervous System and Arrhythmogenesis

There is a substantial body of information suggesting that peripheral sympathetic neural structures are primarily involved in mediating the autonomic nervous system influence on ventricular electrical stability. For example, it has been shown that the profibrillatory effects of central nervous system stimulation can be prevented by cardiac sympathectomy or by administration of sympatholytic drugs (Corr et al., 1978; Corr and Sharma, 1982; Elharrar et al., 1979; Hockman et al., 1966; Manning and Peiss, 1960; Rosen et al., 1971; Sheridan et al., 1980; Stewart et al., 1980; Manning and Cotten, 1962; Rosen et al., 1977). The direct effects of sympathetic neural influences can be demonstrated by electrical stimulation of the stellate ganglia (Figure 2-1). In normal animals, stimulation of cardiac sympathetic efferent fibers markedly lowers the vulnerable period threshold (Han et al., 1964) and increases the incidence of spontaneous VF during myocardial ischemia (Harris et al., 1971). Conversely, stellate ganglionectomy increases the VF threshold (Schwartz et al., 1976a), reduces susceptibility to cardiac arrhythmias during coronary artery occlusion (Schwartz et al., 1976b), and increases the capacity of the coronary arterial bed to dilate (Schwartz and Stone, 1977) (Figs. 2-2 and 2-3).

The specific involvement of α-adrenergic receptors in neurally induced arrhythmias is not well understood. This relates, in part, to the complexity of their influences, which include both direct actions on myocardial excitable properties (Rosen et al., 1971) and indirect effects on insulin secretion (Majid et al., 1970), platelet aggregability (Pfister and Imhof, 1977), and coronary hemodynamic function (Mohrman and Feigl, 1978; Schwartz and Stone, 1977). The latter consideration may be of particular import in view of growing evidence implicating coronary vasospasm as a factor in the genesis of lethal arrhythmias (Maseri et al., 1979).

By contrast β-adrenergic receptors appear to be involved directly in mediating neurally induced vulnerability (Matta et al., 1976b; Rosenfeld et al., 1978; Verrier and Lown, 1977). Our group and others have demonstrated this using a variety of experimental models. For example, β-adrenergic blockade has been shown to prevent stress induced vulnerability to VF during classical (Verrier and Lown, 1977) and instrumental (Matta et al., 1976b) conditioning as well as during elicitation of an anger-like state (Verrier et al., 1982).

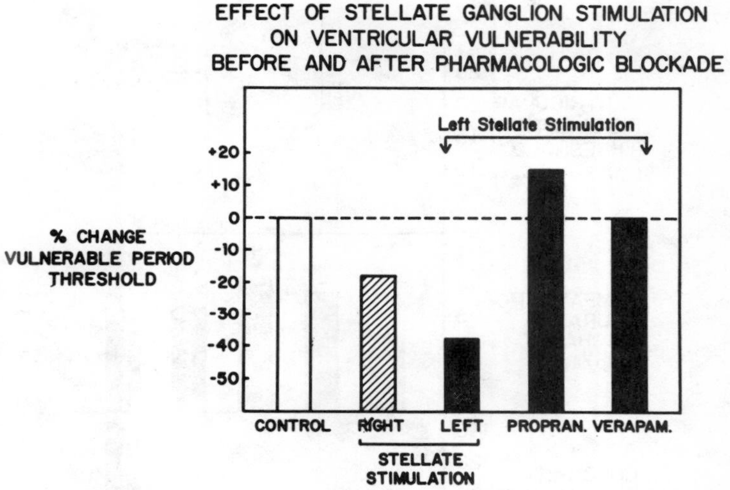

2-1 Effect of stellate ganglion stimulation on ventricular vulnerability before and after pharmacologic blockade. Left stellate ganglion stimulation exerted a predominant effect on the vulnerable period threshold, but a substantial effect was also produced by right stellate stimulation. The decrease in threshold induced by sympathetic stimulation was abolished by β-adrenergic blockade with propranolol (0.25 mg/kg) or verapamil infusion (0.01 mg/kg/min for 15 min) (Verrier and Lown, 1978a).

Skinner and co-workers (1975), however, have been unable to demonstrate a protective effect of β-adrenergic blockade against stress induced fibrillation. They found that whereas adaptation of pigs to a laboratory environment protected against VF during coronary artery obstruction, β-adrenergic blockade with propranolol was completely ineffective in protecting unadapted animals. It remains unclear whether the failure of propranolol to protect against ventricular fibrillation resulted from inadequate blockade of adrenergic inputs to the heart or to other effects, such as the unmasking of the constrictor influence of unopposed α-receptors on coronary vascular smooth muscle. The latter hypothesis is suggested by recent clinical experience. Kern et al. (1983) have demonstrated in patients with coronary artery disease that propranolol potentiates the coronary vasoconstrictor response to the reflex activation of the sympathetic nervous system which occurs during the cold pressor test.

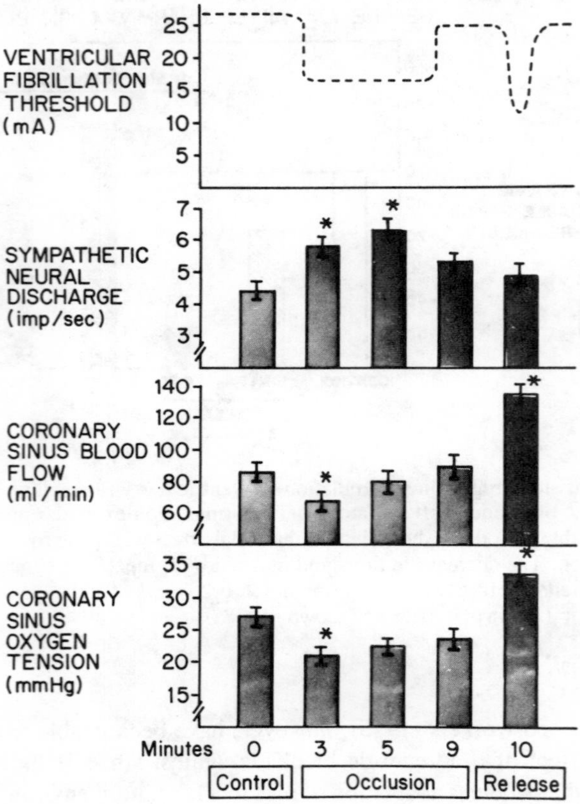

2-2 Effects of a 10-min period of left anterior descending coronary artery occlusion and release on neural sympathetic activity, coronary sinus blood flow, and oxygen tension. A schematic representation of the time course of changes in ventricular fibrillation threshold is also displayed. Left anterior descending coronary artery occlusion results in a consistent activation of sympathetic preganglionic fibers which corresponds with the period of maximal increase in vulnerability to ventricular fibrillation. The concomitant changes in coronary sinus blood flow and reperfusion are also displayed. *$p < 0.05$ compared to control period (Lombardi et al., 1983).

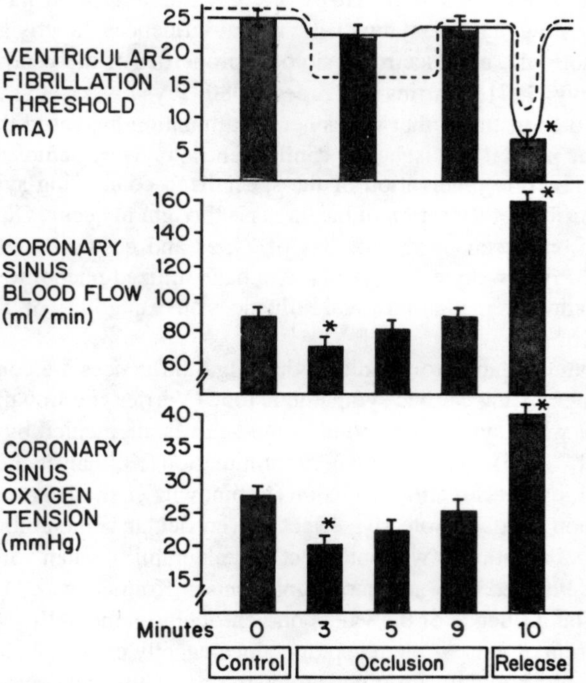

2-3 Effects of bilateral stellectomy on ventricular fibrillation threshold, coronary sinus blood flow, and oxygen tension changes induced by a 10-min period of coronary artery occlusion and release. Stellectomy provides complete protection during coronary artery occlusion without influencing the pattern of change of coronary sinus blood flow and oxygen tension. In contrast, stellectomy enhances the susceptibility to ventricular fibrillation during release-reperfusion. The reactive hyperemic response is also enhanced (see Fig. 3-1). The dashed and solid lines represent the schematized vulnerability threshold changes in neurally intact and stellectomized dogs, respectively. * $p < 0.05$ compared to control period (Lombardi et al., 1983).

Parasympathetic Nervous System and Cardiac Arrhythmias

The prevailing view had been that vagal innervation did not extend to the ventricular myocardium. Clinical teaching had been in accord with this perception. If a tachycardia responded to cholinergic measures, the site of impulse formation was judged to be supraventricular. However, considerable data have now been amassed indicating that parasympathetic neural influences directly affect the inotropic, chronotropic, and electrophysiologic properties of the ventricles (Kent et al., 1974; Levy, 1971; Martins and Zipes, 1980; Prystowsky et al., 1981). Kent et al. (1974) demonstrated that vagus nerve stimulation increased the VF threshold in both the normal and ischemic canine ventricle. They demonstrated, moreover, the cholinergic innervation of the specialized conducting system through which the antifibrillatory action of the vagus is thought to occur. Our understanding has been enhanced by the studies of Zipes and co-workers (Martins and Zipes, 1980; Prystowsky et al., 1981) who have utilized phenol to delineate the anatomical pathways mediating vagal influences on excitability of the normal and ischemic heart.

Results from this laboratory indicate that vagal influences are contingent upon the level of preexisting cardiac sympathetic tone (Verrier and Lown, 1978b). We observed that when sympathetic tone to the heart is augmented by thoracotomy (Kolman et al., 1975), sympathetic nerve stimulation (Kolman et al., 1975; Matta et al., 1976a), or catecholamine infusion (Rabinowitz et al., 1976), simultaneous vagal activation exerts a protective effect on ventricular vulnerability (Fig. 2-4). Vagus nerve stimulation is without effect on vulnerability when adrenergic input to the heart is blocked by β-adrenergic antagonists (Kolman et al., 1975; Yoon et al., 1977). The influence of the vagus on ventricular vulnerability appears to be due to activation of muscarinic receptors, since vagally mediated changes in vulnerability are prevented by atropine administration. Muscarinic agents have been shown both to inhibit the release of norepinephrine from sympathetic nerve endings (Levy, 1971; Levy and Blattberg, 1976) and to attenuate the response to norepinephrine at receptor sites by cyclic nucleotide interactions (Watanabe and Besch, 1974, 1975; Watanabe et al., 1977, 1981).

There is evidence indicating that sympathetic-parasympathetic interactions also modulate myocardial electrical stability in the conscious state (Lown and Verrier, 1976; Verrier and Lown, 1980). This is supported by studies in which relatively small doses of atropine (0.05 mg/kg) were employed to block selectively vagal efferent activity to the heart. When animals were exposed to an aversive environment where catecholamine levels were elevated, vagal efferent blockade resulted in a substantial 50% reduction in the vulnerable period threshold (Fig. 2-5). In a nonstressful setting where plasma catecholamine levels were low, vagal blockade

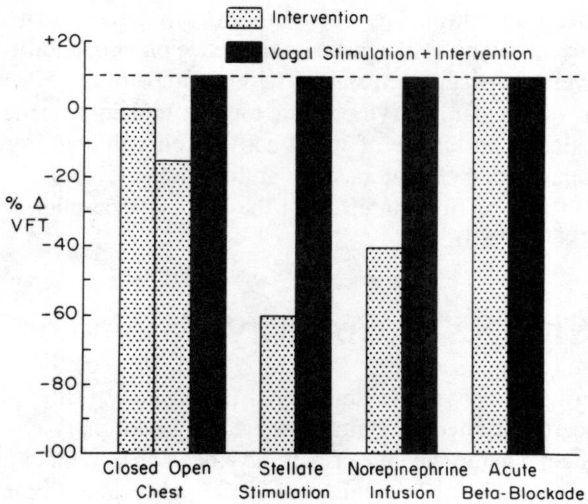

2-4 Influence of vagal stimulation in the presence of various levels of adrenergic tone. The vagal effect on ventricular fibrillation threshold (VFT) is demonstrable only when neural or humoral activity is increased (Lown and Verrier, 1976).

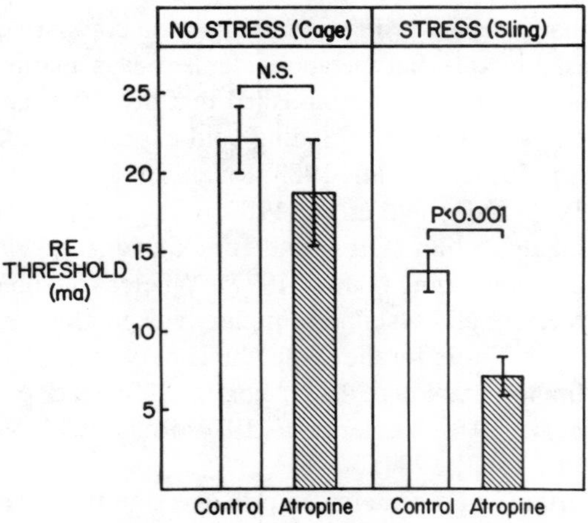

2-5 Influence of atropine (0.05 mg/kg) on repetitive extrasystole (RE) threshold in conscious dogs exposed to nonaversive and aversive environments. In the aversive setting, blockade of vagal efferent activity with atropine substantially reduced the vulnerable period threshold, indicating an enhanced propensity for ventricular fibrillation. In the nonstressful setting, where adrenergic activity was low, no effect of the drug was evident. Heart rate was maintained constant during cardiac electrical testing by ventricular pacing (Verrier and Lown, 1981).

was without effect on ventricular vulnerability (Verrier and Lown, 1980). Thus, tonic vagal activity can exert a significant influence on vulnerability to VF in the conscious as well as anesthetized state. The magnitude of the effect is related to the level of prevailing cardiac sympathetic tone. It remains uncertain, however, whether the salutary influence of vagal activity on vulnerability results from sympathetic-parasympathetic interactions at the cardiac level (Levy, 1971; Levy and Blattberg, 1976) or from an effect at the coronary vascular smooth muscle level (Feigl, 1969, 1983).

Role of Changes in Coronary Vasomotor Tone

Coronary artery spasm has been implicated increasingly in the provocation of transient myocardial ischemia. Primary decreases in coronary blood flow independent of systemic hemodynamic effects have been observed not only in variant angina (Oliva et al., 1973; Chierchia et al., 1980; Hillis and Braunwald, 1978), but also in classic and unstable angina (Hillis and Braunwald, 1978; Deanfield et al., 1983; Maseri et al., 1978a, 1979; Luchi et al., 1979). Deanfield and coworkers (1983) reported recurrent episodes of ST segment depression during ambulatory monitoring in patients with stable angina. These were not correlated with changes in heart rate and were shown to be associated with myocardial ischemia. They concluded that transient primary impairment in coronary artery blood flow rather than increased myocardial metabolic demand was a common stimulus for myocardial ischemia. It has been established that diverse events or stimuli can lead to coronary vasoconstriction including cold exposure (Mudge et al., 1976, 1979; Ricci et al., 1979; Kern et al., 1983; Raizner et al., 1980), exercise (Hillis and Braunwald, 1978; Deanfield et al., 1983; Luchi et al., 1979; Yasue et al., 1979), myocardial infarction (Oliva and Breckinridge, 1977; Maseri et al., 1978b), and verbal conditioning (Lown, 1977). Whereas the precise mechanisms responsible for excessive and sustained coronary vasomotion are unclear, several studies indicate a central role for the sympathetic nervous system (Mohrman and Feigl, 1978; Buffington and Feigl, 1981; Feigl, 1983; Mark et al., 1972; Pitt et al., 1967; Orlick et al., 1978; Vatner et al., 1974; Ross, 1976; Verrier and Lown, 1984; Verrier et al., 1982, 1984).

Excitation of certain brain centers can provoke significant coronary vasoconstriction (Pasyk et al., 1981; Pasyk and Pitt, 1983; Pitt et al., 1982). Pasyk et al. (1981, 1983) have shown that injection of opioids into the lateral cerebral ventricles of conscious dogs produces profound and sustained coronary vasoconstriction that is abolished by α-adrenergic blockade. These investigators have also obtained preliminary evidence that opiate-induced vasopressin release may be associated with coronary artery spasm in man (Pitt et al., 1982). They found increased serum arginine vasopressin in both spontaneous and ergonovine-induced coronary artery spasm. They postulate that endogenous arginine vasopressin in conjunction with local vascular hypersensitivity is implicated in the pathogenesis of coronary artery spasm.

Central nervous system γ-aminobutyric acids (GABA) receptors may also affect coronary vascular tone and cardiac rhythm (Gillis, 1982; Gillis et al., 1980). Gillis and co-workers (DiMicco et al., 1977; Segal et al., 1981; Segal and Gillis, 1983) have found that administration of the GABAergic antagonist picrotoxin into the lateral cerebral ventricle of chloralose-anesthetized cats produces coronary artery constriction, ST segment elevation, and ventricular arrhythmias. These effects are blocked by pretreatment with the GABA receptor agonist muscimol. Peripheral sympathetic nervous system ablation by surgical means or by injection of α-adenoreceptor drugs also prevents the alterations in coronary vascular tone and cardiac rhythm.

The cold pressor test has been employed as a nonpharmacologic means for provoking coronary artery spasm (Mudge et al., 1976, 1979; Ricci et al., 1979; Kern et al., 1983; Raizner et al., 1980). Mudge and co-workers (1976) have found that hand immersion in cold water produces coronary vasoconstriction, ST segment elevation, and chest pain in patients with coronary disease but not in normal individuals. The constrictor response is prevented by α-adrenergic blockade with phentolamine (Mudge et al., 1976) and augmented by β-adrenergic blockade with propranolol (Kern et al., 1983). Potentiation of the coronary vasoconstrictor response by propranolol is thought to be mediated by unopposed α-adrenergic vasomotor tone (Kern et al., 1983).

What is the basis for the differing coronary vasomotor responses to the cold pressor challenge in normal subjects versus those with ischemic heart disease? Mudge and colleagues (1976) have proposed the following hypothesis to explain this finding. In the normal heart, constriction of large coronary vessels in response to a neurogenic stimulus can be compensated for by metabolically mediated vasodilation of small coronary vessels. However, in the diseased coronary vascular bed, coronary vasodilation downstream to the occlusion is already maximal to maintain resting flow at normal levels. Under these conditions, a vasoconstrictor stimulus cannot be offset and results in increased vascular resistance. The results of our recent study support this hypothesis. Whereas behavioral stress produces vasodilation in the normal dog's coronary circulation, profound vasoconstriction results in animals with prior coronary artery stenosis (Verrier et al., 1984).

We examined this effect of coronary artery stenosis on vascular responsiveness during behavioral stress in dogs which were instrumented to determine left circumflex coronary artery blood flow, aortic blood pressure, and coronary vascular resistance before and after coronary artery stenosis (Verrier et al., 1984). The stress model consisted of inducing an anger-like state by food-access denial. In the absence of coronary artery stenosis, provocation of anger increased coronary artery blood flow by 147% and *decreased* coronary vascular resistance by 38%. During mechanical stenosis with an encircling cuff, there was no significant change in coronary blood flow, and coronary vascular resistance *increased* by 33%, indicating a *substantial* vasoconstrictor response to stress. Thus, as proposed by Mudge and co-workers (1976), the presence of a coronary artery obstruction does alter significantly the coronary vascular response to neurogenic stimuli. These observations carry profound scientific and clinical implications which deserve further exploration.

We examined whether behaviorally induced changes in vulnerability to fibrillation are mediated by alterations in coronary vasomotor tone (Verrier and Lown, 1984; Verrier et al., 1982). Several stress states, elicited by passive-aversive conditioning or induction of anger by food-access denial, significantly augmented myocardial blood flow. However, myocardial oxygen extraction was increased concomitantly (Verrier et al., 1982), suggesting possible inadequacy in myocardial perfusion. The basis for this phenomenon was elucidated by administering the calcium antagonist nifedipine which induces coronary vasodilatation. While nifedipine prevented the stress induced increase in myocardial oxygen extraction, it did not affect the lowering in vulnerable period threshold for ventricular fibrillation. In contrast, induction of β-adrenergic blockade with metoprolol did not influence the changes in oxygen extraction, whereas it did prevent the fall in vulnerable period threshold. Thus, increased vulnerability to ventricular fibrillation in the normal heart during behavioral stress is due to the direct effects of catecholamines on myocardial β-adrenergic receptors rather than to alterations in myocardial perfusion.

These observations, however, do not preclude the possibility that in the presence of compromised coronary circulation, behaviorally induced arrhythmogenesis may be mediated by coronary malperfusion. Recent findings indicate that this may indeed be the case. In the presence of a critical coronary artery stenosis, provocation of the anger-like state produces substantial vasoconstriction even though the accompanying sinus tachycardia and systemic hypertension indicate increased cardiac metabolic demand (Verrier et al., 1984). This inappropriate coronary vasoconstriction may contribute to the enhanced vulnerability to VF observed during biobehavioral stress.

Role of Alterations in Platelet Function

Intracoronary platelet aggregation may provide an important mechanism whereby neural factors predispose to cardiac arrhythmias. The induction of platelet aggregation in animals with adenosine diphosphate causes both myocardial infarction and lethal arrhythmias (Haft et al., 1972). Pathologic studies in patients who have died suddenly have shown platelet microthrombi and platelet aggregates in numbers far greater than in those whose deaths were not sudden (Schwartz and Gerrity, 1975; Jorgensen et al., 1968; Haerem, 1974).

Recent methodologic advances have made possible a detailed study of the effects of platelet aggregation on ventricular electrical stability. Folts et al. (1976) have demonstrated that a critical coronary artery stenosis may induce a gradual decline of coronary blood flow over 5–10 min which is followed by an abrupt (usually <5 s) recovery of flow to the initial level. These changes may lead to ST segment elevation and may reduce the vulnerable period threshold for ventricular fibrillation (Kowey et al., 1981). Considerable evidence implicates aggregation and disaggregation of platelets in these phenomena (Folts et al., 1976; Kowey et al., 1981; Folts and Rowe, 1977). Various antiplatelet drugs such as aspirin, sulfinpyrazone, and prostacyclin have been shown to prevent the cyclical changes in coronary arterial blood flow and the concomitant electrophysiologic alterations (Kowey et al., 1981; Folts and Rowe, 1977). Furthermore, Folts et al. (1976, 1982) have been able to capture platelet plugs distal to the stenosis. It has been observed that infused catecholamines frequently induce the flow changes in unresponsive animals (Folts and Rowe, 1978). It was uncertain, however, whether spontaneous fluctuations in autonomic nervous system activity can alter the pattern of cyclical coronary arterial blood flow changes during partial stenosis.

To help resolve this issue, we performed a study on chloralose-anesthetized dogs in which the effects of bilateral vagotomy and stellectomy were examined during partial stenosis of the left circumflex coronary artery (Raeder et al., 1982). Vagotomy reduced the frequency of coronary blood flow (CBF) oscillations but not the magnitude of the flow changes. Bilateral cervical stellectomy reduced both the frequency of CBF changes and their magnitude. In five dogs in which cyclical CBF changes were reduced or abolished by decentralizing the stellate ganglia, electrical stimulation of the main body of the left ganglion evoked or enhanced the oscillation in two dogs, had no distinct effect in two dogs, and elicited no response in one dog (Figs. 2-6 and 2-7). A 5-min infusion of epinephrine provoked the CBF changes in all animals for a period of 5–10 min. Blockade of muscarinic receptors by atropine resulted in a significant attenuation of flow changes, which may at least in part have been due to a direct effect of atropine on platelets. The conclusion was that cardiac sympathetic tone significantly influences the CBF pattern during critical coronary artery stenosis.

Alterations in platelet function may also provide an important mechanism whereby behavioral stress conduces to cardiac arrhythmias. Haft and Fani (1973) demonstrated that stress induces intracoronary aggregation of platelets in rats following heat and electric shock stress. Pathologic examination of the heart revealed partial or total occlusion of coronary vessels by platelet thrombi and fibrin deposits. Examination of the hearts of monkeys following shock avoidance stress by Corley et al. (1977) revealed myofibrillar degeneration, myocytolysis, and fuchsinophilia. Similar cardiac pathology has resulted from electric shock, in-

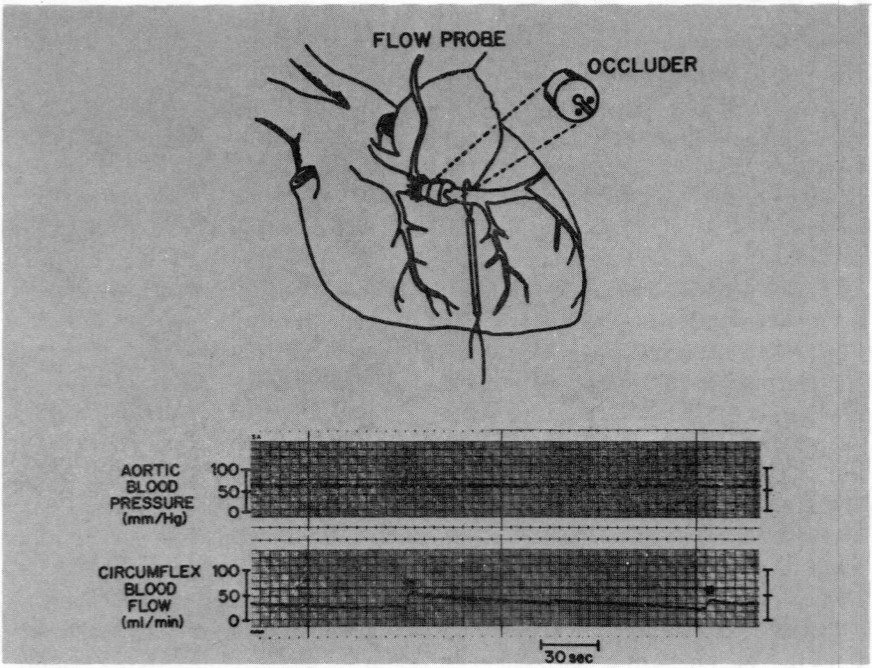

2-6 Schematic representation of the partial coronary artery occlusion model (upper panel). The cyclical changes in blood flow induced by aggregation and disaggregation of platelets are also depicted (lower panel). Note that blood pressure remains unchanged despite significant oscillations in coronary arterial blood flow (Raeder et al., 1982).

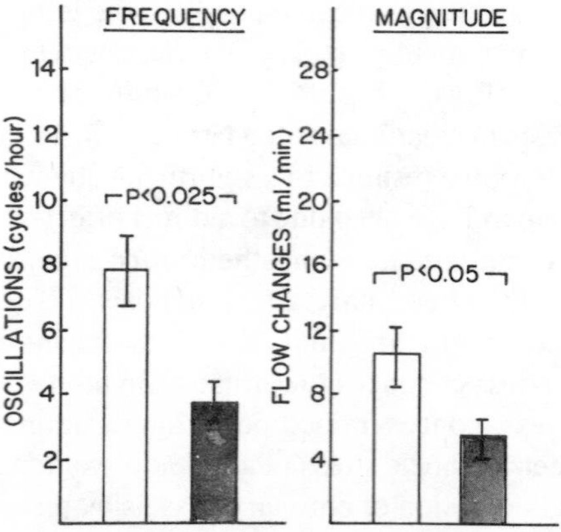

2-7 Influence of bilateral stellectomy on spontaneous oscillations in coronary arterial blood flow during partial stenosis in nine dogs (Raeder et al., 1982).

tense light and sound, and audiopresentation to rats of a rat-cat fight (Raab, 1966).

The exact role of enhanced platelet aggregability in stress induced ventricular electrical instability remains to be defined.

Final Comments

The above-cited studies underscore the importance of neural factors in the genesis of cardiac arrhythmias. It is evident, moreover, that multiple intermediary mechanisms are involved. These include direct effects on myocardial excitable properties and indirect influences mediated through alterations in coronary vasomotor tone and platelet aggregability. The parasympathetic nervous system exerts its effect largely by opposing the action of the adrenergic inputs to the heart.

These observations suggest that an important strategy for clinical management of malignant ventricular arrhythmias will require lessening cardiac sympathetic drive while enhancing vagal tone. We and others have initiated studies to determine whether neurochemical agents which induce such a pattern of autonomic neural outflow may thereby protect against ventricular arrhythmias (Table 2-1). To date, the results have been most encouraging and provide support for the concept that containment of neurophysiologic triggers may indeed provide a powerful therapeutic tool.

Table 2-1 Current Approaches for Containment of Neural Triggers for Malignant Ventricular Arrhythmias (Verrier and Lown, 1984).

Central
- Decreasing cardiac sympathetic tone
  - Neurochemical agents (Falk et al., 1981; Gillis, 1982; Rabinowitz and Lown, 1978; Skinner and Verrier, 1982; Wurtman and Fernstrom, 1975)
  - Dietary "precursor therapy" (Wurtman and Fernstrom, 1975)
- Increasing vagal tone
  - Digitalis drugs (Brooks et al., 1979)
  - Exercise conditioning (Billman et al., 1983; Stone et al., 1983)

Peripheral
- Adrenergic receptor blockade (Beta-blocker Heart Attack Study Group, 1981; Corr and Sharma, 1982; Hjalmarson et al., 1981; Norwegian Multicenter Study Group, 1981; Skinner and Verrier, 1982)
- Stellectomy (Schwartz, 1978, 1980; Schwartz et al., 1976a, 1976b; Stone et al., 1983)
- Calcium channel blockade (Stone and Antman, 1983; Stone et al., 1980; Verrier et al., 1983; Zipes and Gilmour, 1982)

Acknowledgments

Supported in part by grants HL-28387 and HL-07776 from the National Heart, Lung and Blood Institute, National Institutes of Health, United States Public Health Service, Bethesda, Maryland, and by The Rappaport International Program in Cardiology.

The authors express their appreciation to Sandra S. Verrier for her editorial assistance and to Marian Cordaro for typing the manuscript.

References

Beta-blocker Heart Attack Study Group. 1981. The Beta-blocker heart attack trial. JAMA 246:2073–2074.

Billman, G.E., Schwartz, P.J., and Stone, H.L. 1983. The effects of daily exercise on susceptibility to sudden cardiac death: Protection from ventricular fibrillation. Fed Proc 42:586.

Brooks, W.W., Verrier, R.L., and Lown, B. 1979. Digitalis drugs and vulnerability to ventricular fibrillation. Eur J. Pharmacol 57:69–78.

Buffington, C.W., and Feigl, E.O. 1981. Adrenergic coronary vasoconstriction in the presence of coronary stenosis in the dog. Circ Res 48:416–423.

Chierchia, S., Brunelli, C., Simonetti, I., Lazzari, M., and Maseri, A. 1980. Sequence of events in angina at rest: Primary reduction in coronary flow. Circulation 61:759–768.

Corley, K.C., Shiel, F.O'M., Mauck, H.P., Clark, L.S., and Barber, J.H. 1977. Myocardial degeneration and cardiac arrest in squirrel monkey: physiological and psychological correlates. Psychophysiology 14:322–328.

Corr, P.B., Penkoske, P.A., and Sobel, B.E. 1978. Adrenergic influences on arrhythmias due to coronary occlusion and reperfusion. Br Heart J 40:62–70.

Corr, P.B., and Sharma, A.D. 1982. Alpha- versus beta-adrenergic influences on dysrhythmias induced by myocardial ischaemia and reperfusion. In: A. Zanchetti, ed. Advances in Beta-blocker Therapy II, pp. 163–180. Amsterdam: Excerpta Medica.

Deanfield, J.E., Maseri, A., Selwyn, A.P., Ribeiro, P., Chierchia, S., Krikler, S., and Morgan, M. 1983. Myocardial ischaemia during daily life in patients with stable angina: Its relation to symptoms and heart rate changes. Lancet 2:753–758.

DiMicco, J.A., Prestel, T., Pearle, D.L., and Gillis, R.A. 1977. Mechanism of cardiovascular changes produced in cats by activation of the central nervous system with picrotoxin. Circ Res 41:446–451.

Elharrar, V., Watanabe, A.M., Molello, J., Besch, H.R., Jr., and Zipes, D.P. 1979. Adrenergically mediated ventricular fibrillation in probucol-treated dogs: Roles of alpha and beta adrenergic receptors. Pace 2:435–443.

Falk, R.H., DeSilva, R.A., and Lown, B. 1981. Reduction in vulnerability to ventricular fibrillation by bromocriptine, a dopamine agonist. Cardiovasc Res 15:175–180.

Feigl, E.O. 1969. Parasympathetic control of coronary blood flow in dogs. Circ Res 25:509–519.

Feigl, E.O. 1983. Coronary physiology. Physiol Rev. 63:1–205.

Folts, J.D., Crowell, E.B., and Rowe, G.G. 1976. Platelet aggregation in partially obstructed vessels and its elimination with aspirin. Circulation 54:365–370.

Folts, J.D., Gallagher, K., and Rowe, G.G. 1982. Blood flow reductions in stenosed canine coronary arteries: vasospasm or platelet aggregation? Circulation 65:248–255.

Folts, J.D., and Rowe, G.G. 1977. Letter. Circulation 56:333.

Folts, J.D., and Rowe, G.G. 1978. Platelet aggregation in stenosed coronary arteries: Mechanism of sudden death? Am J Cardiol 41:425.

Gillis, R.A. 1982. Neurotransmitters involved in the central nervous system control of cardiovascular function. In: O.A. Smith, R.A. Galosy, and S.M. Weiss, eds. Circulation, Neurobiology, and Behavior. pp. 41–53. New York: Elsevier Science Publishing Co.

Gillis, R.A., DiMicco, J.A., Williford, D.J., Hamilton, B.L., and Gale, K.N. 1980. Importance of CNS GABAergic mechanisms in the regulation of cardiovascular function. Brain Res Bull 5:303-315.

Haerem, J. 1974. Platelet aggregates and mural microthrombi in early stages of acute, fatal coronary disease. Thromb Res 5:243–249.

Haft, J.I., and Fani, K. 1973. Intravascular platelet aggregation in the heart induced by stress. Circulation 47:353–358.

Haft, J.I., Gershengorn, K., Kranz, P.D., and Oestreicher, R. 1972. Protection against epinephrine-induced myocardial necrosis by drugs that inhibit platelet aggregation. Am J Cardiol 30:838–843.

Han, J., Garcia de Jalon, P., and Moe, G.K. 1964. Adrenergic effects on ventricular vulnerability. Circ Res 14:516–524.

Harris, A.S., Otero, H., and Bocage, A.J. 1971. The induction of arrhythmias by sympathetic activity before and after occlusion of a coronary artery in the canine heart. J Electrocardiol 4:34–43.

Hillis, L.D., and Braunwald, E. 1978. Coronary-artery spasm. N Engl J Med 299:695–702.

Hjalmarson, Å., Elmfeldt, D., Herlitz, J., Holmberg, S., Málek, I., Nyberg, G., Rydén, L., Swedberg, K., Vedin, A., Waagstein, F., Waldenström, A., Waldenström, J., Wedel, H., Wilhelmsen, L., and Wilhelmsson, C. 1981. Effect on mortality of metoprolol in acute myocardial infarction. Lancet 2:823–827.

Hockman, C.H., Mauck, H.P., Jr., and Hoff, E.C. 1966. ECG changes resulting from cerebral stimulation. II. A spectrum of ventricular arrhythmias of sympathetic origin. Am Heart J 71:695–700.

Hoff, E.C., Kell, J.F., Jr., and Carroll, M.N., Jr. 1963. Effects of cortical stimulation and lesions on cardiovascular function. Physiol Rev 43:68–114.

Jorgensen, L., Haerem, J., and Chandler, A. 1968. The pathology of acute coronary death. Acta Anaesthesiol Scand Suppl. 29:193–209.

Kent, K.M., Smith, E.R., Redwood, D.R., and Epstein, S.E. 1974. Beneficial electrophysiologic effects of nitroglycerin during acute myocardial infarction. Am J Cardiol 33:513–516.

Kern, M.J., Ganz, P., Horowitz, J.D., Gaspar, J., Barry, W.H., Lorell, B.H., Grossman, W., and Mudge, G.H., Jr. 1983. Potentiation of coronary vasoconstriction by beta-adrenergic blockade in patients with coronary artery disease. Circulation 67:1178–1185.

Kolman, B.S., Verrier, R.L., and Lown, B. 1975. The effect of vagus nerve stimulation upon vulnerability of the canine ventricle: Role of sympathetic-parasympathetic interactions. Circulation 52:578–585.

Korteweg, G.C.J., Boeles, J.T.F., and Ten Cate, J. 1957. Influence of stimulation of some subcortical areas on electrocardiogram. J Neurophysiol 20:100–107.

Kowey, P.R., Verrier, R.L., Lown, B., and Handin, R.I. 1981. The effects of nitroglycerin on intracoronary platelet aggregation and ventricular vulnerability during partial coronary stenosis. Am J Cardiol 47:489.

Levy, M.N. 1971. Sympathetic-parasympathetic interactions in the heart. Circ Res 29:437–445.

Levy, M.N., and Blattberg, B. 1976. Effect of vagal stimulation on the overflow of norepinephrine into the coronary sinus during cardiac sympathetic nerve stimulation in the dog. Circ Res 38:81–85.

Lombardi, F., Verrier, R.L., and Lown, B. 1983. Relationship between sympathetic neural activity, coronary dynamics, and vulnerability to ventricular fibrillation during myocardial ischemia and reperfusion. Am Heart J 105:958–965.

Lown, B. 1977. Verbal conditioning of angina pectoris during exercise testing. Am J Cardiol 40:630–634.

Lown, B., and Verrier, R.L. 1976. Neural activity and ventricular fibrillation. N Engl J Med 294:1165–1170.

Lown, B., Verrier, R.L., and Rabinowitz, S.H. 1977. Neural and psychologic mechanisms and the problem of sudden cardiac death. Am J Cardiol 39:890–902.

Luchi, R.J., Chahine, R.A., and Raizner, A.E. 1979. Coronary artery spasm. Ann Intern Med 91:441–449.

Majid, P.A., Saxton, C., Dykes, J.R.W., Galvin, M.C., and Taylor, S.H. 1970. Autonomic control of insulin secretion and the treatment of heart failure. Br Med J 4:328–334.

Manning, J.W., and Cotten, M.DeV. 1962. Mechanism of cardiac arrhythmias induced by diencephalic stimulation. Am J Physiol 203:1120–1124.

Manning, J.W., Jr., and Peiss, C.N. 1960. Cardiovascular responses to electrical stimulation in the diencephalon. Am J Physiol 198:366–370.

Mark, A.L., Abboud, F.M., Schmid, P.G., Heistad, D.D., and Mayer, H.E. 1972. Differences in direct effects of adrenergic stimuli on coronary, cutaneous, and muscular vessels. J Clin Invest 51:279–287.

Martins, J.B., and Zipes, D.P. 1980. Epicardial phenol interrupts refractory period responses to sympathetic but not vagal stimulation in canine left ventricular epicardium and endocardium. Circ Res 47:33–40.

Maseri, A., L'Abbate, A., Baroldi, G., Chierchia, S., Marzilli, M., Ballestra, A.M., Severi, S., Parodi, O., Biagini, A., Distante, A., and Pesola, A. 1978b. Coronary vasospasm as a possible cause of myocardial infarction. A conclusion derived from the study of "preinfarction" angina. N Engl J Med 299:1271–1277.

Maseri, A., L'Abbate, A., Chierchia, S., Parodi, O., Severi, S., Biagini, A., Distante, A., Marzilli, M., and Ballestra, A.M. 1979. Significance of spasm in the pathogenesis of ischemic heart disease. Am J Cardiol 44:788–792.

Maseri, A., Severi, S., De Nes, M., L'Abbate, A., Chierchia, S., Marzilli, M., Ballestra, A.M., Parodi, O., Biagini, A., and Distante, A. 1978a. "Variant" angina: one aspect of a continuous spectrum of vasospastic myocardial ischemia. Pathogenetic mechanisms, estimated incidence and clinical and coronary arteriographic findings in 138 patients. Am J Cardiol 42:1019–1035.

Matta, R.J., Lawler, J.E., and Lown, B. 1976b. Ventricular electrical instability in the conscious dog. Effects of psychologic stress and beta adrenergic blockade. Am J Cardiol 38:594–598.

Matta, R.J., Verrier, R.L., and Lown, B. 1976a. Repetitive extrasystole as an index of vulnerability to ventricular fibrillation. Am J Physiol 230:1469–1473.

Mohrman, D.E., and Feigl, E.O. 1978. Competition between sympathetic vasoconstriction and metabolic vasodilation in the canine coronary circulation. Circ Res 42:79–86.

Mudge, G.H., Jr., Goldberg, S., Gunther, S., Mann, T., and Grossman, W. 1979. Comparison of metabolic and vasoconstrictor stimuli on coronary vascular resistance in man. Circulation 59:544–550.

Mudge, G.H., Jr., Grossman, W., Mills, R.M., Jr., Lesch, M., and Braunwald, E. 1976. Reflex increase in coronary vascular resistance in patients with ischemic heart disease. N Engl J Med 295:1333–1337.

Norwegian Multicenter Study Group, 1981. The timolol-induced reduction in mortality and reinfarction in patients surviving acute myocardial infarction. N Engl J Med 304:801–807.

Oliva, P.B., and Breckinridge, J.C. 1977. Arteriographic evidence of coronary arterial spasm in acute myocardial infarction. Circulation 56:366–374.

Oliva, P.B., Potts, D.E., and Pluss, R.G. 1973. Coronary arterial spasm in Prinzmetal angina: documentation by coronary arteriography. N Engl J Med 288:745–751.

Orlick, A.E., Ricci, D.R., Alderman, E.L., Stinson, E.B., and Harrison, D.C. 1978. Effects of alpha adrenergic blockade upon coronary hemodynamics. J Clin Invest 62:459–467.

Pasyk, S., and Pitt, B. 1983. Central opiate induced ventricular arrhythmias in the conscious dog. Circulation 68:III249.

Pasyk, S., Walton, J., and Pitt, B. 1981. Central opioid mediated coronary and systemic vasoconstriction in the conscious dog. Circulation 64:IV41.

Pfister, B., and Imhof, P.R. 1977. Inhibition of adrenaline-induced platelet aggregation by the orally administered alpha-adrenergic receptor blocker phentolamine (Regitine®). Eur J Clin Pharmacol 11:7–10.

Pitt, B., Elliott, E.C., and Gregg, D.E. 1967. Adrenergic receptor activity in the coronary arteries of the unanesthetized dog. Circ Res 21:75–84.

Pitt, B., Pasyk, S., Walton, J., and Grekin, R. 1982. Endogenous arginine vasopressin release in patients with coronary artery spasm. Circulation 66:II88.

Prystowsky, E.N., Jackman, W.M., Rinkenberger, R.L., Heger, J.J., and Zipes, D.P. 1981. Effect of autonomic blockade on ventricular refractoriness and atrioventricular nodal conduction in humans. Evidence supporting a direct cholinergic action on ventricular muscle refractoriness. Circ Res 49:511–518.

Raab, W. 1966. Emotional and sensory stress factors in myocardial pathology. Am Heart J 72:538–564.

Rabinowitz, S.H., and Lown, B. 1978. Central neurochemical factors related to serotonin metabolism and cardiac ventricular vulnerability for repetitive electrical activity. Am J Cardiol 41:516–522.

Rabinowitz, S.H., Verrier, R.L., and Lown, B. 1976. Muscarinic effects of vagosympathetic trunk stimulation on the repetitive extrasystole (RE) threshold. Circulation 53:622–627.

Raeder, E.A., Verrier, R.L., and Lown, B. 1982. Influence of the autonomic nervous system on coronary blood flow during partial stenosis. Am Heart J 104:249–253.

Raizner, A.E., Chahine, R.A., Ishimori, T., Verani, M.S., Zacca, N., Jamal, N., Miller, R.R., and Luchi, R.J. 1980. Provocation of coronary artery spasm by the cold pressor test. Hemodynamic, arteriographic and quantitative angiographic observations. Circulation 62:925–932.

Ricci, D.R., Orlick, A.E., Cipriano, P.R., Guthaner, D.F., and Harrison, D.C. 1979. Altered adrenergic activity in coronary arterial spasm: Insight into mechanism based on study of coronary hemodynamics and the electrocardiogram. Am J Cardiol 43:1073–1079.

Rosen, M.R., Gelband, H., and Hoffman, B.F. 1971. Effects of phentolamine on electrophysiologic properties of isolated canine Purkinje fibers. J Pharmacol Exp Ther 179:586–593.

Rosen, M.R., Hordof, A.J., Ilvento, J.P., and Danilo, P., Jr. 1977. Effects of adrenergic amines on electrophysiological properties and automaticity of neonatal and adult canine Purkinje fibers. Evidence for alpha- and beta-adrenergic actions. Circ Res 40:390–400.

Rosenfeld, J., Rosen, M.R., and Hoffman, B.F. 1978. Pharmacologic and behavioral effects on arrhythmias that immediately follow abrupt coronary occlusion: A canine model of sudden coronary death. Am J Cardiol 41:1075–1082.

Ross, G. 1976. Adrenergic responses of the coronary vessels. Circ Res 39:461–465.

Satinsky, J., Kosowsky, B., Lown, B., and Kerzner, J. 1971. Ventricular fibrillation induced by hypothalamic stimulation during coronary occlusion. Circulation 44:II60.

Schwartz, C., and Gerrity, R. 1975. Anatomical pathology of sudden unexpected cardiac death. Circulation 52:III18–III26.

Schwartz, P.J. 1978. Unilateral stellectomy and dysrhythmias. Circ Res 43:939–940.

Schwartz, P.J. 1980. The long QT syndrome. In: H.E. Kulbertus and H.J.J. Wellens, eds. Sudden Death. pp. 358–378. The Hague: Martinus Nijhoff.

Schwartz, P.J., Snebold, N.G., and Brown, A.M. 1976a. Effects of unilateral cardiac sympathetic denervation on the ventricular fibrillation threshold. Am J Cardiol 37:1034–1040.

Schwartz, P.J., and Stone, H.L. 1977. Tonic influence of the sympathetic nervous system on myocardial reactive hyperemia and on coronary blood flow distribution in dogs. Circ Res 41:51–58.

Schwartz, P.J., Stone, H.L., and Brown, A.M. 1976b. Effects of unilateral stellate ganglion blockade on the arrhythmias associated with coronary occlusion. Am Heart J 92:589–599.

Segal, S.A., and Gillis, R.A. 1983. Blockade of CNS GABAergic tone causes sympathetic-mediated coronary constriction in cats. Fed Proc 42:1122.

Segal, S.A., Pearle, D.L., and Gillis, R.A. 1981. Coronary spasm produced by picrotoxin in cats. Eur J Pharmacol 76:447–451.

Sheridan, D.J., Penkoske, P.A., Sobel, B.E., and Corr. P.B. 1980. Alpha adrenergic contributions to dysrhythmia during myocardial ischemia and reperfusion in cats. J Clin Invest 65:161–171.

Skinner, J.E., Lie, J.T., and Entman, M.L. 1975. Modification of ventricular fibrillation latency following coronary artery occlusion in the conscious pig. The effects of psychological stress and beta-adrenergic blockade. Circulation 51:656–667.

Skinner, J.E., and Verrier, R.L. 1982. Task force report on sudden cardiac death and arrhythmias. In: O.A. Smith, R.A. Galosy, and S.M. Weiss, eds. Circulation, Neurobiology, and Behavior. pp. 309–316. New York: Elsevier Science Publishing Co., Inc.

Stewart, J.R., Burmeister, W.E., Burmeister, J., and Lucchesi, B.R. 1980. Electrophysiologic and antiarrhythmic effects of phentolamine in experimental coronary artery occlusion and reperfusion in the dog. J Cardiovasc Pharmacol 2:77–91.

Stone, H.L., Billman, G.E., and Schwartz, P.J. 1983. Exercise and sudden death. In: H.E. Kulbertus and H.J.J. Wellens, eds. The First Year after a Myocardial Infarction. New York: Futura.

Stone, P.H., and Antman, E.M. 1983. Calcium Channel Blocking Agents in the Treatment of Cardiovascular Disorders. New York: Futura.

Stone, P.H., Antman, E.M., Muller, J.E., and Braunwald, E. 1980. Calcium channel blocking agents in the treatment of cardiovascular disorders. Part 2: Hemodynamic effects and clinical applications. Ann Intern Med 93:886–904.

Vatner, S.F., Higgins, C.B., and Braunwald, E. 1974. Effects of norepinephrine on coronary circulation and left ventricular dynamics in the conscious dog. Circ Res 34:812–823.

Verrier, R.L. 1980. Neural factors and ventricular electrical instability. In: H.E. Kulbertus and H.J.J. Wellens, eds. Sudden Death. pp. 137–155. Netherlands: Martinus Nijhoff.

Verrier, R.L., Calvert, A., and Lown, B. 1975. Effect of posterior hypothalamic stimulation on ventricular fibrillation threshold. Am J Physiol 228:923–927.

Verrier, R.L., Hagestad, E.L., and Lown, B. 1984. Behaviorally induced coronary vasoconstriction in dogs with critical coronary artery stenosis. Fed Proc 43:1003.

Verrier, R.L., Lombardi, F., and Lown, B. 1982. Restraint of myocardial blood flow during behavioral stress. Circulation 66:II258.

Verrier, R.L., and Lown, B. 1977. Effects of left stellectomy on enhanced cardiac vulnerability induced by psychologic stress. Circulation 55/56:III80.

Verrier, R.L., and Lown, B. 1978a. Influence of neural activity on ventricular electrical stability during acute myocardial ischemia and infarction. In: E. Sandøe, D.G. Julian, and J.W. Bell, eds. Management of Ventricular Tachycardia: Role of Mexiletine. pp. 133–150. Amsterdam: Excerpta Medica (International Congress Series No. 458).

Verrier, R.L., and Lown, B. 1978b. Sympathetic-parasympathetic interactions and ventricular electrical stability. In: P.J. Schwartz, A.M. Brown, A. Malliani, and A. Zanchetti, eds. Neural Mechanisms in Cardiac Arrhythmias. pp. 75–85. New York: Raven Press.

Verrier, R.L., and Lown, B. 1981. Autonomic nervous system and malignant cardiac arrhythmias. In: H. Weiner, M.A. Hofer, and A.J. Stankard, eds. Brain, Behavior, and Bodily Disease. pp. 273–291. New York: Raven Press.

Verrier, R.L., and Lown, B. 1984. Behavioral stress and cardiac arrhythmias. Annu Rev Physiol 46:155–176.

Verrier, R.L., Raeder, E., and Lown, B. 1983. Use of calcium channel blockers after myocardial infarction: Potential cardioprotective mechanisms. In: H.E. Kulbertus and H.J.J. Wellens, eds. The First Year After a Myocardial Infarction. pp. 341–352. New York: Futura.

Watanabe, A.M., and Besch, H.R., Jr. 1974. Cyclic adenosine monophosphate modulation of slow calcium influx channels in guinea pig hearts. Circ Res 35:316–324.

Watanabe, A.M., and Besch, H.R., Jr. 1975. Interaction between cyclic adenosine monophosphate and cyclic guanosine monophosphate in guinea pig ventricular myocardium. Circ Res 37:309–317.

Watanabe, A.M., Hathaway, D.R., Besch, H.R., Jr., Farmer, B.B., and Harris, R.A. 1977. Alpha-adrenergic reduction of cyclic adenosine monophosphate concentrations in rat myocardium. Circ Res 40:596–602.

Watanabe, A.M., Lindemann, J.P., Jones, L.R., Besch, H.R., Jr., and Bailey, J.C. 1981. Biochemical mechanisms mediating neural control of the heart. In: F.M. Abboud, H.A. Fozzard, J.P. Gilmore, and D.J. Reis, eds. Disturbances in Neurogenic Control of the Circulation. pp. 189–203. Bethesda, MD: American Physiological Society.

Wurtman, R.J., and Fernstrom, J.D. 1975. Control of brain monoamine synthesis by diet and plasma amino acids. Am J Clin Nutr 28:638–647.

Yasue, H., Omote, S., Takizawa, A., Nagao, M., Miwa, K., and Tanaka, S. 1979. Exertional angina pectoris caused by coronary arterial spasm: Effects of various drugs. Am J Cardiol 43:647–652.

Yoon, M.S., Han, J., Tse, W.W., and Rogers, R. 1977. Effects of vagal stimulation, atropine, and propranolol on fibrillation threshold of normal and ischemic ventricles. Am Heart J 93:60–65.

Zipes, D.P., and Gilmour, R.J., Jr. 1982. Calcium antagonists and their potential role in the prevention of sudden coronary death. Ann NY Acad Sci 382:258–288.

Chapter 3

Anatomical, Biochemical, and Electrophysiologic Evidence for Parasympathetic Innervation of the Ventricle

John C. Bailey, Richard J. Kovacs, and David P. Rardon

Introduction

The effects of sympathetic nerve stimulation or sympathetic agonists on the electrophysiologic properties of the heart have been well known for many years. These effects are generally thought to favor the development of cardiac arrhythmias, especially in the clinical setting of acute myocardial ischemia. Conversely, cardiac β-adrenoreceptor blocking agents are antiarrhythmic, and the use of these antagonists following myocardial infarction reduces mortality in certain circumstances, although the protection these agents provide may not be due to their antiarrhythmic properties.

Only more recently have the effects of vagal stimulation and muscarinic cholinergic agonists on the electrical properties of the mammalian ventricle been recognized, yet the clinical significance of these interventions remains unproven. Nevertheless, numerous lines of evidence suggest that alteration of muscarinic cholinergic tone exerts substantial effects on ventricular electrical function. It is the purpose of this chapter to review the evidence for vagal input and vagal effects on the ventricles of man and animals. For further details, the reader should refer to reviews by Higgins et al. (1973), Zipes et al. (1981), and Rardon and Bailey (1983a,b).

Evidence Indicating the Presence of Vagus Nerve, Acetylcholine, Acetylcholine Synthesis, and Muscarinic Cholinergic Receptors in Mammalian Ventricle

If the vagus nerves exert effects on ventricular function, then there should be evidence of innervation of the ventricles by these nerves. Early anatomical studies failed to demonstrate vagal fibers in association with ventricular myocardium or the His-Purkinje specialized conducting system (Nonidez, 1943). On the other hand, other investigators report morphologic evidence for vagus nerve fibers in the ventricle. For example, Napolitano et al. (1965), using electron microscopic techniques, demonstrated the presence of neural elements in ventricular tissue that persisted following total cardiac excision and reimplantation. Cardiac excision would necessarily require that the postganglionic sympathetic and preganglionic parasympathetic nerves to the heart be transected. Although the study by Napolitano could not distinguish between sympathetic or parasympathetic nerves, only the postganglionic divisions of the vagus nerve (the intrinsic cardiac nerves) should remain following complete transection of the extrinsic cardiac nerves. Kent and colleagues (1974) demonstrated that the specialized intraventricular conducting systems of both man and dog were richly innervated by cholinergic nervous tissue as judged by dense staining of acetylcholinesterase (AChE) in these regions. In contrast, ventricular myocardium appeared sparsely innervated by vagal fibers. Following ablation of canine cardiac cholinergic fibers by injection of vinblastine, specific AChE activity was markedly diminished or absent, indicating cholinergic denervation. Certain electrophysiologic effects on the ventricle of vagal stimulation were abolished following vinblastine, and these investigators marshalled evidence indicating that these electrophysiologic effects of vagal stimulation persisted following adrenergic denervation or depletion of norepinephrine with 6-hydroxydopamine. Jacobowitz and colleagues (1967) likewise demonstrated the presence of cholinergic nerves in ventricular tissue of guinea pigs by using the technique of specific staining for AChE. In both studies cited above, the atria were more richly innervated by cholinergic nerves than were the ventricles.

The presence of acetylcholine in ventricular myocardium of cat hearts was reported by Brown (1976) using mass spectrometric techniques. He demonstrated that cat atria contained at least three times the amount of acetylcholine as did the ventricles. Following bilateral cervical vagotomy, acetylcholine content of the left cardiac chambers and the interventricular septum did not fall, whereas acetylcholine content of the right cardiac chambers fell significantly. The reasons for this disparity following vagotomy are not apparent.

Roskoski et al. (1975) measured the activity of choline acetyltransferase in guinea pig. This enzyme, present in the heart only in the parasympathetic nerves, catalyzes synthesis of acetylcholine from acetylcoenzyme A and choline. These investigators demonstrated bioenzyme in all cardiac chambers in the following order of decreasing activity: right atrial appendage, right ventricle; left atrial appendage and left ventricle nearly equal (expressed as nanomoles per min per g).

The presence of muscarinic cholinergic receptors in homogenates of heart cells from guinea pigs, rats, and rabbits was demonstrated by Fields and colleagues (1978). They used radiolabeled [^{3}H]quinuclidinyl benzilate, a ligand with specific, high affinity for muscarinic cholinergic receptors, to identify and characterize muscarinic cholinergic receptors in various regions of the hearts of these mammalian species. They demonstrated that the atria contained six to nine times more of these receptors per g of protein than the ventricles, although ventricular tissue, because of its greater weight, contained approximately 60% of the total number of cardiac muscarinic cholinergic receptors.

Evidence Indicating that the Vagus Nerves Exert Electrophysiologic Effects on the Ventricle

Despite the notion, until recently the majority opinion, that the vagus nerves exerted no effects on the heart below the atrioventricular junction, numerous studies in the early literature indicate that vagal stimulation elicits electrophysiologic alterations in the ventricle (for a review, see Scherf and Schott, 1973). More recently, Eliakim and colleagues (1961) demonstrated that acetylcholine slowed the rate of discharge of idioventricular pacemakers following establishment of complete atrioventricular block in dogs, an effect also observed during vagal stimulation in dogs following His bundle transaction, sympathectomy, and adrenalectomy (Gonzáles-Serrato and Alanís, 1962). Fisch and co-workers (1964) demonstrated in dogs that acetylcholine injected into the aortic root increased the amplitude of the electrocardiographic T wave and suggested that the neurotransmitter increased the rate of repolarization of ventricular myocardial cells. Early microelectrode studies from our laboratories (Bailey et al., 1972) demonstrated that acetylcholine suppressed the rate of spontaneous phase 4 depolarization in cells of the canine bundle of His and proximal bundle branches, an effect also observed in the more peripheral Purkinje network (Tse et al., 1976). In our own experience, acetylcholine effects little if any change in action potential duration of otherwise untreated guinea pig ventricular myocytes or canine cardiac Purkinje fibers, although other investigators report acetylcholine-induced action potential duration prolongation in dog cardiac Purkinje fibers (Gadsby et al., 1978) and shortening in guinea pig ventricular myocytes (Ochi and Hino, 1978).

A now well-recognized effect of acetylcholine is to antagonize potently the effects of simultaneous β-adrenergic stimulation on ventricular function (Levy, 1971). Inui and Imamura (1977) demonstrated that acetylcholine antagonized isoproterenol-dependent action potentials and contractions. We reported that acetylcholine antagonized isoproterenol-induced action potential shortening in normally polarized canine cardiac Purkinje fibers and abolished slow responses induced by isoproterenol in potassium-depolarized canine cardiac Purkinje fibers (Bailey et al., 1979). The effects of acetylcholine were blocked by atropine. Biegon and Pappano (1980) demonstrated similar effects of acetylcholine in embryonic avian ventricles.

We have also demonstrated that muscarinic cholinergic stimulation produces significant negative chronotropic effects on guinea pig cardiac Purkinje fibers independent of the presence of simultaneous β-adrenergic stimulation (Rardon and Bailey, 1983a). In control guinea pig Purkinje fibers, physostigmine elicited a negative chronotropic response that was similar to the response to physostigmine observed in Purkinje fibers from guinea pigs following pretreatment with reserpine. Similarly, adrenergic blockade did not affect action potential duration prolongation of sheep cardiac Purkinje fibers treated with acetylcholine (Carmeliet and Ramon, 1980).

In other experiments, we have examined the effects of acetylcholine on feline atrial and ventricular action potential parameters before and after bilateral cervical vagotomy (Kovacs and Bailey, 1983). In control cats, acetylcholine elicited, as expected, a concentration-dependent decrease in atrial action potential duration. Ventricular action potential duration was unaffected by the choline ester. Following bilateral cervical vagotomy, the effects of acetylcholine on atrial action potential durations were exaggerated. In ventricular myocardium following vagotomy, acetylcholine produced a concentration-dependent shortening of action potential duration. The effects of acetylcholine were abolished by atropine, indicating that the site of action of acetylcholine was the muscarinic cholinergic receptor.

In intact animals subjected to experimental coronary artery occlusion, vagus nerve stimulation is protective against ventricular fibrillation. Kent et al. (1973) demonstrated, in nonischemic dogs during constant ventricular pacing, that vagal stimulation increased substantially the ventricular pacing, that vagal stimulation increased substantially the ventricular fibrillation threshold, whether or not the vagi were intact or decentralized. These investigators also demonstrated similar effects of vagal stimulation following coronary ligation. They concluded that the protection afforded by vagal stimulation was due to vagally induced heart rate slowing, as well as a direct effect on the ventricle of heightened vagal tone. Corr and Gillis (1974) demonstrated, in cats following coronary artery ligation, that administration of atropine or bilateral cervical vagotomy increased the incidence of spontaneous ventricular fibrillation even though the heart rate was held constant by cardiac pacing. These authors concluded that the presence of efferent vagal tone per se reduced the incidence of ventricular fibrillation. Myers et al. (1974) also determined that vagal stimulation during acute ischemia in dogs protected against spontaneous ventricular fibrillation, an effect that was independent of any change in heart rate.

Implications of Muscarinic Cholinergic Innervation of Human Ventricular Myocardium

The previous sections of this chapter have reviewed some of the evidence indicating the presence and functional significance of vagal innervation of the ventricles of numerous species. In man and animals, vagally induced changes in sinoatrial node, atrial, or atrioventricular node function would be expected to alter secondarily certain electrophysiologic properties of the ventricles. However, very little information is known regarding the effects of vagal stimulation, resulting in release of acetylcholine in the vicinity of muscarinic cholinergic receptors located on human ventricular cells. To the extent that vagal innervation of and actions on the ventricles may be similar in man and animals, then one might speculate that parasympathetic effects on ventricular electrical function might be profound, especially in circumstances such as acute myocardial ischemia when sympathetic tone is high. These speculations, however, await appropriate testing. The experiments that are necessary to prove a clinically important role for the vagus nerves in modifying electrophysiologic properties of the human ventricle may prove to be exceedingly difficult, considering technical and ethical constraints, but the few studies now available encourage the hope that more evidence will be forthcoming. Prystowsky et al. (1981), using standard catheter techniques for invasive electrophysiologic testing, demonstrated that elimination of muscarinic cholinergic tone by administration of atropine during simultaneous β-adrenergic receptor blockade, significantly shortened effective and functional refractory periods in human ventricles. Waxman and Wald (1977) have reported termination of ventricular tachycardia in man by potent vagal stimulation. More recently, Waxman et al. (1981) have described an instance of ventricular tachycardia that could be induced or aborted depending on the level of existing vagal tone.

Summary

Compelling evidence from numerous disciplines forces the conclusion that the vagus nerves are present in the ventricles of man and animals, and that both direct and indirect effects of muscarinic cholinergic stimulation can be demonstrated in ventricular tissue of animals. We anticipate that human experimentation will continue to reveal a clinically significant role for the vagus nerves in modulating the electrophysiologic properties of the ventricle of man.

Acknowledgments

Supported in part by the Herman C. Krannert Fund, grants HL06308 and HL07182 from the National Heart, Lung, and Blood Institute, National Institutes of Health, Bethesda, Maryland, and the American Heart Association, Indiana Affiliate, Inc.

References

Bailey, J.C., Greenspan, K., Elizari, M.V., Anderson, G.J., and Fisch, C. 1972. Effects of acetylcholine on automaticity and conduction in the proximal portion of the His-Purkinje specialized conduction system of the dog. Circ Res 30:210–216.

Bailey, J.C., Watanabe, A.M., Besch, H.R., Jr., and Lathrop, D.A. 1979. Acetylcholine antagonism of the electrophysiological effects of isoproterenol on canine cardiac Purkinje fibers. Circ Res 44:378–383.

Biegon, R.L., and Pappano, A.J. 1980. Dual mechanism for inhibition of calcium dependent action potentials by acetylcholine in avian ventricular muscle: relationship to cyclic AMP. Circ Res 46:353–362.

Brown, O.M. 1976. Cat heart acetylcholine: structural proof and distribution. Am J Physiol 231:781–785.

Carmeliet, E., and Ramon, J. 1980. Electrophysiological effects of acetylcholine in sheep cardiac Purkinje fibers. Pflügers Arch Ges Physiol 387:197–205.

Corr, P.B., and Gillis, R.A. 1974. Role of the vagus nerves in the cardiovascular changes induced by coronary occlusion. Circulation 49:86–97.

Eliakim, M., Bellet, S., Elias, T., and Muller, O. 1961. Effect of vagal stimulation and acetylcholine on the ventricle. Circ Res 9:1372–1379.

Fields, J.Z., Roeske, W.R., Morkin, E., and Yamamura, H.I. 1978. Cardiac muscarinic cholinergic receptors. Biochemical identification and characterization. J Biol Chem 253:3251–3258.

Fisch, C., Knoebel, S.B., and Feigenbaum, H. 1964. Effect of acetylcholine and potassium on repolarization of the heart. J Clin Invest 43:1769–1775.

Gadsby, D.C., Witt, A.L., and Cranefield, P.F. 1978. The effects of acetylcholine on the electrical activity of canine cardiac Purkinje fibers. Circ Res 43:29–35.

Gonzáles-Serrato, H., and Alanís, J. 1962. La accion de los nervios cardiacos y de la acetilcolina sobre el automatismo del corazon. Acta Physiol Lat Am 12:139–152.

Higgins, C.B., Vatner, S.F., and Braunwald, E. 1973. Parasympathetic control of the heart. Pharmacol Rev 25:119–155.

Inui, J., and Imamura, H. 1977. Effects of acetylcholine on calcium-dependent electrical and mechanical responses in the guinea-pig papillary muscle partially depolarized by potassium. Naunyn-Schmied Arch Pharmacol 299:1–7.

Jacobowitz, D.M., Cooper, T., and Barner, H.B. 1967. Histochemical and chemical studies of the localization of adrenergic and cholinergic nerves in normal and denervated cat hearts. Circ Res 20:289–298.

Kent, K.M., Epstein, S.E., Cooper, T., and Jacobowitz, D.M. 1974. Cholinergic innervation of the canine and human ventricular conducting system: anatomic and electrophysiologic considerations. Circulation 50:948–955.

Kent, K.M., Smith, E.R., Redwood, D.R., and Epstein, S.E. 1973. Electrical stability of acutely ischemic myocardium. Influences of heart rate and vagal stimulation. Circulation 47:291–298.

Kovacs, R.J., and Bailey, J.C. 1983. Exaggerated cardiac electrophysiological effects of acetylcholine following bilateral cervical vagotomy in the cat. Circulation 68(abstr):154.

Levy, M.N. 1971. Sympathetic-parasympathetic interactions in the heart. Circ Res 29:437–445.

Myers, R.W., Pearlman, A.S., Hyman, R.M., Goldstein, R.A., Kent, K.M., Goldstein, R.E., and Epstein, S.E. 1974. Beneficial effects of vagal stimulation and bradycardia during experimental acute myocardial ischemia. Circulation 49:943–947.

Napolitano, L.M., Willman, V.L., Hanlon, C.R., and Cooper, T. 1965. Intrinsic innervation of the heart. Am J Physiol 208:455–458.

Nonidez, J. 1943. The structure and innervation of the conductive system of the heart of the dog and rhesus monkey, as seen with a silver impregnation technique. Am Heart J 26:577–597.

Ochi, R., and Hino, N. 1978. Depression of slow inward current by acetylcholine in mammalian ventricular muscle. Proc Japan Acad 54B:474–477.

Prystowsky, E.N., Jackman, W.M., Rinkenberger, R.L., Heger, J.J., and Zipes, D.P. 1981. Effect of autonomic blockade on ventricular refractoriness and atrioventricular nodal conduction in humans. Evidence supporting a direct cholinergic action on ventricular muscle refractoriness. Circ Res 49:511–518.

Rardon, D.P., and Bailey, J.C. 1983a. Direct effects of cholinergic stimulation on ventricular automaticity in guinea pig myocardium. Circ Res 52:105–110.

Rardon, D.P., and Bailey, J.C. 1983b. Parasympathetic effects on electrophysiological properties of cardiac ventricular tissue. J Am Coll Cardiol 2:1200–1215.

Roskoski, R., Schmid, P.G., Mayer, H.E., and Abboud, F.A. 1975. In vitro acetylcholine biosynthesis in normal and failing guinea pig hearts. Circ Res 36:547–552.

Scherf, D., and Schott, A. 1973. Extrasystoles and Allied Arrhythmias. pp. 487–527. London: William Heinemann Medical Books Ltd.

Tse, W.W., Han, J., and Yoon, M. 1976. Effect of acetylcholine on automaticity of canine Purkinje fibers. Am J Physiol 230:116–119.

Waxman, M.B., Staniloff, H., and Wald, R.W. 1981. Respiratory and vagal modulation of ventricular tachycardia. J Electrocardiol 14:83–89.

Waxman, M.B., and Wald, R.W. 1977. Termination of ventricular tachycardia by an increase in cardiac vagal drive. Circulation 56:385–391.

Zipes, D.P., Martins, J.B., Ruffy, R., Prystowsky, E.N., Elharrar, V., and Gilmore, R.F. 1981. Roles of autonomic innervation in the genesis of ventricular arrhythmias. In: F.M. Abboud, H.A. Fozzard, J.P. Gilmore, and D.J. Reis, eds. Disturbances in Neurogenic Control of the Circulation. pp. 225–250. Bethesda, MD: American Physiological Society.

EDITOR'S NOTES

Mechanisms of Arrhythmias and Antiarrhythmic Drug Action

In his thought-provoking introduction to the discussion on mechanisms of arrhythmias, Dr. Paul Cranefield reminds us from the start that our understanding of the mechanisms of arrhythmias, at least at the basic level, depends heavily upon the experimental models chosen for study. In this regard, his point about the complex nature of even "simple" models should not be overlooked. It is critical to step back occasionally and reflect more thoroughly on what models actually tell us or, equally important, what the limitations of a particular model might be. On the other hand, the quest for more "clinically relevant" animal models must continue. As we increase our sophistication in studying more closely the ultimate model, man himself, various possibilities arise for making effective comparisons between results in experimental models and those obtained in man. Such examples include electrophysiologic studies on transplanted hearts, as well as animal models of programmed electrical stimulation utilizing protocols comparable to those employed in man. Thus, while the search for more clinically relevant models must continue, Dr. Cranefield's point about placing data obtained from particular models in an appropriate perspective, considering both the viable predictions one obtains from such a model as well as its inherent limitations, seems a very appropriate reminder.

The detailed discussion of electrophysiologic mechanisms of cardiac arrhythmias by Dr. Wit is both a reflection of existing theories regarding major mechanisms of arrhythmias as well as an interpretation of the impact of more recent data. Concerning the former aspect, current theories of the mechanisms of arrhythmias largely confirm the original proposal by Hoffman and Cranefield that arrhythmias result from either abnormalities of impulse initiation, impulse conduction, or a combination of both. On the other hand, Dr. Wit's amplification of these original concepts brings these basic assumptions into sharper focus by the addition of more recent data. For example, it is now apparent that, at least at the basic level, abnormal impulse generation can be achieved by normal or abnormal automatic mechanisms as well as triggered activity related to after-depolarizations. The concept of after-depolarizations, although initially discussed several years ago, only now appears to be prevailing, perhaps since many of these abnormalities have been found to be caused by pathophysiologic alterations that exist in the presence of myocardial ischemia, a consequence of coronary artery disease.

Although after-depolarization-related arrhythmias can be easily demonstrated in a variety of experimental settings, it remains to be clinically proven whether such arrhythmias result from these abnormalities. In contrast, ample clinical support has been developed for the concept of abnormal impulse conduction and reentry. In fact, the original concept proposed by Mines, some seven decades ago, has actually been proven and, indeed, expanded. Regarding the latter point, the leading circle hypothesis can be considered an important advance in our understanding of the reentrant process in both atrial and ventricular tissue which can be interpreted from a clinical point of view. In addition, more recent research relating such electrophysiologic concepts to pathophysiologic and anatomic structures may be of particular importance since this complex relationship may lead to a better explanation for the interpatient arrhythmia variability and the variable severity of arrhythmias observed in patients with seemingly comparable cardiac disease. Thus we are being consistently reminded that the complex picture arising from the research level may indeed reflect the many perturbations that may occur clinically. Current methodologies and techniques available at the clinical level are, however, unable to effectively differentiate among such mechanisms, which limits, in part, our assessment of arrhythmic events. A more accurate understanding and prediction of the mechanisms of arrhythmias is important, both to correctly diagnose a particular arrhythmia and to guide the practitioner in choosing the appropriate medical treatment. This dynamic process in the discovery of arrhythmia genesis is likely to continue to challenge existing and evolving theories for some time to come.

The chapter by Verrier and Hagestad emphasizes the critical modulation that the central nervous system imposes on the abnormal physiologic mechanisms elucidated by Dr. Wit. One is, therefore, immediately reminded that cardiac arrhythmias cannot be diagnosed or analyzed only by their electrophysiology but that modulating influences, in this case from the central nervous system, also must be considered. The pathophysiologic process that leads to abnormal impulse generation or conduction can thus be significantly altered or modulated by both the sympathetic or parasympathetic nervous system. The impact of this modulation may be particularly significant during the early stages of myocardial ischemia, when electrical abnormalities leading to sudden death are known to occur. Considering the complexity of the individual organs involved, one can appreciate the difficulties in studying the neural impact on cardiac arrhythmias based upon the myriad effects produced by individual alterations of either organ systems. Of particular note was the discussion of the role of changes in coronary vasomotor tone produced by autonomic manipulations. In addition to its direct effects on myocardial electrophysiologic properties, the changing coronary vasomotor tone may, in addition, produce transient ischemia, which could lead to exacerbation of arrhythmias. Thus, in the final analysis, existing arrhythmias must be fully interpreted and appreciated not only from an electrophysiologic or electrocardiographic viewpoint, but with regard to the underlying hemodynamic manifestations and the balance between sympathetic and parasympathetic outflow. In particular, the potential relevance of the sympathetic nervous system acting as a "trigger" to initiate an imbalance in the ionic or electrophysiologic milieu may be an important critical factor to consider in arrhythmogenesis. The concept of neurally mediated mechanisms of cardiac arrhythmias has implications for drug therapy; therefore, effective drug treatment is critically dependent on our improved understanding of this interaction.

In his final comments, Dr. Verrier noted that, based on his assessment of neural mechanisms and cardiac arrhythmias, an important strategy for clinical management of malignant ventricular arrhythmias may require lessening cardiac sympathetic drive while enhancing parasympathetic tone. Considering the known patterns of innervation and functional impact of the sympathetic nervous system, therapeutic approaches tend to mainly focus on modulating sympathetic drive. One reason for emphasizing such an approach may have been the relative paucity of data demonstrating the presence and functional significance of the parasympathetic nervous system in the functioning ventricle. Dr. Bailey and his colleagues effectively amplify this concept of parasympathetic innervation of the ventricle and its impact therein. To date the data regarding parasympathetic innervation is, however, largely based on studies utilizing animal models. Although the results strongly suggest that similar considerations apply to human situations, the actual manifestations of the presumed parasympathetic innervation regarding electrophysiologic properties and arrhythmias remain to be fully elucidated. However, evidence from limited clinical studies suggests that the clinical impact may be apparent under specific situations. Furthermore, data has not been fully developed and appreciated regarding the impact of myocardial infarction in disrupting or altering the manifestation of either sympathetic or parasympathetic innervation. Recent studies by several investigators have alluded to the impact of disrupting such innervation as far as the development of arrhythmias is concerned. Thus a basic and functional understanding of the parasympathetic innervation of the ventricle is vital to completely interpret and appreciate the autonomic influence on ventricular function, ventricular pathophysiology, and cardiac arrhythmias.

B. Mechanisms of Antiarrhythmic Drug Action

Chapter 4

Cellular Electrophysiologic Mechanisms of Antiarrhythmic Drug Action

Michael R. Rosen and Peter Danilo, Jr.

Introduction

The purpose of this discussion is to review the mechanisms whereby antiarrhythmic drugs modify the cellular electrophysiologic properties of cardiac fibers, and how these changes in turn modify or terminate cardiac arrhythmias. To do this, first we will review the mechanisms responsible for arrhythmias, and then we will demonstrate how these may be affected by individual drugs.

Abnormalities of Impulse Propagation

During normal sinus rhythm, sinus node impulse initiation is followed by activation of the specialized conducting system and myocardium in an ordered fashion. In a variety of situations, abnormal propagation or reentry may occur; sometimes as the result of disease and sometimes as the result of an anatomical abnormality, such as an A-V bypass tract.

Figure 4-1 demonstrates a classic model for reentry described by Schmitt and Erlanger (1928). For reentry to occur in this situation, there are several prerequisites. First, a site of unidirectional conduction block is required. Second, a pathway must be present through which the retrogradely propagating impulse can travel at a velocity sufficiently slow to permit refractoriness to terminate in the tissues into which the retrograde impulse is propagating. If the conditions of timing, conduction velocity, and termination of refractoriness are not met, reentry will not occur (Moe, 1975; Wit and Cranefield, 1978). Moreover, it has been demonstrated that for many reentrant rhythms, critical sinus or extrinsic pacemaker cycle lengths can be identified at which the rhythm can be initiated (or terminated) reproducibly (Wellens, 1978; Josephson and Seides, 1979).

There are a number of means whereby a drug may modify or terminate reentry. One very simple way is by changing cardiac rate. Such a change in rate can result

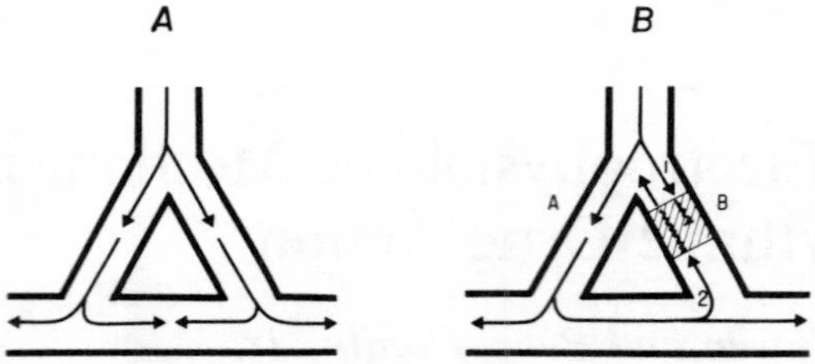

4-1 Schmitt and Erlanger model of reentry. Panel A is a model for normal conduction in a section of the heart. Activation proceeds from the distal Purkinje system (top of panel), through two terminal Purkinje fibers, to the myocardium. Panel B shows an area of depressed and depolarized tissue (cross-hatched) in fiber B. Antegrade activation proceeds through site 1 and conducts slowly and then is blocked in the depressed section. Normal antegrade activation proceeds through fiber A, and approaches the depressed segment in a retrograde direction through site 2. It propagates slowly through the depressed segment in a retrograde direction and then reenters the proximal conducting system.

in several changes in the reentrant pathway, two of which are explored in Figure 4-2. Panel A demonstrates the model for reentry. At a given heart rate, we see that fibers in the conducting system, although not firing spontaneously, are undergoing some degree of phase 4 depolarization (a); there is a very slow conduction through a depressed segment (cross-hatched area), and reentry (b). In panel B, sinus rate has slowed considerably. Depending on the effect of the drug on phase 4 depolarization in the Purkinje system, one of two possible effects on conduction may be seen. If phase 4 is unchanged, the membrane may be depolarized further at the time of action potential initiation and conduction may be slowed further (solid line in a) or may fail completely. Alternatively, if the drug depresses phase 4 depolarization (broken line in a) then conduction velocity may actually increase. Regardless of the effect of the drug on phase 4, the slowing of sinus rate will be accompanied by a prolongation of repolarization and refractoriness (Rosen, 1979). Hence, as sinus rate decreases, determinants of both refractoriness and conduction velocity may change. As a result, the critical timing requirements for reentry may not be met and the arrhythmia may cease.

Another possibility is explored in Figure 4-2C. Here sinus rate increases, resulting in an acceleration of repolarization (b). However, elsewhere in the conducting system, the action potential is initiated at a higher level of membrane potential and may propagate more rapidly (a). Again, the critical timing requirement for reentry may not be met, and the arrhythmia may terminate.

These illustrations indicate how a drug-induced change in rate can upset the balance of conduction velocity and refractoriness required for reentry, thereby suppressing the arrhythmia. There are many ways in which pharmacologic agents can modify sinus rate. β-blocking drugs, such as propranolol, reduce the rate of sinus node depolarization through blockade of sympathetic effects on the sinus

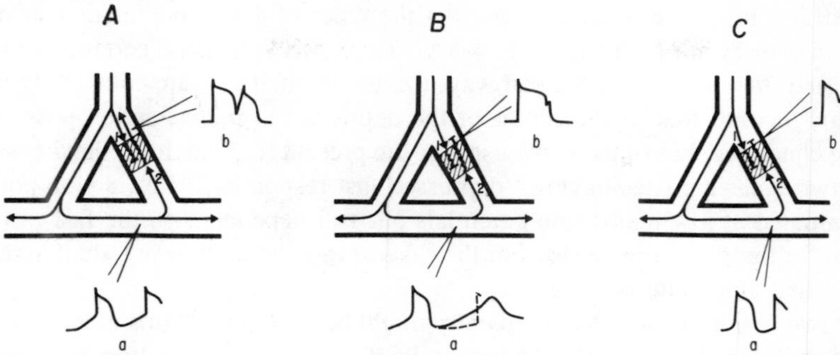

4-2 Examples of the modification of reentry by changing heart rate. Panel A, reentry model. As in Figure 4-1, there is a depressed (cross-hatched) segment in which there is antegrade conduction block and slow retrograde propagation. "a" is an action potential at a distal subendocardial site in which there is phase 4 depolarization, but at the rate at which the heart is beating, there is no automaticity at site "a." "b" is an action potential in the proximal conducting system showing that the reentrant impulse arrives after the termination of refractoriness, permitting further propagation. Panel B shows the result of a slowing of cardiac rate. If a drug both slows rate and decreases the slope of phase 4 depolarization (broken trace in "a"), then conduction may proceed more rapidly. The slowing of rate prolongs repolarization, and with this refractoriness, at site "b" such that the reentrant impulse now arrives before the effective refractory period is completed, and retrograde conduction fails. Another variation on the model would occur if as rate slowed the slope of phase 4 depolarization in "a" did not change (solid trace). In this instance, conduction velocity would slow further, or conduction might fail, resulting in another change in the relationship between refractoriness and conduction, and again terminating reentry. In panel C, cardiac rate has increased and the slope of phase 4 at site "a" is overdrive-suppressed, resulting in an acceleration of conduction of the action potential. Although the effect of the acceleration of heart rate is to accelerate repolarization and shorten the refractory period at "b," the velocity of propagation has increased sufficiently that the retrograde impulse arrives at "b" before the effective refractory period terminates and reentry ceases. It must be emphasized that all three panels here are models that demonstrate the interaction between cardiac rate, repolarization and conduction in the generation of reentry. As models, they are oversimplified and do not demonstrate additional changes in conduction and refractoriness that may occur as a drug acts to modify cardiac rate, repolarization, and conduction.

pacemaker (Rosen, 1979). The slow channel blocker, verapamil, can slow the rate of sinus impulse initiation through depression of phase 4 depolarization in the sinus node (Wit and Cranefield, 1974). Drugs which increase vagal effects on the heart, such as edrophonium, may decrease the slope of phase 4 depolarization and the rate of impulse initiation in the sinus node; whereas vagolytic drugs, such as atropine, may speed sinus rate (Hoffman and Cranefield, 1960).

Many of the antiarrhythmic drugs that suppress reentry can do so even if overall heart rate is unchanged. This occurs as the result of the direct effects of drugs on the action potentials at various sites in the reentrant pathway. To explore these drug effects fully, we first shall consider the types of action potentials that may occur in a reentrant pathway (Fig. 4-3A). Here, we will make certain assumptions: first, that in much of the pathway, the action potentials are completely normal (a); second, that in the center of the depressed segment, action potentials having characteristics of the slow response are present (c); and third, that between these two areas are sites having "depressed fast responses," i.e., action potentials initiated at low membrane potentials but still dependent on the fast inward current for their occurrence (b). For the sake of this illustration, we shall assume as well that sinus rate is unvarying.

The two major means whereby reentry might be abolished in this model are explored in Figure 4-3, B and C. In Figure 4-3B, the action of the drug has been to improve antegrade propagation, thereby removing the site of unidirectional block and restoring a normal activation pattern. Such an effect might be achieved most readily if a drug were to hyperpolarize the depolarized tissues in the depressed segments (b,c), and provide a basis for the fast response action potential again to occur. It is uncertain whether any antiarrhythmic drugs act in this way clinically. However, in certain experimental settings, phenytoin, lidocaine, and propranolol may exert such an effect. Considering phenytoin, at $(K^+)_o$ = 3 mM, low concentrations of drug have been found to increase resting potential, $\dot{V}_{max}$, and conduction velocity in atrial and Purkinje fibers, especially in instances where mechanical trauma, low temperatures, or digitalis have been used initially to depolarize the fibers (Rosen et al., 1974; Bigger et al., 1968; Strauss et al., 1968; Bassett et al., 1970). The mechanism(s) responsible for these effects of phenytoin have not as yet been determined. Lidocaine, too, can hyperpolarize cardiac fibers (Gadsby and Cranefield, 1977; Arnsdorf and Mehlman, 1978). This effect has

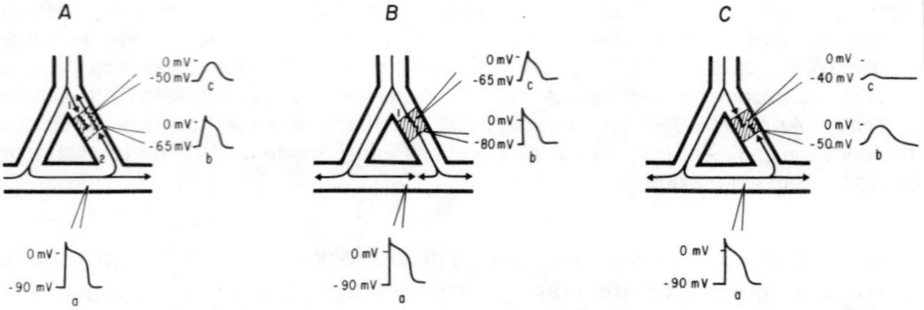

4-3 Means for suppression of reentry. In this model, the following assumptions are made (panel A): The action potentials in much of the conduction system are normal (a); slow responses are occurring in the depressed segment (c); and at intermediate sites, there are depressed fast responses (b). In panel B are the results that might be seen if a drug were to hyperpolarize the depressed tissues at b and c. Here, antegrade conduction has resumed and there is no reentry. In panel C are the results that might be seen if a drug were to further depolarize or otherwise depress the depressed tissues at b and c. As a result, there is now bidirectional conduction block and suppression of reentry.

been attributed to a drug-induced decrease in steady-state Na^+ current (Colatsky, 1982). A similar effect is described for propranolol (Arnsdorf and Mehlman, 1978). Whether this is due to an action like that of lidocaine on steady-state Na^+ current is not known. Another possibility is that propranolol may exert a minor stimulatory effect at the β-receptor (Hermsmeyer et al., 1982), thereby hyperpolarizing depressed fibers.

An additional means whereby a drug might improve antegrade propagation is if depressed conduction occurs in the setting of a low activation voltage secondary to phase 4 depolarization (Fig. 4-4). In this instance, any drug that decreases the slope of phase 4 depolarization might improve conduction, even if the drug is, in its own right, a depressant of conduction. Such an effect has been demonstrated for procainamide (Singer et al., 1967). It is understood that in the presence of procainamide, conduction at the higher activation voltage is not as rapid as it might have been at the same voltage were procainamide not present; nonetheless, it is far faster than it was at the lower activation voltage in the absence of procainamide. The point to be made using this particular example is that, even if a drug is known to depress phase 0 of the action potential and conduction velocity, its ability to depress phase 4 may counterbalance the effect on the action potential upstroke and enhance conduction.

Another means to terminate reentry is through depression of conduction and the induction of bidirectional conduction block (Fig. 4-3C). Here, again, we will assume an unchanging heart rate. Just where the locus of bidirectional block occurs in the example in Figure 4-3 will depend in part on the mechanism of action of the

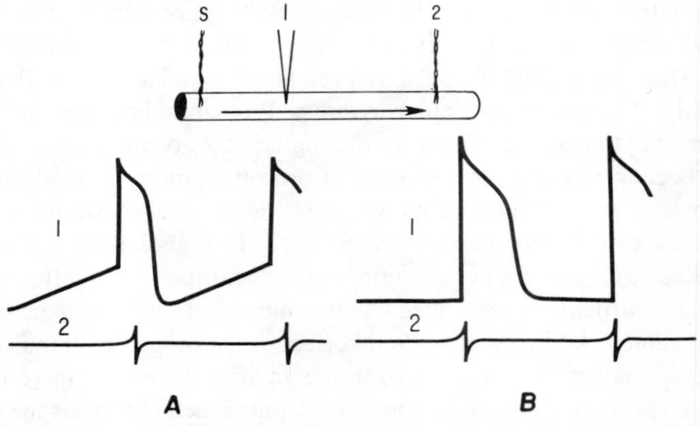

4-4 Effects of depressing the slope of phase 4 on conduction. The experimental model is shown in the upper panel. A Purkinje fiber bundle is stimulated at one end (S). Microelectrode (1) and surface electrogram (2) recordings are made and displayed on the lower panels. In panel A, there is marked phase 4 depolarization and conduction, measured from the upstroke of the action potential to the electrogram, is slow. In panel B, a drug such as procainamide has depressed the slope of phase 4, and conduction now proceeds more rapidly.

drug administered. For example, quinidine depresses the rapid inward current in fibers having the fast response (Hoffman, 1958; Vaughan Williams and Szekeres, 1961) as well as the depressed fast response action potential (Hondeghem, 1976). As a result, it would be anticipated to depress conduction at both sites a and b. Still another means whereby quinidine depresses conduction is through displacement of threshold potential to more positive voltages, thereby reducing the excitability of cardiac fibers (Hoffman et al., 1975). This ability of quinidine to depress conduction in fibers having normal action potentials is reflected in its action on the electrocardiogram: therapeutic concentrations of quinidine routinely prolong both the P-R interval and QRS duration.

In addition to its action on normal and depressed fast responses, quinidine exerts a minor action on the slow response action potential (Nawrath, 1981). This might be expected to result in depression of conduction at site c in Figure 4-3C, as well. Hence, quinidine is a drug having a rather nonspecific effect on conduction, depressing it in normal and depolarized tissues. This also provides a basis for quinidine's toxic effects: that is, just as it can depress conduction to the point of inducing bidirectional block in pathways that previously were reentrant, it also can sufficiently depress conduction at other previously normal sites to the point of inducing unidirectional block and reentry.

In addition to slowing conduction, quinidine also prolongs repolarization and refractoriness (Vaughan Williams, 1958). Considering Figure 4-3C again, this provides another means for inducing bidirectional block, as it increases the interval during which cardiac fibers are protected from the propagation of premature beats. Although the prolongation of refractoriness is beneficial, the prolongation of repolarization may not be so. The basis for making this statement is explored in Figure 4-5. In Fig. 4-5A, we consider a fiber with a short action potential duration and effective refractory period. Premature impulse "a" will propagate slowly and is likely to induce an arrhythmia. Premature impulse "b" also may induce an arrhythmia; but, based on the higher level of membrane potential at which it occurs, it would be expected to propagate more normally than "a." Moreover, any impulse that occurs before full repolarization would be expected to induce an R on T phenomenon on the ECG. In Figure 4-5B, a drug such as quinidine has prolonged repolarization and refractoriness. The effective refractory period is sufficiently prolonged that the impulse at "a" no longer can propagate. This represents an antiarrhythmic effect of the drug. The impulse at "b," however, occurs before full repolarization and after the end of the effective refractory period. It may now induce an R on T phenomenon and has the capability of inducing a more dangerous arrhythmia than it did in Fig. 4-5A. This represents a toxic effect of the drug.

Summing up the actions of quinidine, then, in the presence of an unchanging cycle length its actions are many, including the depression of conduction in normal and depolarized tissues, the prolongation of repolarization, and the ability to suppress or induce arrhythmias.

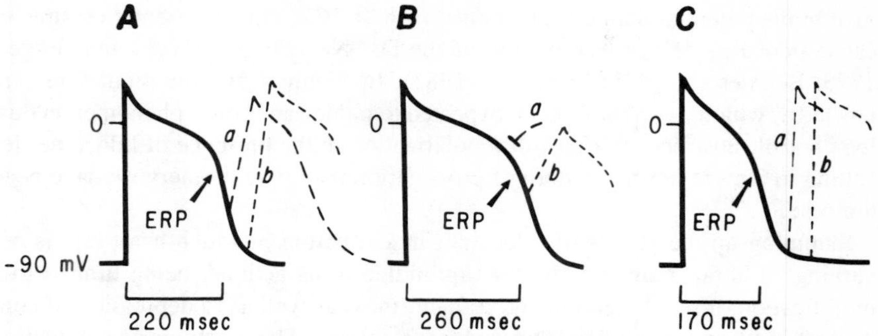

4-5 Relationships between the effective refractory period (ERP) and conduction of premature beats ("a" and "b"). In panel A, both "a" and "b" occur after ERP has terminated. "a" is at a lower membrane potential and propagates slowly and "b" is at a higher membrane potential and propagates less slowly. In panel B, a drug has prolonged action potential duration and the ERP. Propagation of "a" now is blocked. "b" occurs at a less negative membrane potential than in panel B and now propagates more slowly. In panel C, a drug has accelerated repolarization and shortened the ERP. "a" and "b" now occur at higher membrane potentials and propagate more normally.

Let us contrast this type of drug effect with those of two drugs that are more specific than quinidine in their actions: lidocaine and verapamil. Lidocaine is, like quinidine, a local anesthetic. Unlike quinidine, lidocaine induces only small decreases in $\dot{V}_{max}$, has no effect on threshold potential, and has no significant effect on conduction in the normal ventricular specialized conducting system and myocardium (Davis and Temte, 1969; Bigger and Mandel, 1970). Relating this to the electrocardiogram, lidocaine routinely does not alter the P-R interval or QRS complex. Lidocaine also has no effect on the slow response. In contrast, lidocaine markedly depresses the $\dot{V}_{max}$ of fibers having the depressed fast response (Brennan et al., 1978). The reason for this greater selectivity of lidocaine for depolarized fibers is that it apparently has an increased binding affinity for the inactivated Na^+ channels that occur at low levels of membrane potential (Hondeghem and Katzung, 1980; Gintant et al., 1983). Lidocaine's depressant effect on $\dot{V}_{max}$ also increases as pH is lowered, because lidocaine is ionized increasingly as pH decreases (Nattel, et al., 1981; Grant et al., 1980). Hence, in situations where ischemia has resulted in a reduced membrane potential and acidosis, lidocaine will depress $\dot{V}_{max}$ and conduction to a far greater extent than in normal tissues.

Unlike quinidine, lidocaine accelerates repolarization and reduces the duration of the effective refractory period. The acceleration of repolarization is believed to result from block of Na^+ entry through those Na^+ channels that remain open during the plateau (Colatsky, 1982; Carmeliet and Saikawa, 1982). However, the duration of refractoriness is prolonged relative to that of the action potential. As a result, the earliest premature beat that can propagate occurs at a higher level of membrane potential than during control (Fig. 4-5C). This apparently occurs because lidocaine delays reactivation of the fast Na^+ channel (Weld and Bigger, 1975; Bean et al., 1981; Lee et al., 1981). In Figure 4-5C, the premature beat labeled a, which would have been expected to induce an R on T phenomenon during control, now occurs after full repolarization in the presence of lidocaine, resulting in a more normal pattern of propagation than would otherwise have been the case.

Summing up the effects of lidocaine, in a situation in which heart rate is not varying: it is far more specific than quinidine in its actions, being limited to a modification of repolarization and refractoriness as well as to depression of conduction in fibers having the depressed fast response. These actions on conduction and repolarization in a reentrant pathway can be expected to modify the critical relationship of conduction and refractoriness required for reentry to occur.

Verapamil provides us with another example of drug specificity. This drug has only minor effects on the normal and depressed fast response action potentials and on the effective refractory period of fibers in the ventricle (Rosen et al., 1974; Singh and Vaughan Williams, 1972). However, concentrations having no effect on the fast response can completely abolish the slow response in ventricular and atrial fibers (Cranefield et al., 1974). Because sinus and A-V nodal potentials are a type of slow response, verapamil can depress impulse initiation and propagation at both these sites as well (Wit and Cranefield, 1974). As a result, therapeutic concentrations can slow sinus rate and prolong the P-R interval. However, they do not routinely affect QRS duration.

Summing up our consideration of reentry, using the model of unidirectional block and retrograde propagation, changes in several variables that modify refractoriness and/or conduction can alter the timing in a reentrant circuit and abolish it. We also have seen that the drugs which exert such effects may vary widely in their selectivity and their mechanisms of action. We will not consider other models for reentry here. Suffice it to say that the ability of drugs to modify conduction and repolarization and refractoriness in these models also will provide an antiarrhythmic effect.

There is one factor that requires further consideration here. This relates to the effects of heart rate on the ability of a drug to suppress an arrhythmia. In most of the examples of drug effect, above, we assumed an unvarying heart rate. Yet, this is not the case in many tachycardias, which may vary in their rates in an individual at different times as well as vary in their rates from individual to individual.

To consider further the interaction of heart rate and drug action, we will review the phenomenon of the ''use dependence'' of a drug's action (Hondeghem and Katzung, 1980; Hondeghem and Katzung, 1977) (Fig. 4-6). The model of use dependence suggests that fast Na^+ channels in the cell membrane may exist in resting (R), activated (A), and inactivated (I) states. Both association (k) and dissociation (l) rate constants, which differ for the R, A, and I states as well as for individual drugs, determine the affinity of the drug for the receptor (channel) site.

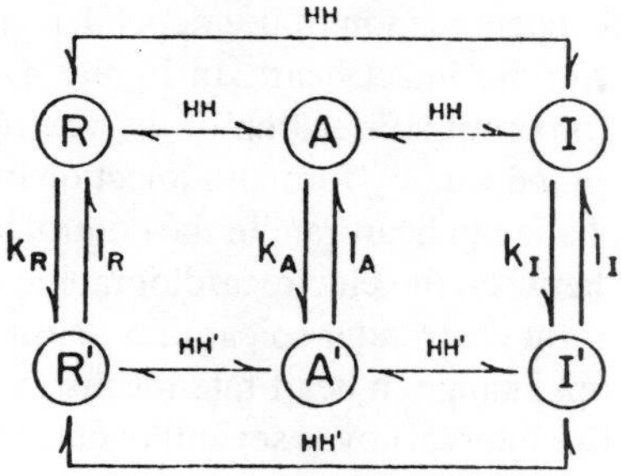

4-6 A model of the Na^+ channel for the description of antiarrhythmic drug action. R, A, and I indicate the resting, activated, and inactivated states of the channel when not occupied by drug. The resting, activated, and inactivated states of the drug-occupied channel are represented as R′, A′, and I′. Channels move between states by Hodgkin-Huxley (HH) kinetics: k and l are association and dissocation rate constants for drug interaction with the sodium channels in each of the states. Constants are characteristic for each drug (reproduced from Hondeghem and Katzung (1980), by permission).

Drugs which interact mainly with activated channels will bind with these channels during the action potential upstroke. The greater the affinity of the drug for the channel, the more rapidly block will occur. Because increasing block of the fast Na^+ channel develops with each action potential until a steady-state effect is reached, this type of block is referred to as "use-dependent."

In the inactivated state, the constants k and l for some drugs, such as lidocaine, are relatively long. As a result, little channel blocking occurs here, nor is there much removal of drug. During repolarization, there is normal removal of inactivation of those channels that are not bound by drug; however, the removal of inactivation of the drug-associated channels is delayed. On return to the resting state, there is more rapid removal of drug from the drug-associated channels, as the constants k and l are smaller than during inactivation, and, therefore, drug affinity is reduced (Nattel et al., 1981; Grant et al., 1980; Chen et al., 1975).

Summing up, the phenomenon of use dependence introduces a cardiac rate-related variable to the actions of antiarrhythmic drugs, based on the affinity of a drug for the fast channel. Most of the fast channel blockade develops during phase 0 of the action potential. At low heart rates, many channels that are blocked during phase 0 may become unblocked during phase 4. However, as heart rate increases, the ability of channels to become unblocked during phase 4 is reduced, and so increasing numbers of channels accumulate in the inactivated state. As a result, the increase in heart rate is accompanied by an ever-increasing depression of $\dot{V}_{max}$ and conduction.

We must stress that the phenomenon of use dependence occurs not only in isolated cardiac fibers, but in the intact heart. In Figure 4-7 are records from the heart of an intact dog. To permit stimulation of the ventricle at slow rates, complete heart block has been induced by formalin injection of the His bundle. In the upper panel, an abrupt change in heart rate in the control state induces no change in an interval measured between the electrocardiographic Q wave and an electrogram recorded from the right ventricular epicardium. However, in the presence of quinidine, the same abrupt change in heart rate results in a change in conduction (prolongation of the Q-EG interval) over several cycles. This is an example of a use-dependent change in conduction. In the lower panel is shown the dV/dt of the electrogram record. During control, this does not change despite changes in cardiac cycle length. However, following abrupt decreases in cycle length in the presence of quinidine, there are decreases in dV/dt as well.

Abnormalities of Impulse Initiation

We will consider abnormal impulse initiation as resulting from either automatic mechanisms or afterdepolarizations. In reviewing automaticity, we must stress the diversity of situations under which automatic impulse initiation is seen. Using specialized conducting and the muscle fibers of the ventricle as our example, in fully polarized tissues (membrane potential > -80 mv), only the specialized fibers will develop automatic rhythms. These rhythms, which result from phase 4 depolarization, are induced in turn by the accumulation of positive charge within the cell during phase 4. There is some argument at present as to whether phase 4 depolarization here results primarily from an outward current carried by K^+ that diminishes in magnitude (i_{k_2}) (Noble, 1975), or from an inward current carried by Na^+ (i_f) (DiFrancesco, 1981). Regardless of the cause, this rhythm is characterized by a slow rate (usually $\leq$ 40/min in the absence of catecholamines) and by the ability to be overdrive-suppressed.

In contrast, at very low membrane potentials (i.e., ≤ -50 mv) both specialized and myocardial cells can generate automatic rhythms. Here, the rhythm tends to occur at a faster rate and results from an inward current carried by Na^+ and/or Ca^{2+} during phase 4 (Dangman and Hoffman, 1980; Toda, 1970). This rhythm tends not to be overdrive-suppressible. The reason for the change from overdrive suppression at high membrane potentials to failure to suppress at low membrane potentials appears to be the following: at high membrane potentials, overdrive pacing results in increased Na^+ entry into the fiber per unit time. This Na^+ entry provides an important stimulus for Na^+/K^+ pumping and hyperpolarizes the fiber. At membrane potentials ≤ -50 mv, the action potentials tend to be slow responses which carry in less Na^+ than the fast responses at high membrane potentials. As a result, there is little or no added stimulus for Na^+/K^+ pump-

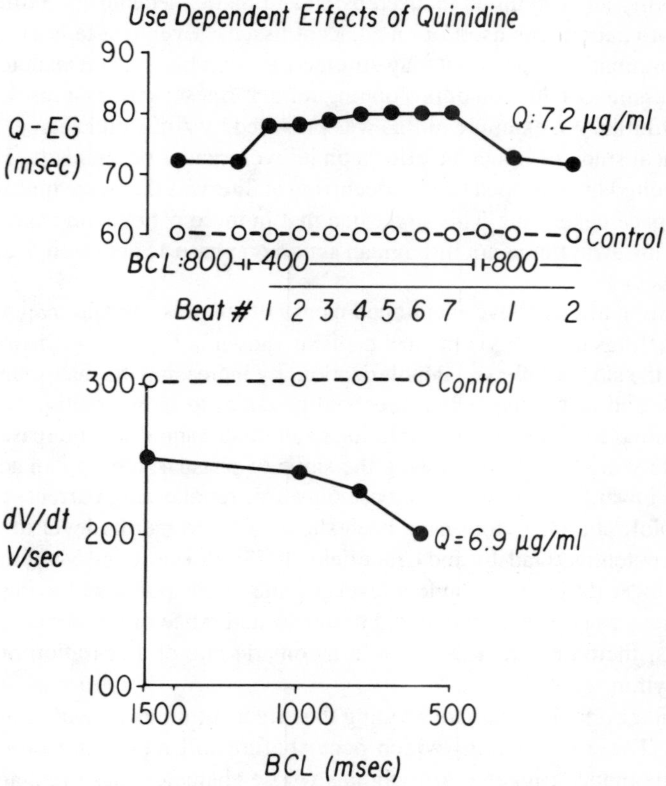

4-7 Use-dependent effects of quinidine in an intact canine heart. Upper panel: Q-electrogram interval plotted as a function of drive cycle length (BCL). Unfilled circles: control. Changing the pacing cycle length from 800–400 ms does not change the Q-EG interval of 60 ms. Filled circles, quinidine, 7.2 μg/ml. At the cycle length of 800 ms, the Q-EG interval now is 72 m. When cycle length is abruptly shortened to 400 ms for seven beats conduction slows. It accelerates again when the drive cycle length is increased to 800 ms. Lower panel: The dV/dt of the electrogram is plotted as a function of steady-state drive cycle length. During control, dV/dt is constant at 300 v/s from CL 1600–500 ms (unfilled circles). At quinidine, 6.9 μg/ml, (filled circles), dV/dt is reduced at all cycle lengths, and is lowest at the shortest cycle length.

ing. It must be stressed that at membrane potentials between the two extremes we have been discussing (−50 and −80 mv) there are intermediate degrees of overdrive suppression (Hoffman and Dangman, In Press; Vassalle, 1977).

To modify an arrhythmia induced by an automatic mechanism, a drug may act on the automatic focus itself or on adjacent tissues. Even if it fails to have an effect on automaticity, per se, it may still increase exit block from an automatic site (by depressing conduction or prolonging refractoriness) and, as a result, suppress the arrhythmia. An example of this was provided by Aravandikshan et al. (1977) in a clinical study of lidocaine effects on idioventricular pacemakers. Here, lidocaine resulted in "dropped beats" occurring at intervals that were multiples of the original pacemaker rate. This suggested that in these patients lidocaine was suppressing the arrhythmia not through an action on phase 4, but through an increase in exit block.

In addition to this above-mentioned means of suppressing automaticity, antiarrhythmic drugs may act via the mechanisms shown in Figure 4-8. In brief, by decreasing the slope of phase 4 depolarization, by increasing the maximum diastolic potential, and/or by displacing threshold potential to more positive voltages the time required for phase 4 depolarization to attain threshold will increase and automatic rate will slow. In depressing the slope of phase 4, a drug can act either to decrease inward current or to increase outward, repolarizing current. Lidocaine, propranolol, and phenytoin have been shown to increase the level of maximum diastolic potential (Gadsby and Cranefield, 1977; Arnsdorf and Mehlman, 1978). With all these drugs, fibers at low levels of membrane potential having abnormal automaticity may be hyperpolarized to the normal range of membrane potentials. With this, there may be a decrease in automatic rate or a cessation of the automatic rhythm.

A similar effect is seen in evaluating the effects of drugs on early afterdepolarizations. These oscillations which occur before full repolarization of the cell membrane induce triggered arrhythmias whose characteristics often are difficult to distinguish from those of abnormal automaticity. It is likely that the same maneuvers that modify abnormal automaticity will suppress early afterdepolarization-induced triggered rhythms as well. Certainly, both lidocaine and procainamide have been shown to hyperpolarize preparations having such activity, thereby abolishing it (Arnsdorf, 1971).

Delayed afterdepolarizations have been studied in more detail than early afterdepolarizations. Most investigations have centered around those induced in Purkinje fibers by digitalis (Rosen et al., 1973; Ferrier et al., 1973) and those induced in atrium (Hashimoto and Moe, 1973; Hordof et al., 1978; Mary-Rabine et al., 1980) or coronary sinus (Wit and Cranefield, 1971) by digitalis or catecholamines. The mechanisms for these have been reviewed elsewhere in this volume (see Chapter 1). Suffice it to say, for the purpose of this discussion, that they appear to result from an overload of intracellular Ca^{2+} (presumably released from

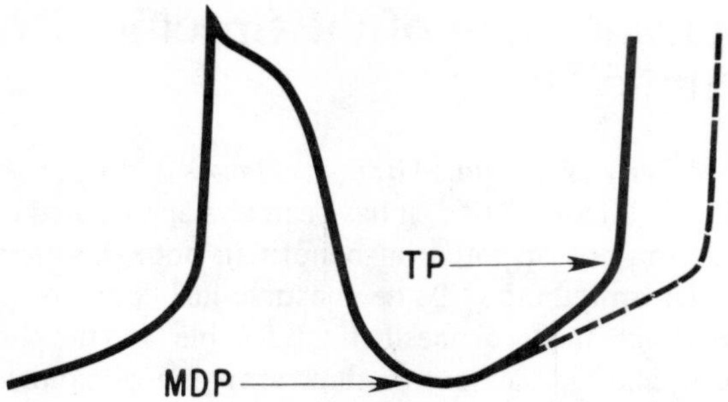

4-8 An automatic fiber is shown here. An antiarrhythmic drug may slow automatic rate by displacing the maximum diastolic potential (MDP) to more negative values, the threshold potential (TP) to more positive values, and/or by decreasing the slope of phase 4 (broken lines).

the sarcoplasmic reticulum) which, in turn, increases the monovalent cation conductance of the membrane and induces an oscillatory inward current. Based on this information, a delayed afterdepolarization should be suppressed by any agent that either decreases inward current carried by Na^+ or Ca^{2+}, and/or that increases outward, repolarizing current carried by K^+. With this in mind it might be predicted that a number of drugs would suppress delayed afterdepolarizations, and this is, in fact, the case. Most studies have been performed in Purkinje fibers having digitalis-induced delayed afterdepolarizations. In these studies, agents which depress inward Na^+ current, such as lidocaine (Rosen and Danilo, 1980), agents which depress inward Ca^{2+} current such as verapamil (Rosen et al., 1974; Rosen and Danilo, 1980), or Mn^{2+} (Ferrier and Moe, 1973); and agents which increase repolarizing current, such as procainamide (Hewett and Rosen, 1980) all have been shown to suppress delayed afterdepolarizations. β-blocking concentrations of propranolol will not alter digitalis-induced delayed afterdepolarizations unless catecholamine is present as well as digitalis; however, higher concentrations of propranolol, in the local anesthetic range, will do so even in the absence of catecholamines (Hewett and Rosen, 1982).

Summing up this information on abnormal impulse initiation, we have seen that a number of different effects of antiarrhythmic drugs can contribute to suppression of an arrhythmia. These means may be indirect, aimed at limiting the spread of electrical activity from an ectopic focus, through the modification of conduction velocity or refractoriness, or they may be more direct, through an action on the arrhythmogenic mechanism itself.

Further Consideration of the Specificity of Antiarrhythmic Drugs

Although the specificity of individual drugs or classes of drugs has long been recognized (Vaughan Williams, 1970), it has been less appreciated that such differences in drug action are of potential benefit in both the diagnosis and the treatment of cardiac arrhythmias. To demonstrate just how this might occur, we will consider two drugs, the local anesthetic, lidocaine, and the phenothiazine derivative, ethmozin, and their actions on three arrhythmogenic mechanisms: normal automaticity, abnormal automaticity, and delayed afterdepolarizations. The cellular electrophysiologic actions of the drugs on these mechanisms are summarized in Table 4-1. In brief, lidocaine in therapeutic concentrations suppresses both delayed afterdepolarizations and normal automaticity (presumably through decreasing inward current carried by Na^+), but has no effect on abnormal automaticity. In contrast, therapeutic concentrations of ethmozin suppress abnormal automaticity and delayed afterdepolarizations, but have no effect on normal automaticity. The mechanisms responsible for ethmozin's actions are not yet known. If one were to apply this information to the study of arrhythmias in an intact animal model (or patient) and could rule out reentry as a cause, then one might use the matrix in Table 4-1 to help identify whether the rhythm was induced by normal automaticity (in which case lidocaine but not ethmozin would be effective), abnormal automaticity (in which case ethmozin but not lidocaine would be effective), or delayed afterdepolarizations (in which case both would be effective). This has been done, in a canine model in which an accelerated idioventricular rhythm was induced by formalin injection of the His bundle (Ilvento et al., 1982). The accelerated idioventricular rhythm persists for the first 1–3 days after heart block, and subsequently, only the slow idioventricular rhythm is seen. Hence, this particular model provides one with an opportunity to study the effects of different antiarrhythmic drugs on two different arrhythmogenic mechanisms. As shown in Figure 4-9, the slow idioventricular rhythm is readily suppressed by lidocaine, but not ethmozin, whereas the accelerated rhythm (Fig. 4-10B) is suppressed by ethmozin, but not lidocaine. These results indicate that using a simple

Table 4-1 Actions of Therapeutic Concentrations of Lidocaine and Ethmozin on Three Arrhythmogenic Mechanisms.*

	Normal automaticity	Abnormal automaticity	Delayed afterdepolarizations
Lidocaine	+	–	+
Ethmozin	–	+	+

*Results from isolated tissue studies using normal or low $(K^+)_o$ to induce normal automaticity, Ba^{2+} or infarction to induce abnormal automaticity, and digitalis to induce delayed afterdepolarizations.

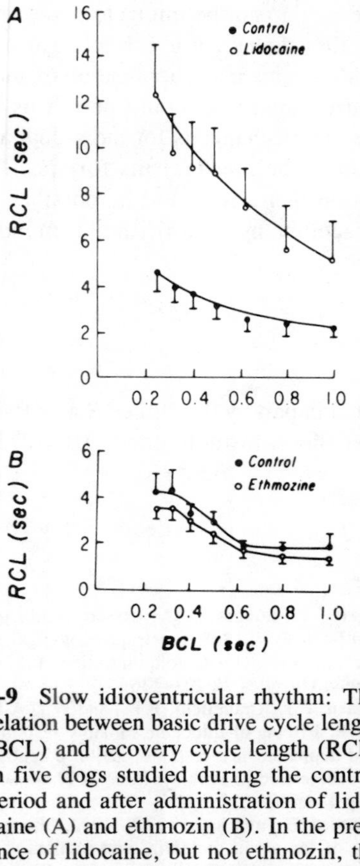

4-9 Slow idioventricular rhythm: The relation between basic drive cycle length (BCL) and recovery cycle length (RCL) in five dogs studied during the control period and after administration of lidocaine (A) and ethmozin (B). In the presence of lidocaine, but not ethmozin, the rhythm is markedly overdrive-suppressed. (Modified from Ilvento et al., 1982.)

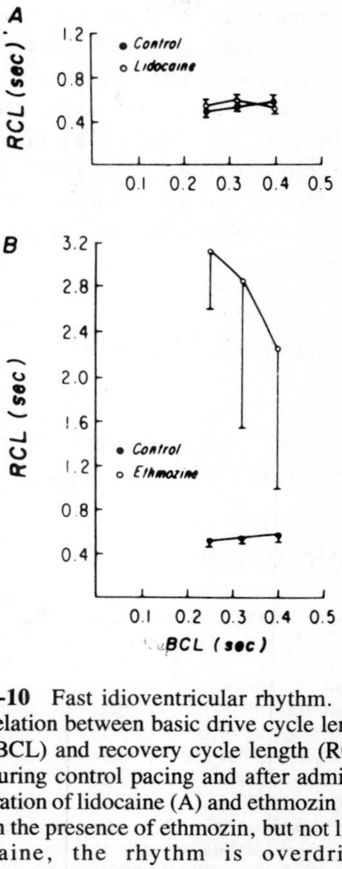

4-10 Fast idioventricular rhythm. The relation between basic drive cycle length (BCL) and recovery cycle length (RCL) during control pacing and after administration of lidocaine (A) and ethmozin (B). In the presence of ethmozin, but not lidocaine, the rhythm is overdrive-suppressed. (Modified from Ilvento et al., 1982.)

matrix, such as that in Table 4-1, consisting of drugs whose effects are disparate, at least in part, can help us understand the mechanism for an arrhythmia. In this case, the results suggest the slow rhythm is the result of normal automaticity (which has been verified in microelectrode studies); whereas the accelerated rhythm is the result of abnormal automaticity (which is yet to be tested conclusively).

We must stress that the above-mentioned results do not permit us to make any firm conclusions about mechanism. However, they do help us to formulate an approach that should be promising in the future development and application of antiarrhythmic drugs. Very simply, the use of drug matrices should permit us to define more specifically than now is possible the mechanisms for individual arrhythmias. Further, once more is known about the mechanisms for specific arrhythmias and the actions of various drugs on them, it should be possible to provide more specific, and successful, pharmacotherapy for arrhythmias in individual patients.

Acknowledgments

Certain of the studies referred to were supported in part by the United States Public Health Service, National Heart, Lung and Blood Institute grants HL-12738 and HL-28223.

References

Aravindakshan, V., Kuo, C-S., and Gettes, L.S. 1977. Effects of lidocaine on escape rate in patients with complete atrioventricular block. Am J Cardiol 40:177–183.

Arnsdorf, M.F. 1977. The effect of antiarrhythmic drugs on triggered sustained rhythmic activity in cardiac Purkinje fibers. J Pharmacol Exp Ther 201:689–700.

Arnsdorf, M.F., and Mehlman, D.J. 1978. Observations on the effects of selected antiarrhythmic drugs on mammalian cardiac Purkinje fibers with two levels of steady-state potential: influences of lidocaine, phenytoin, propranolol, disopyramide and procainamide on repolarization, action potential shape and conduction. J Pharmacol Exp Ther 207:983–991.

Bassett, A.L., Bigger, J.T., Jr., and Hoffman, B.F. 1970. 'Protective' action diphenylhydantoin on canine Purkinje fibers during hypoxia. J Pharmacol Exp Ther 173:336–343.

Bean, B.P., Cohen, C.J., and Tsien, R.W. 1981. Lidocaine binding to resting and inactivated cardiac sodium channels. Biophys J 33:208.

Bigger, J.T., and Mandel, W.T. 1970. Effect of lidocaine on transmembrane potentials of ventricular muscle and Purkinje fibers. J Clin Invest 49:63–77.

Bigger, J.T., Strauss, H.C., Bassett, A.L., and Hoffman, B.F. 1968. Electrophysiological effects of diphenylhydantoin on canine Purkinje fibers. Circ Res 22:221–236.

Brennan, F.J., Cranefield, P.F., and Wit, A.L. 1978. Effects of lidocaine on slow response and depressed fast response action potentials of canine cardiac Purkinje fibers. J Pharmacol Exp Ther 204:312–324.

Carmeliet, E., and Saikawa, T. 1982. Shortening of the action potential and reduction of pacemaker activity by lidocaine quinidine and procainamide in sheep cardiac Purkinje fibers: an effect on Na or K currents? Circ Res 50:257–272.

Chen, C.M., Gettes, L.C., and Katzung, B.G. 1975. Effects of lidocaine and quinidine on steady-state characteristics and recovery kinetics (dv/dt) max in guinea pig ventricular myocardium. Circ Res 37:20–29.

Colatsky, T. 1982. Mechanisms of action of lidocaine and quinidine on action potential duration in rabbit cardiac Purkinje fibers: an effect on steady-state sodium currents? Circ Res 50:17–27.

Cranefield, P.F., Aronson, R.S., and Wit, A.L. 1974. Effect of verapamil on the normal action potential and on a calcium-dependent slow response of canine Purkinje fibers. Circ Res 34:204–213.

Dangman, K., and Hoffman, B.F. 1980. Effects of nifedipine on electrical activity of cardiac cells. Am J Cardiol 46:1059–1067.

Dangman, K.H., and Hoffman, B.F. 1983. Antiarrhythmic effects of ethmozin in cardiac Purkinje fiber: Suppression of automaticity and abolition of triggering. J Pharm Exp Therap 227:578–586.

Danilo, P., Jr., Langan, W.B., Rosen, M.R., and Hoffman, B.F. 1977. Effects of the phenothiazine analog EN 313 on ventricular arrhythmias in dogs. Eur J Pharmacol 45:127–139.

Davis, L.D., and Temte, J.V. 1969. Electrophysiological actions of lidocaine on canine ventricular muscle and Purkinje fibers. Circ Res 24:639–655.

DiFrancesco, D. 1981. A new interpretation of the pace-maker current in calf Purkinje fibers. J Physiol 314:359–376.

Ferrier, G.R., and Moe, G.K. 1973. Effect of calcium on acetylstrophanthidin-induced transient depolarizations in canine Purkinje tissue. Circ Res 35:508–515.

Ferrier, G.R., Saunders, J., and Mendez, C. 1973. Cellular mechanism for the generation of ventricular arrhythmias by acetylstrophanthidin. Circ Res 32:610–617.

Gadsby, D.C., and Cranefield, P.F. 1977. Two levels of resting potential in cardiac Purkinje fibers. J Gen Physiol 70:725–746.

Gintant, G., Hoffman, B.F., and Naylor, R.E. 1983. The influence of molecular form on the interactions of local anesthetic-type antiarrhythmic agents with canine cardiac Na^+ channel. Circ Res 52:735–746.

Grant, A.O., Strauss, L.J., Wallace, A.G., and Strauss, H.C. 1980. The influence of pH on the electrophysiologic effects of lidocaine in guinea pig ventricular myocardium. Circ Res 47:542–550.

Hashimoto, K., and Moe, G.K. 1973. Transient depolarizations induced by acetylstrophanthidin in specialized tissues of dog atrium and ventricle. Circ Res 32:618–624.

Hermsmeyer, K., Mason, R., Griffen, S., and Becker, P. 1982. Rat cardiac muscle single cell automaticity responses to α- and β-adrenergic agonists and antagonists. Circ Res 51:532–537.

Hewett, K., and Rosen, M.R. 1980. Effects of ethmozin and procainamide on ouabain-induced afterdepolarizations. Fed Proc 39:966.

Hewett, K., and Rosen, M.R. 1982. β-adrenergic modulation of digitalis-induced delayed afterdepolarizations and triggered activity. Am J Cardiol 49:913.

Hoffman, B.F. 1958. The action of quinidine and procainamide on single fibers of dog ventricle and specialized conducting system. Ann Acad Brasil Cienc 29:365–368.

Hoffman, B.F., and Cranefield, P.F. 1960. Electrophysiology of the Heart. New York: McGraw-Hill.

Hoffman, B.F., and Dangman, K. Are arrhythmias caused by automatic impulse generation? In: P. Paes de Carvalho, M. Lieberman, and B. Hoffman, eds. Normal and Abnormal Conduction in the Heart. New York: Futura Press. In Press.

Hoffman, B.F., Rosen, M.R., and Wit, A.L. 1975. Electrophysiology and pharmacology of cardiac arrhythmias. VII. Cardiac effects of quinidine and procainamide. Am Heart J 90:117–122.

Hondeghem, L.M. 1976. Effects of lidocaine, phenytoin and quinidine on ischemic canine myocardium. J Electrocardiol 9:203–209.

Hondeghem, L.M., and Katzung, B.G. 1977. Time and voltage-dependent interactions of antiarrhythmic drugs with cardiac sodium channels. Biochim Biophys Acta 474:373–398.

Hondeghem, L.M., and Katzung, B.G. 1980. Test of a model of antiarrhythmic drug action: effects of quinidine and lidocaine on myocardial conduction. Circulation 61:1217–1224.

Hordof, A.J., Edie, R., Malm, J.R., Hoffman, B.F., and Rosen, M.R. 1976. Electrophysiological properties and response to pharmacologic agents of fibers from diseased human atria. Circulation 54:774–779.

Hordof, A.J., Spotnitz, H., Mary-Rabine, L., Edie, R., and Rosen, M.R. 1978. The cellular electrophysiologic effects of digitalis on human atrial fibers. Circulation 57:223–229.

Ilvento, J.P., Provet, J., Danilo, P., Jr., and Rosen, M.R. 1982. Fast and slow idioventricular rhythms in the canine heart: A study of their mechanism using antiarrhythmic drugs and electrophysiologic testing. Am J Cardiol 49:1909–1916.

Josephson, M.E., and Seides, S.F. 1979. Clinical Cardiac Electrophysiology. Techniques and Interpretations. Philadelphia: Lea and Febiger.

Lee, K.S., Hume, Jr., Giles, W., and Brown, A.M. 1981. Sodium current depression by lidocaine and quinidine in isolated ventricular cells. Nature 291:325–327.

Mary-Rabine, L., Hordof, A.J., Danilo, P., Malm, J.R., and Rosen, M.R. 1980. Mechanisms for impulse initiation in isolated human atrial fibers. Circ Res 47:267–277.

Moe, G.K. 1975. Evidence for reentry as a mechanism for cardiac arrhythmias. Rev Physiol Biochem Pharmacol 72:56–66.

Nattel, S., Elharrar, V., Zipes, D., and Bailey, J.C. 1981. pH-dependent electrophysiological effects of quinidine and lidocaine on canine cardiac Purkinje fibers. Circ Res 48:55–61.

Nawrath, H. 1981. Action potential, membrane currents and force of contraction in mammalian heart muscle fibers treated with quinidine. J Pharmacol Exp Ther 216:176–182.

Noble, D. 1975. The Initiation of the Heart Beat. Oxford: Clarendon Press.

Rosen, M.R. 1979. Cardiac drugs. In: M.I. Ferrer, ed. Current Cardiology. pp. 259–303. Boston: Houghton-Mifflin.

Rosen, M.R., and Danilo, P. 1980. Effects of tetrodotoxin, lidocaine, verapamil and AHR-2666 on ouabain-induced delayed afterdepolarization in canine Purkinje fibers. Circ Res 46:117–124.

Rosen, M.R., Danilo, P., Jr., Alonso, M.B., and Pippenger, C.E. 1974. Effects of therapeutic concentrations of diphenylhydantoin on transmembrane potentials of normal and depressed Purkinje fibers. J Pharmacol Exp Ther 197:594–604.

Rosen, M.R., Ilvento, J.P., Gelband, H., and Merker, C. 1974. Effects of verapamil on electrophysiologic properties of canine Purkinje fibers. J Pharmacol Exp Ther 189:414–421.

Rosen, M.R., Merker, C. Gelband, H., and Hoffman, B.F. 1973. Effects of ouabain on phase 4 of Purkinje fiber transmembrane potentials. Circulation 47:681–689.

Schmitt, F.O., and Erlanger, J. 1928. Directional differences in the conduction of the impulse through heart muscle and their possible relation to extrasystolic and fibrillary contractions. Am J Physiol 87:326–347.

Singer, D.H., Strauss, H.C., and Hoffman, B.F. 1967. Biphasic effects of procainamide on cardiac conduction. Bull NY Acad Med 43:1194–1195.

Singh, B.N., and Vaughan Williams, E.M. 1972. A fourth class of antidysrhythmic action? Effect of verapamil on ouabain toxicity, on atrial and ventricular intracellular potentials, and on other features of cardiac function. Cardiovasc Res 6:109–119.

Strauss, H.C., Bigger, J.T., Bassett, A.L., and Hoffman, B.F. 1968. Actions of diphenylhydantoin on the electrical properties of isolated rabbit and canine atria. Circ Res 23:463–477.

Toda, N. 1970. Barium-induced automaticity in relation to calcium ions and norepinephrine in the rabbit left atrium. Circ Res 27:45–57.

Vassalle, M. 1977. The relationship among cardiac pacemakers: overdrive suppression. Circ Res 41:269–277.

Vaughan Williams, E.M. 1958. The mode of action of quinidine on isolated rabbit atria interpreted from intracellular potential electrodes. Br J Pharmacol 13:276–287.

Vaughan Williams, E.M. 1970. Classification of antiarrhythmic drugs. In: E. Sandoe, E. Flensted-Jensen, and K. Olesen, eds. Symposium on Cardiac Arrhythmias. pp. 449–469. Sodertalje, Sweden: AB Astra.

Vaughan Williams, E.M., and Szekeres, L. 1961. A comparison of tests of antifibrillatory action. Br J Pharmacol 17:424–432.

Weld, F.M., and Bigger, J.T., Jr. 1975. Effect of lidocaine on the early inward transient current in sheep cardiac Purkinje fibers. Circ Res 37:630–639.

Wellens, H.J.J. 1978. Value and limitations of programmed electrical stimulation of the heart in the study and treatment of tachycardias. Circulation 57:845–853.

Wit, A.L., and Cranefield, P. 1974. Effect of verapamil on the sinoatrial and atrioventricular nodes of the rabbit and the mechanism by which it arrests reentrant atrioventricular nodal tachycardia. Circ Res 35:413–425.

Wit, A.L., and Cranefield, P.F. 1977. Triggered and automatic activity in the canine coronary sinus. Circ Res 41:435–445.

Wit, A.L., and Cranefield, P.F. 1978. Reentrant excitation as a cause of cardiac arrhythmias. Am J Physiol 235:H1–H17.

Chapter 5

Relationship Between Arrhythmogenic Mechanisms and Drug Actions

Gary J. Anderson

Introduction

Thirty years ago, the clinician confronted with cardiac arrhythmias had but a few drugs from which to select. The increase in the numbers of drugs available for arrhythmia suppression has been paralleled by an increased number of proposed potential mechanisms for arrhythmogenesis. The increasing numbers of drugs available for arrhythmia suppression led Vaughan Williams (1970) to formulate a drug classification system based on their intracellular electrophysiologic effects. This classification system has proven useful and, despite minor modifications (Singh and Vaughan Williams, 1972), it has remained widely used, although an alternative classification system has been suggested based upon arrhythmogenic mechanisms (Gettes, 1979).

With any classification system, the clinician is confronted with several apparent limitations. The first of these is that the response of any given arrhythmia is not entirely predictable by the class of drug. This relates to the fact that the classification system of Vaughan Williams categorizes antiarrhythmic drugs, not responses to arrhythmias. Conversely, attempts to classify prototype drugs and relate the drug to the antiarrhythmic response have a benefit of the correlation of the drug to a cardiac arrhythmia, but do not provide a unified approach to the drugs. It is tempting to rise to the opportunity on this occasion to write another classification system, but reality dictates that another classification system should be an improvement rather than an addition, a charge which is difficult to achieve. Rather it is the intent of this paper to review the classification system of Vaughan Williams and to relate this system to the emerging mechanisms of arrhythmogenesis. Recently, several new mechanisms for arrhythmogenesis have been raised with electrophysiologic support for their potential contribution to both supraventricular and ventricular arrhythmias. With the emergence of these new theories for arrhythmogenesis, both the old and new antiarrhythmic drugs take on new and broadened dimensions for their presumed mechanisms.

The Classification System and Cardiac Arrhythmias

The classification system of Vaughan Williams is based on the drug-induced electrophysiologic effects. These effects, in turn, are presumed to have a specific mechanism of action to account for the suppression of a given cardiac arrhythmia. It is presumed that the clinician is cognizant of "the" specific arrhythmogenic mechanism which is operative. Unfortunately, specific mechanisms are not clinically determined with ease, if at all. Therefore, the classification system based on the electrophysiologic responses of cardiac cells is only presumptively related to an antiarrhythmic action. Moreover, a review of the drug classification system reveals that there are a multiplicity of cellular responses affecting each component of the action potential. Since the electrophysiologic responses dramatically differ between drug class and even within the same drug class, it is difficult to ascribe a specific membrane effect to the suppression of an inciting arrhythmogenic mechanism. A second issue of concern is that the classical models for arrhythmogenesis (primarily automaticity and reentry) are oversimplifications and the interaction between mechanisms and drug is more complex. In the past few years, new potential mechanisms for cardiac arrhythmias have been suggested. This chapter will describe some of the various effects of antiarrhythmic drugs on different aspects of both new and old arrhythmia models. For the sake of brevity and at the expense of clarity, the reader is encouraged to review the cited references regarding these newer proposed models for arrhythmogenesis.

A review of the basic electrophysiologic mechanisms for cardiac arrhythmias is revealing in that there is no unanimity of opinion that any single mechanism is responsible. Three basic principles for arrhythmogenesis have been described and include: (a) automaticity, (b) reentry, and (c) reexcitation (see Table 5-1). The more recent literature, however, has expanded upon these and more variations on these mechanisms have been offered. For instance, automaticity now encompasses triggered automaticity, reflection, parasystole with entrainment, and delayed afterdepolarizations. The more simple classical concepts of reentry have given way to more complex mechanisms often encompassing more than a single mechanism. The clinician unfortunately cannot clearly deduce the operative mechanism at the bedside.

Classical Reentry

The early reports of Mines (1913) described reentry as an impulse which, once initiated, resulted in excitation of the tissue twice, thus "reentering" the tissue. This mechanism requires slow conduction and unidirectional block (Fig. 5-1),

Table 5-1 Theories for Extrasystoles.

Reentrant excitation
Circus movement
Leading circle
Automaticity
"Normal" automaticity
Triggered automaticity
Parasystole
(with and without entrainment)
Delayed afterdepolarizations
Reflection
Reexcitation

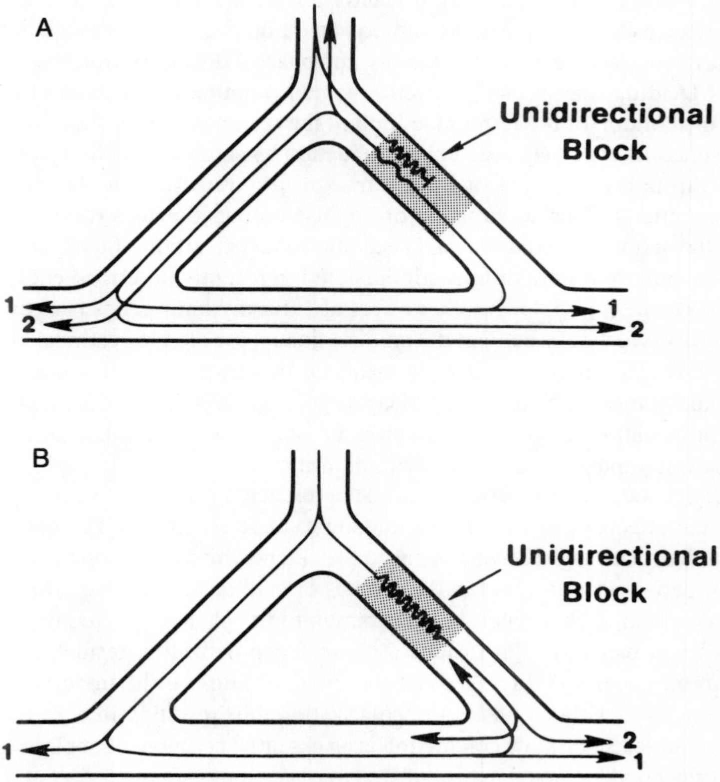

5-1 Reentrant conduction in Purkinje fibers may occur via two mechanisms. Unidirectional conduction block may occur (panel A) and reentry may occur by retrograde conduction. Slow orthograde conduction with retrograde unidirectional conduction block may also induce reentry. (Stippled area indicates regions of depressed conduction; beats 1 and 2 refer to the "normal" and reentrant beat, respectively.)

and the model has been applied to both contractile myocardium (Mines, 1913), as well as the specialized conducting system (Cranefield et al., 1973). The slow conduction model has received much attention, in part attributable to the ease of study of Purkinje fibers as well as the known relationship of ischemia to slow and fragmented conduction (Boineau and Cox, 1973). The relationship of the drug classification system to this model and its various permutations is somewhat complex even within a single drug class. This is related to the fact that there are many physiologic facets which contribute to reentrant excitation. Drug-induced changes in the electrophysiologic properties of the cells may occur in the abnormal and/or normal tissues resulting in abolition of the reentrant impulse. A class IA drug increases action potential duration and decreases excitability and may affect the reentrant circuit in a significantly different fashion than a class IB drug which decreases action potential duration (see Fig. 5-2A) even though both drugs may have similar effects on excitability and phase 4 depolarization. For instance, a class IA drug may prolong action potential duration of the normal fiber and result in abolition of the retrograde limb of the reentrant circuit. In contradistinction, a class IB drug may accelerate conduction by shortening action potential duration through a segment of long refractoriness resulting in abolition of the reentrant circuit. This acceleration of impulse propagation as a result of shortening of the action potential may also account for acceleration of tachyarrhythmias when an antiarrhythmic drug is administered, a recently described entity (Allessie, 1977) (see Fig. 5-1). Another effect of antiarrhythmic drugs is a decrease in excitability which may convert the unidirectional block to bidirectional block (see Fig. 5-2A). This effect is primarily mediated by directional differences in action potential amplitude and impulse propagation. These directional differences in impulse propagation remain a mechanism by which the classical reentrant theory may be interrupted by an antiarrhythmic drug.

Although the above description has been restricted primarily to class IA and IB drugs, the effects of other drugs belonging to class II, III, and IV should not be disregarded. Although it is unclear as to the extent which adrenergically mediated phase 4 depolarization plays in the genesis of cardiac arrhythmias, β-adrenergic blockade could alter adrenergic contribution to the physiologic requirements for the reentrant pathway. For instance, phase 4 depolarization results in a loss of membrane potential during diastole. β-blockade would in turn diminish adrenergically mediated phase 4 depolarization thus resulting in cells remaining more negative. Since slow conduction is an essential component of classical reentry and slow conduction is in turn related to reduced membrane potential, abolishing the adrenergic contribution to phase 4 depolarization would result in a relative hyperpolarization and acceleration of conduction. Similarly, a class III drug by affecting action potential duration would act in a fashion similar to a class IA drug. Class IV drugs would act on the classical reentrant model primarily through their effect on slow conduction. Loss of transmembrane potential, especially in

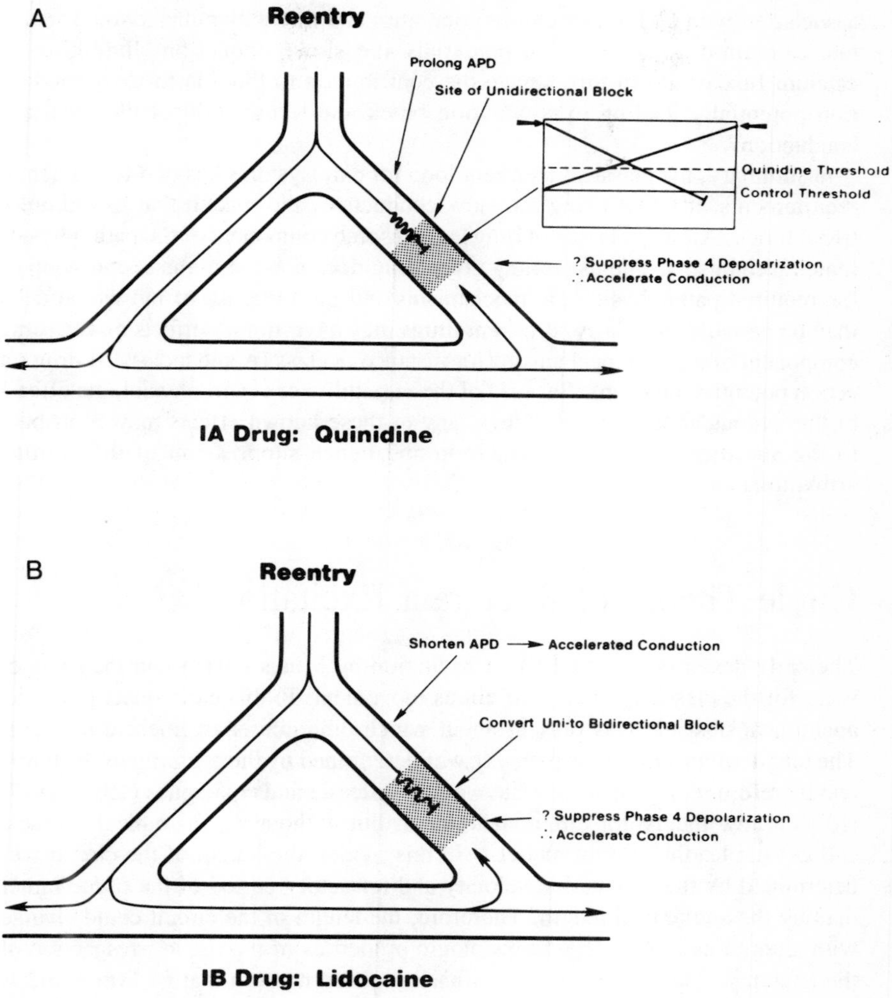

5-2 A, possible effects of quinidine on a typical reentrant loop. Effects of quinidine on excitability are shown to the right. Impulse propagation from left to right undergoes decremental conduction and the impulse falls below threshold. In the opposite direction, the stimulating efficacy of impulse conduction remains suprathreshold, thereby establishing unidirectional conduction. The administration of quinidine would elevate the threshold and result in conversion to bidirectional block as stimulating efficacy would fall below threshold in both directions (see text). B, effect of class IB drug on a typical reentrant pathway. Effects include conversion of uni- to bidirectional conduction block and suppression of phase 4 depolarization which would result in acceleration of conduction. Either conduction acceleration or shortening of refractory period could result in abolition of a reentrant pathway. APD, action potential duration.

association with high extracellular potassium and catecholamines, would facilitate calcium-dependent action potentials and slow conduction. Inhibition of calcium flux would in turn negate the contribution to this ion to slow conduction potentially leading to conduction block and termination of the reentrant conduction.

In summary, the classical reentrant loop for extrasystoles has two fundamental requirements, the first being the slow conduction, the second that of unidirectional block. All four classes of drugs affect some component of the pathophysiologic mechanisms. The use of any given drug does not assure the suppression of the required pathophysiologic mechanisms and the response of individual cells may be variable. Similarly, different drugs may have similar effects on the same component of a given mechanism (for instance, a class IA and a class III drug on action potential duration). Because of the variability of electrophysiologic effects of the various antiarrhythmic drugs, any of these known effects may contribute to the abolition of the reentrant loop and hence suppression of the cardiac arrhythmia.

Circle Theory of Reentrant Excitation

The early descriptions of reentrant excitation by Mines (1913) laid the groundwork for the classical concept of circus movement. In this early description, an anatomical obstacle was present about which the circus movement developed. The length of the circuitous pathway was determined by the anatomy of the tissue and therefore remained fixed. The work of Allessie and colleagues (1973, 1977) led to a new theory for circus movement, but without an anatomical obstacle called ''the leading circuit model.'' In this model, the length of the circuit was determined by the conduction velocity and refractory period of the tissue rather than by the anatomical length. Therefore, the length of the circuit could change with alterations in the electrophysiologic properties of the tissue irrespective of the anatomy. This model was significantly different from that of Mines and is summarized in Figure 5-3. The important feature of this model is its critical dependence upon electrophysiologic properties and its response to antiarrhythmic drugs may differ from the model of Mines (1913) (Fig. 5-4).

Allessie characterized some of the differences in response of the two models using different interventions. Tetrodotoxin (TTX) was shown to have a greater effect on the tachycardia in the ring model than in the intact left atrium (leading circuit model) (see Fig. 5-5A). In contradistinction, carbamylcholine slowed the sinus rhythm, accelerated the tachycardia in the intact left atrium (leading circle model), and had little effect on the reentrant tachycardia in the ring model (see Fig. 5-5B).

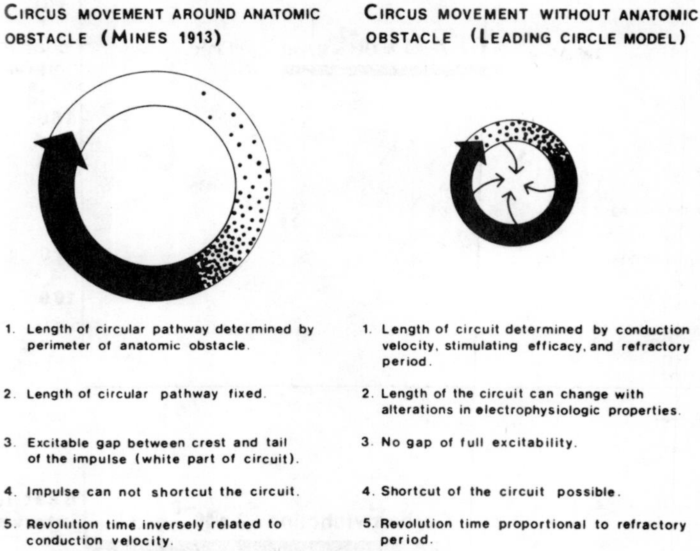

CIRCUS MOVEMENT AROUND ANATOMIC OBSTACLE (MINES 1913)
CIRCUS MOVEMENT WITHOUT ANATOMIC OBSTACLE (LEADING CIRCLE MODEL)
1. Length of circular pathway determined by perimeter of anatomic obstacle.
2. Length of circular pathway fixed.
3. Excitable gap between crest and tail of the impulse (white part of circuit).
4. Impulse can not shortcut the circuit.
5. Revolution time inversely related to conduction velocity.
1. Length of circuit determined by conduction velocity, stimulating efficacy, and refractory period.
2. Length of the circuit can change with alterations in electrophysiologic properties.
3. No gap of full excitability.
4. Shortcut of the circuit possible.
5. Revolution time proportional to refractory period.

5-3 Comparison between the Mines and Allessie models for circus movement. (From Allessie, 1977. Figure reprinted by permission.)

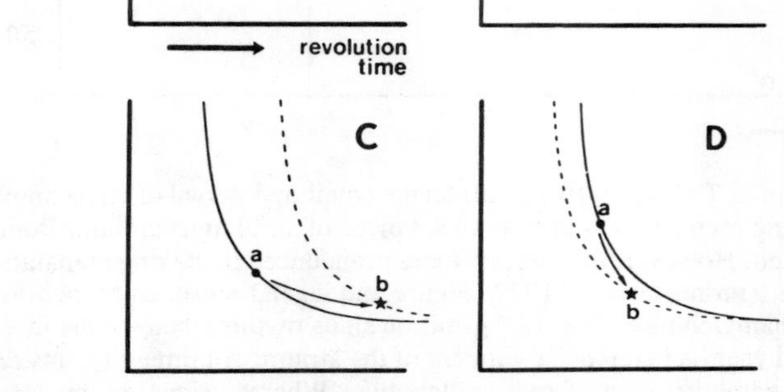

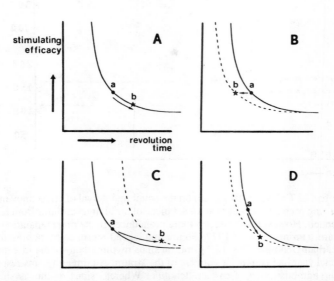

5-4 Comparison of the properties of circus movement with and without the involvement of a central atomic obstacle. (From Allessie, 1977. Figure and legend reprinted by permission.)

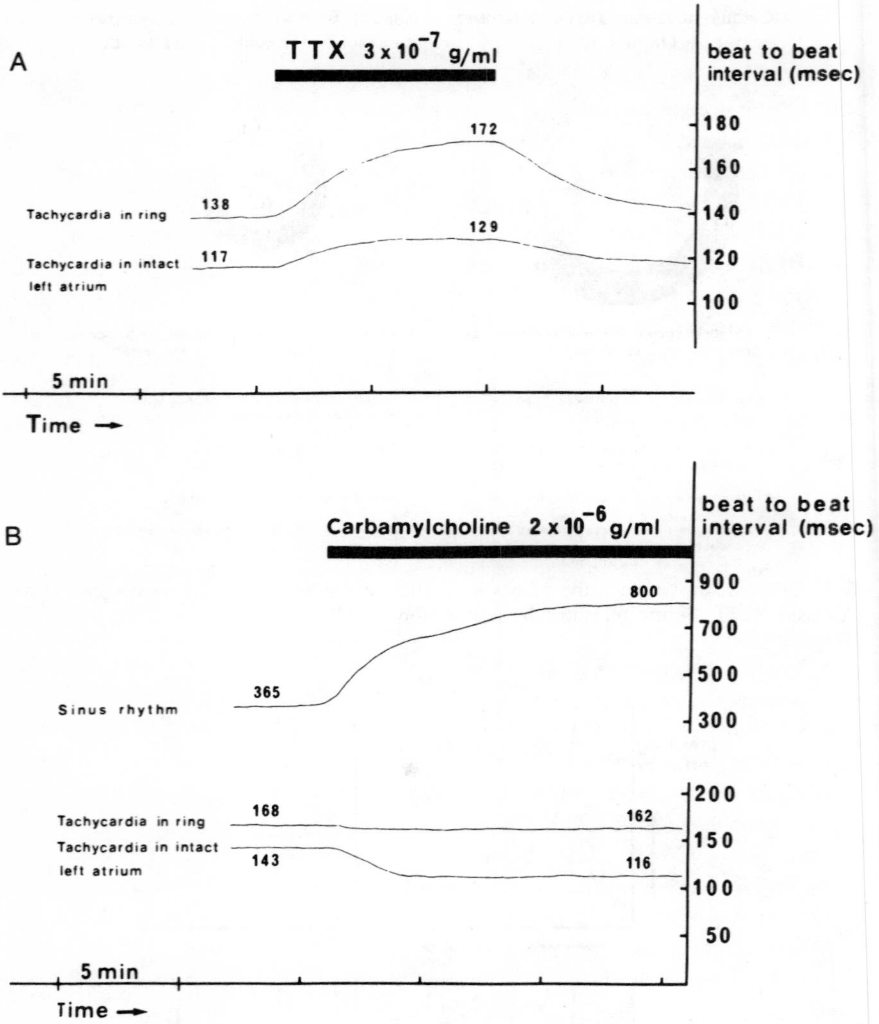

5-5 A, effect of TTX (3×10^{-7} g/ml) on the coupling interval of circus movement tachycardia in a ring preparation and in an intact piece of atrial myocardium. Both tachycardias are decelerated. However, the effect is more pronounced in the ring preparation than in the intact atrium. (From Allessie, 1977. Figure and legend reprinted by permission.) B, the effect of carbamylcholine (2×10^{-6} g/ml) on sinus rhythm, tachycardia in a ring preparation, and tachycardia in an intact segment of the atrium. All three rhythms respond differently to the administration of carbamylcholine. Whereas sinus rhythm is slowed down and the tachycardia in the intact atrium is accelerated, the circus movement in the ring of atrial muscle is hardly influenced. (From Allessie, 1977. Figure and legend reprinted by permission.)

These studies indicated that reentrant excitation in these two models respond differently to alterations in their electrophysiologic properties. Similarly, it would be anticipated that antiarrhythmic drugs would have different effects, although the effects are speculative and the above-noted studies only suggest the anticipated responses. A similarity does exist between the leading circle model and the classical reentrant model. In both cases, the premature beat initiating a tachycardia must encounter a zone of unidirectional block. Since unidirectional block is affected both by change in excitability as well as action potential duration, drugs which affect either of these parameters might have similar responses in both models. The conversion of unidirectional block to bidirectional block or to bidirectional conduction would result in abolition of the reentrant pathway in either model. Class IA drugs would slow revolution time (and hence the tachycardia) by both decreasing the stimulating efficacy as well as shifting the strength duration curve to the right (see Fig. 5-4, panel C).

Automaticity

Automaticity has been defined classically as a property of cardiac cells, more or less limited to the specialized conducting system whose transmembrane potential spontaneously depolarizes until it attains threshold, thereby resulting in a propagated action potential. Spontaneous diastolic depolarization may either be a normal property of cardiac cells (such as the sinus node or escape mechanisms within the A-V junction) or may be pathophysiologically enhanced such as the so-called "automatic" tachyarrhythmias. These include arrhythmias such as accelerated junctional rhythm in the presence of inferior wall infarction, nonparoxysmal junctional tachycardia with cardiac glycoside toxicity, and the so-called "slow" ventricular tachycardias.

However, the description of the so-called delayed afterdepolarizations (Davis, 1973; Ferrier et al., 1973; Rosen et al., 1975) (oscillatory afterpotentials, transient depolarizations, etc.) introduced new potential electrophysiologic mechanisms for tachyarrhythmias. Early descriptions of delayed afterdepolarizations demonstrated that a reduction in calcium concentration in the perfusate reduced the amplitude of the delayed afterpotentials. However, a detailed study of the effects of most antiarrhythmic drugs on these phenomena is not available at this time. Recent studies by Wasserstrom and Ferrier (1982) have demonstrated that both quinidine and phenytoin reduce the amplitude of the oscillatory afterpotential. When false tendons were exposed to acetylstrophanthin (1.6×10^{-7} M) oscillatory afterpotentials were induced which were suppressed (but not completely) by phenytoin (1.2×10^{-5} M). In contrast, acetylstrophanthin-induced afterpotentials were suppressed by quinidine (3.2×10^{-6} M) but were still observed after 50 min exposure to that concentration. Wasserstrom and Ferrier speculated that both phenytoin and quinidine induced their effects on oscillatory afterpotentials possibly by their local anesthetic properties, resulting in a shift in the sodium-calcium equilibrium which in turn reduces intracellular calcium concentration. This effect would lead to a reduction in the digitalis-induced oscillatory afterpotentials. In addition, the local anesthetics might reduce the amount of calcium released by the sarcoplasmic retriculum. It is not clear, however, whether or not these agents directly decrease the slow inward current.

Parasystole with Entrainment

Parasystole with entrainment encompasses the concept that an automatic parasystolic focus is affected electrotonically by the normal (sinus) beats. Based upon an electrophysiologic in vitro model, Jalife and Moe (1979) demonstrated that a parasystolic cycle length was modulated by the arrival time of an electrotonic subthreshold impulse. When electrotonic effects (presumably similar to sinus beats with entrance block) occurred early in the cycle length of the parasystolic focus, the parasystolic rate was slowed. When the electrotonic effect (sinus) occurred late in the parasystolic cycle length, the parasystolic beat was accelerated. This led Moe and his colleagues to postulate that a parasystolic rhythm could be entrained by the sinus to appear as coupled ventricular extrasystoles (Moe et al., 1977). This model, while complex in its presentation, demonstrates several fundamental principles of arrhythmogenesis. The first is that parasystole is due to automaticity with unidirectional block at the interface between parasystolic focus and the normal tissue. The second principle is that electrotonic interaction modifies the intrinsic rate of the ectopic (parasystolic) pacemaker. The reader is referred to the publications of these authors for a more extensive explanation of the models and their implications. It had been suggested by these authors that parasystole with entrainment might represent a commonly encountered arrhythmogenic mechanism (Moe et al., 1977). Although proof of this is difficult, a subsequent study supported this point of view (Anderson, 1983b).

With regard to antiarrhythmic agents, the effects on this model are not proven, but there may be several. As with any parasystole, drugs which affect conduction velocity or depress membrane responsiveness (typically the class I drugs) could convert the unidirectional block surrounding the parasystolic focus to bidirectional conduction block. This, in turn, would result in abolition of the arrhythmia without necessarily modifying pacemaker focus. In addition, class I drugs which suppress phase 4 depolarization would be expected to slow the parasystolic rate as with any automatic focus. With specific reference to the model proposed by Moe and co-workers (1977), the effects of antiarrhythmic drugs are more complex. Since the expression of extrasystoles secondary to parasystole with entrainment is the function of the ratio of ectopic pacemaker cycle length to the sinus node cycle length, drugs which affect either or both would alter the expression of extrasystoles. Drugs which depress phase 4 depolarization of the ectopic pacemaker (such as class I drugs or in instances where catecholamine-induced phase 4 is present) slow the ectopic pacemaker cycle length and increase the ratio of ectopic to sinus cycle length (Fig. 5-4). As the ectopic pacemaker cycle length to sinus node cycle length approaches 2.5, the extrasystoles might be more prevalent followed by a gradual disappearance of extrasystoles. In contradistinction, a slowing of the sinus rate might further enhance the frequency of extrasystoles. In summary, the interaction between the ectopic pacemaker cycle length and sinus node cycle length are the principle determinants of the expression of the extrasystole in this model. Drugs which affect either the sinus node cycle length, ectopic pacemaker cycle length, or both would therein modify the prevalence and appearance of extrasystoles and their relative timing to the sinus beat.

Another model, bearing some similarity to the above-noted model, has been described by Antzelevitch and colleagues (1980) as the "reflection model." It is similar to the above-described parasystolic model in that a parasystolic focus is present and initiates an impulse which is reflected from a sinus beat into the parasystolic focus and back to the more normal tissue. Transmission of the parasystolic beat through reflection requires normal exiting conduction of electronic interaction of the parasystolic focus and the normal tissue. The effects of antiarrhythmic drugs would be similar to those found in the parasystole with entrainment model. Suppression of phase 4 automaticity within the parasystolic focus would reduce the frequency of ectopic beats and possibly convert unidirectional block to bidirectional block, thereby abolishing the arrhythmogenicity of the focus. In addition, if the antiarrhythmic drug affected the electrotonic depolarization, then the ability of the electrotonic interaction to produce a fully propagated action potential within the parasystolic focus would be diminished, thereby eliminating reflection.

The Reexcitation Theory

Acute ischemia has been shown to produce a prompt reduction in the transmembrane resting potential of ischemic cells (Anderson et al., 1983a; Kleber et al., 1978; Janse et al., 1980). This reduction in transmembrane potential renders the ischemic zone positive relative to the normal myocardium during diastole. Ischemia also shortens the action potential in addition to reducing diastolic potential. A shortening of the action potential in ischemic zones may result in a transiently more negative potential in the ischemic zone relative to the normal zone during phases 2 or 3 of the action potential. In this case, the normal zone may become the current source (see Fig. 5-6).

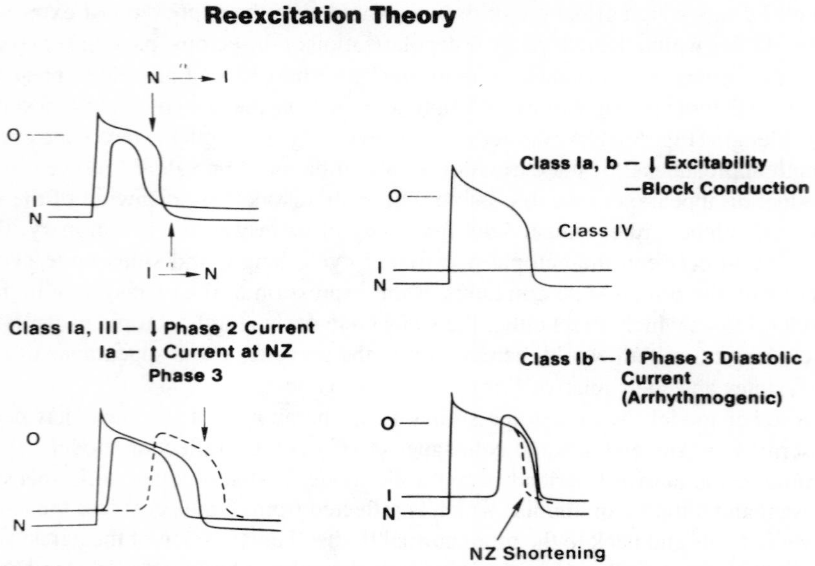

5-6 Potential mechanism for arrhythmogenesis resulting from voltage disparities and current flow. During electrical systole current (α) flow from normal (N) to ischemic (I) zones (Z) and is reversed during diastole (upper left). Phasic current flow resulting from electrical systole would be abolished by induction of inexcitability or conduction block in the ischemic zone (upper right). However, diastolic current flow would persist. Prolongation of the ischemic zone action potential duration would decrease phase 2 current and might be anticipated with a class IA or III drug effect. Shortening of the action potential duration (class IB) might enhance current flow and aggravate an arrhythmia (lower right).

In the reexcitation theory, the proposed mechanism for the induction of arrhythmias is related to the voltage disparity in action potential duration between normal and ischemic zones (Antzelevitch et al., 1980; Kleber et al., 1978). These voltage gradients lead to current sources and sinks and the resulting current flow between these areas may be of sufficient magnitude to induce reexcitation. Any modification which reduces the current flow between zones would, in turn, have a beneficial antiarrhythmic effect. The several mechanisms by which antiarrhythmic drugs potentially abolish an arrhythmogenic mechanism in this model are shown in Figure 5-6. Decreased excitability of tissue or induction of conduction block into an ischemic zone would abolish the influence of the systolic current flow. Since many drugs affect action potential duration, the results would be complex and unpredictable depending upon differential effects between normal and ischemic tissue and the phase of the action potential affected. In addition, a decreased excitability would reduce the stimulating efficacy of current flow.

This model is an attractive mechanism for arrhythmogenesis although it is not new. Understanding the antiarrhythmic mechanisms in this model is indeed complex as there are many factors which might alter the current sources and sinks. However, an antiarrhythmic drug must be delivered to the ischemic zone or at least to the boundary zone to induce its effect. In addition, the normal myocardium has been shown to demonstrate less pronounced electrophysiologic effects than abnormal tissue. Lastly, the effects on excitability and conduction as well as action potential configuration cannot be easily separated. An analysis of this model with regard to antiarrhythmic drugs is therefore very complex and the number of permutations is great. Further research is required both to identify the contribution of current flow to clinical arrhythmias, as well as to delineate mechanisms of antiarrhythmic action.

Summary

The armamentarium of antiarrhythmic drugs currently is expanding at an even more rapid rate than was seen only a few years ago. Clinicians still consider cardiac arrhythmias more or less phenomenologic with little consideration for their potential mechanisms. Even where mechanisms are concerned, they are typically considered in a rather historical (''reentrant'' or ''automatic'') context. Yet despite this, many arrhythmias remain resistant and poorly understood. In part, some of this may be due to a failure of a given arrhythmia to conform to classical concepts including antiarrhythmic therapy response. Perhaps the reason for this is the fact that different arrhythmogenic mechanism(s) are operative. This manuscript calls attention to a perhaps vague and elusive concept, but these new mechanisms cannot be ignored as they may be clinically operative.

References

Allessie, M.A. 1977. Circulating excitation in the heart. Ph.D. Thesis, University of Limburg, Amsterdam, The Netherlands.

Allessie, M.A., Bonke, F.I.M., and Schopman, F.J.G. 1973. Circus movement in rabbit atrial muscle as a mechanism of tachycardia. Circ Res 33:54–62.

Anderson, G.J., and Greenspan, M. 1983b. Ventricular ectopic beats with exit block: A retrospective Holter monitor study. J Electrocardiol 16:133–140.

Anderson, G.J., Reiser, J., Gough, W.B., and Nydegger, C.C. 1983a. Intramyocardial current flow in acute coronary occlusion in the canine heart. J Am Coll Cardiol 1:436–443.

Antzelevitch, C., Jalife, J., and Moe, G.K. 1980. Characteristics of reflection as a mechanism of re-entrant arrhythmias and its relationship to parasystole. Circulation 61:182–191.

Boineau, J.P., and Cox, J.L. 1973. Slow ventricular activation in acute myocardial infarction; Source of re-entrant premature ventricular contractions. Circulation 48:702.

Cranefield, P.F., Wit, A.L., and Hoffman, B.F. 1973. Genesis of cardiac arrhythmias. Circulation 47:190.

Davis, L.D. 1973. The effect of changes in cycle length on diastolic depolarization produced by ouabain in canine Purkinje fibers. Circ Res 32:206.

Ferrier, G.R., Saunders, J.H., and Mendez, C. 1973. A cellular mechanism for the generation of ventricular arrhythmias by acetylstrophanthidin. Cir Res 32:600.

Gettes, L.S. 1979. On the classification of antiarrhythmic drugs. Mod Concepts Cardiovasc Dis 48:13–18.

Jalife, J., and Moe, G.K. 1979. A biologic model of parasystole. Am J Cardiol 43:761–772.

Janse, M.J., van Capelle, F.J.L., Morsink, H., Kleber, A.G., Wilms-Schopman, F., Cardinal, R., d'Alnoncourt, C.N., and Durrer, D. 1980. Flow of "injury" current and patterns of excitation during early ventricular arrhythmias in acute regional myocardial ischemia in isolated porcine and canine hearts. Circ Res 47:151–165.

Kleber, A.G., Janse, M.J., van Capelle, F.J.L., and Durrer, D. 1978. Mechanism and time course of ST and TQ segment changes during acute regional myocardial ischemia in the pig heart determined by extracellular and intracellular recordings. Circ Res 42:603–613.

Mines, R. 1913. On dynamic equilibrium in the heart. J Physiol 46:349.

Moe, G.K., Jalife, J., Mueller, W.J., and Moe, B. 1977. A mathematical model of parasystole and its application to clinical arrhythmias. Circulation 56:968–979.

Rosen, M.R., Wit, A.L., and Hoffman, B.F. 1975. Electrophysiology and pharmacology of cardiac arrhythmias. IV. Cardiac antiarrhythmic and toxic effects of digitalis. Am Heart J 89:391.

Singh, B.N., and Vaughan Williams, E.M. 1972. A fourth class of antidysrhythmic action? Effect of verapamil on ouabain toxicity, on atrial and ventricular intracellular potentials, and on other features of cardiac function. Cardiovasc Res 6:109–119.

Vaughan Williams, E.M. 1970. Classification of antiarrhythmic drugs. In: E. Sandøe, E. Flensted-Jensen, and K.H. Olsen, eds. Symposium on Cardiac Arrhythmias, 1970. pp. 449–501. Sodertalje, Sweden: AB Astra.

Wasserstrom, J.A., and Ferrier, G.R. 1982. Effects of phenytoin and quinidine on digitalis-induced oscillatory afterpotentials, aftercontractions, and inotropy in canine ventricular tissues. J Mol Cell Cardiol 14:725–736.

EDITOR'S NOTES

Mechanisms of Antiarrhythmic Drug Action

The techniques used to study antiarrhythmic drugs in isolated tissue models have identified many mechanisms of antiarrhythmic drug action. Furthermore, the effects elucidated, particularly by the microelectrode technique, have been extensively discussed and summarized as a base of antiarrhythmic drug classification. All antiarrhythmic drugs modify the cellular electrophysiology of cardiac fibers to a varying extent, which may result in the initiation, termination, or perpetuation of the cardiac arrhythmia. Although individual drugs may have multiple actions, certain drugs may, in fact, have a high degree of specificity, whereas others have more global effects. As the excellent chapter by Drs. Rosen and Danilo emphasizes, a nonspecific drug such as quinidine may actually depress arrhythmias by a multiplicity of effects compared to agents such as verapamil or other calcium-blocking agents, which have a more uniform effect due to their specific effect on an ionic current. Alternatively, drug specificity may also be expressed by a preferential effect on depressed versus normal tissue. Lidocaine has been studied and demonstrated to exemplify this type of specificity. A critical point that is emphasized by Drs. Rosen and Danilo concerns the application of drugs with specificity of action in relation to the impact that such drugs may have on the accurate diagnosis of an individual arrhythmia. For example, these authors mention that one may apply the concept of a drug matrix, which employs the specific action of a drug as a means of excluding a particular arrhythmia based upon whether the drug is active or not. Thus, drugs that progress into the patient setting and have a high degree of specificity of action may indeed prove significantly more useful since such drugs may have the added benefit of establishing the diagnosis of cardiac arrhythmias. Unfortunately, at this juncture very few drugs are available that fit the concept of the drug matrix in a clinical setting. As denoted by Drs. Rosen and Danilo, the drug matrix can be applied reasonably well in an experimental setting. However, when considering the diversity of clinical responsiveness to antiarrhythmic drugs, it is not possible, at this point, to apply this concept effectively on a clinical basis, largely due to the lack of available agents having a high degree of specificity of action. Thus, the future holds a significant challenge in regard to developing therapeutic agents that demonstrate specificity of action, not only on a particular tissue type (e.g., atrial versus ventricular), normal or diseased tissue, but also in relation to a particular type of arrhythmic mechanism. The dilemma inherent in answering such a challenge lies, in part, in the inability to appropriately differentiate, at a clinical level, drugs with high-specificity action. The analysis of individual drugs must, therefore, include the impact of multiple arrhythmogenic mechanisms since we are currently unable to precisely identify which mechanisms are clinically operative.

Dr. Anderson has emphasized that the Vaughan Williams classification of antiarrhythmic drugs, although useful, must be viewed in concert with various mechanisms of arrhythmogenesis more recently uncovered. Starting from the original concepts of reentry versus automaticity, Dr. Anderson emphasizes newer considerations for interpreting arrhythmias which have evolved from an inability to effectively explain existing arrhythmias by classic theories. An important consideration regarding his discussion of these newer concepts of arrhythmogenesis relates to the reinterpretation of drug actions demonstrating different responses than what one would predict from the classic theories of drug classification. Indeed, Dr. Anderson argues that one of the reasons that many arrhythmias remain resistant and poorly understood may be their failure to conform to classic concepts, including antiarrhythmic therapy response. In this regard, his conclusion that additional or expanded arrhythmogenic mechanisms must be prospectively considered, conveys an important message to those developing and analyzing novel therapeutic agents, while also expanding background considerations for those analyzing complex arrhythmias at the basic and clinical level. This viewpoint further emphasizes the complexity of arrhythmogenic mechanisms and our limited ability to effectively analyze different mechanisms of arrhythmias at the clinical level.

C. Indices of Antiarrhythmic Drug Efficacy

Chapter 6

Animal Models Used in Testing Antiarrhythmic Agents

Joseph F. Spear and E. Neil Moore

Introduction

Animal models have been crucial to our understanding of the mechanisms of antiarrhythmic action and have contributed to the development of new antiarrhythmic drugs. In human pathology, cardiac arrhythmias are often the result of complex interactions between multiple systems which ultimately contribute to the underlying structural and functional abnormalities responsible for the arrhythmia. In addition, there are a variety of supraventricular and ventricular arrhythmias which have been described. Moreover, their characteristics and causes may in part be peculiar to human physiology and pathology which may not be duplicated exactly in other species. In the face of such complexity, it is obvious that there will be no single animal model which will universally predict antiarrhythmic efficacy of new agents. However, experimental studies using a variety of animal models have expanded our understanding of the mechanisms involved in arrhythmias and how electrophysiologic properties can be manipulated to provide antiarrhythmic action.

In approaching the problem of choosing an appropriate animal model for the electrophysiologic evaluation of an agent, our choice will initially be conditioned by whether a screening model is desired to evaluate antiarrhythmic efficacy and safety or whether the mechanisms of action of an agent primarily are sought. This is not to imply that an animal model suitable for testing efficacy provides no information concerning mechanism of action or vice versa. However, the rationale behind the choice of the animal model will determine its general characteristics with regard to its degree of complexity and its similarity to the human condition.

In evaluating efficacy of an antiarrhythmic agent, the models chosen usually involve intact animals in which the effects of agents can be tested on multiple interacting variables and systems. In such models, the influence of the autonomic nervous system and the interaction of the antiarrhythmic agent with blood-borne components, as well as the influence of circulating metabolites of the agent, may all contribute to its effect. In addition, if an index of efficacy is sought, an ideal animal model should mimic as closely as possible the pathophysiology involved in the human arrhythmic condition.

In contrast, animal models designed to maximize information regarding mechanism of action of an agent, by necessity, must be simple systems in which most of the variables are accessible and controllable experimentally. These are usually in vitro models in which the systems exhibit specific electrophysiologic characteristics which are arrhythmogenic or normal properties which can be manipulated. The effect of an agent in a simple model can be evaluated in the absence of the confounding influences associated with in vivo models. Information derived from such models, by necessity, is specific but incomplete. However, as our knowledge increases concerning cellular mechanisms involved in disturbances of rhythm and how antiarrhythmic drugs modify these characteristics, it becomes easier to infer rationally the potential antiarrhythmic efficacy and safety of an agent by its effect on simple animal systems.

Mechanisms of Arrhythmias

In any logical approach to choosing a model for testing an agent, an understanding of the mechanisms of cardiac arrhythmias exhibited by the model is necessary. In the simplest sense, cardiac arrhythmias are caused by either irregularities in impulse formation, by disturbances in impulse conduction, or by a combination of both of these factors. Recent advances in our understanding of the electrophysiologic basis of arrhythmias has allowed us to categorize these general arrhythmogenic factors in a more specific way. Irregularities of impulse formation can be due to abnormal automaticity, triggered activity, or "focal reexcitation." Triggered activity can be distinguished from abnormal automaticity since, in the former, accelerated firing of impulses is dependent upon an initiating stimulus (Cranefield, 1977; Cranefield and Aronson, 1974). The mechanism involved in focal reexcitation of the myocardium relies on current flowing between depolarized injured tissue and normal tissue (Janse et al., 1980; Katzung et al., 1975).

Abnormalities in impulse conduction responsible for cardiac arrhythmias can be simplified into a consideration of slow conduction and block of the impulse. These two aspects are at the basis of arrhythmogenic mechanisms associated with abnormal conduction, including reentrant excitation (Schmitt and Erlanger, 1928; Allessie et al., 1977; Antzelevitch et al., 1980). Electrophysiologic phenomena contributing to slow conduction and block include the "slow response" in which the current responsible for membrane depolarization is carried by the slow inward current (Aronson and Cranefield, 1973; Cranefield, 1975). Such an action potential may conduct a hundred times slower than normal (Aronson and

Cranefield, 1973). Slow conduction may also occur in tissues with action potentials exhibiting a depressed fast response. In these cells, the fast inward current normally responsible for depolarization in most cardiac tissues is partially inactivated due to a decrease in the level of the resting membrane potential (Brennan et al., 1978; Lazarra and Scherlag, 1980). In addition, since impulse conduction relies on local electrical current flowing in the intracellular and extracellular spaces to depolarize adjacent inactive membrane to threshold, disruptions in cell-to-cell electrical continuity can cause slow conduction and block (Sano et al., 1959; Lieberman et al., 1973). Finally, if membrane excitability or the ease with which a cell can be brought to threshold is depressed, this could also cause slow conduction or block (Peon et al., 1978; Arnsdorf and Bigger, 1975).

Models Used to Screen Compounds for Antiarrhythmic Efficacy

Models used to test efficacy are usually intact animals in which an arrhythmia is induced artificially and an agent is tested for its ability to suppress the arrhythmia. The primary objectives in these types of experiments are not to determine the mechanisms of action of an agent. However, since there is usually information available concerning the particular class of chemical being tested and since much is understood regarding mechanisms of arrhythmias in most in vivo models, general information about a compound's antiarrhythmic mechanism can be obtained. A typical model involves ventricular arrhythmias induced by digitalis toxicity. In these experiments, digitalis or a related compound is injected intravenously until a stable ventricular arrhythmia develops in which a large percentage of the ventricular responses are of ectopic origin (Kastor et al., 1972). Efficacy is measured by the degree to which the ectopy is suppressed by the agent under study (Moore et al., 1978).

Because arrhythmias associated with myocardial infarction are a common clinical finding and may be life threatening, models for evaluating antiarrhythmic efficacy involving experimental coronary artery occlusion have been developed. Following the occlusion of a major coronary artery in dogs, three stages of an arrhythmia occur at specific time intervals following the procedure. Each of these stages of arrhythmia involve slightly different mechanisms. A particular malignant phase occurs within minutes following coronary occlusion. This is characterized by a rapid multifocal ventricular tachycardia which degenerates to ventricular fibrillation in a significant portion of experimental animals (Harris and Rojas, 1943). This period of arrhythmia subsides within the first 30 min to 1 h and is followed 6–24 h later by a second, more benign, phase of monofocal ventricular tachycardia (Harris, 1950). While the early, acute phase of arrhythmia appears to be due to reentry within the ischemic myocardium (Boineau and Cox, 1973), this later phase is due to enhanced automaticity in the subendocardial Purkinje system at the infarcted region (Friedman et al., 1973; Horowitz et al., 1975). It has also been suggested that arrhythmias due to triggered activity can be induced during this period (El-Sherif et al., 1981). The late phase of arrhythmia subsides in approximately 72 h. After the spontaneous arrhythmias disappear, sustained and nonsustained ventricular tachyarrhythmias can still be induced by programmed electrical stimulation. During this chronic phase, the ability to induce arrhythmias by programmed stimulation may persist for weeks or months (Karagueuzian et al., 1979; Michelson et al., 1980; Garan et al., 1980). Antiarrhythmic efficacy can be measured by the degree to which an agent can prevent ventricular fibrillation during the acute phase of occlusion or the degree to which the severity of the arrhythmia is reduced during the late phase or chronic phase.

Antiarrhythmic efficacy has also been quantified in terms of an agent's ability to increase the ventricular fibrillation threshold (Moore and Spear, 1975). In this type of animal model, a controlled and variable intensity of electrical current is applied to the ventricle during the vulnerable period of the cardiac cycle (Wiggers and Wegria, 1940). As the intensity of the current is increased, repetitive ectopic ventricular beats may be induced, and when the intensity of current is sufficient, ventricular fibrillation occurs. The intensity of current at which multiple responses occur or at which fibrillation occurs has been used as a quantitative index of the ''electrical stability'' of the ventricle. Antiarrhythmic efficacy is measured by the degree to which these threshold values can be increased. The mechanism by which electrical current induces repetitive responses and fibrillation appears to involve its ability to set up local microreentrant circuits in the vicinity of the current electrode (Euler and Moore, 1980).

Various models of altered autonomic drive are available to test antiarrhythmic efficacy. Common autonomic manipulations involve arrhythmia induction using psychologic stress (Corgalan et al., 1974; Skinner et al., 1975), unilateral and bilateral stellate ganglion stimulation or ablation (Schwartz et al., 1978; Lucchesi and Hodgeman, 1971), and injection of autonomic agonists or antagonists (Harry et al., 1971; Podzuweit, 1980). Altered autonomic drive can also be used in combination with the previously mentioned animal models.

Finally, a model which has been used as a quick antiarrhythmic screen in the past is the ''chloroform mouse.'' In this model, mice are forced to inhale chloroform. This procedure induces ventricular tachyarrhythmias, probably of autonomic origin, and the animals soon die in ventricular fibrillation. Efficacy of an agent is evaluated in terms of the effective dose necessary to prevent fibrillation (Lawson, 1968; Gupta et al., 1973).

Models of Irregular Impulse Generation

When evaluating an antiarrhythmic compound with the objective of obtaining detailed information concerning its mechanism of action, models are chosen which exhibit a specific mechanism or electrophysiologic property on which the effect of an agent can be tested. Because of the explicit nature of the information which is sought, such models often involve isolated cardiac tissues, superfused in a tissue bath.

Models of abnormal automaticity include isolated cardiac Purkinje fibers whose automaticity has been enhanced by superfusion with toxic doses of digitalis. The early stages of the accelerated automatic rhythm occur in the absence of afterdepolarizations and appear to be due to enhanced diastolic depolarization (Vassalle and Musso, 1976; Vassalle and Bhattacharyya, 1981).

Enhanced diastolic depolarization also occurs in Purkinje fibers removed from the infarcted region of dogs 24 h following coronary occlusion. In this case, fibers are depolarized partially and the rate of spontaneous diastolic depolarization is enhanced (Friedman et al., 1973).

The rate of automaticity of normal Purkinje fibers can be accelerated by superfusion with sympathomimetic agents. Enhanced diastolic depolarization induced by autonomic mediators is a useful model in evaluating the β autonomic blocking potency of antiarrhythmic agents (Hasimoto et al., 1979).

In both Purkinje fibers and ventricular muscle, "slow response" automaticity can be induced if the fibers are depolarized to approximately 55-mv resting potential and the slow inward current is enhanced by exposure of the tissue to catecholamines (Cranefield, 1975; Katzung, 1975). An alternate procedure which produces stable abnormal automaticity is to expose tissues to barium chloride at a concentration between 0.5 and 2 mM. In the latter case, depolarization and automaticity occur due to a reduction in potassium conductance and enhancement of the slow inward current (Hiraoka et al., 1980). In both models, agents which block the slow inward current are effective in suppressing the automacity (Dangman and Hoffman, 1980).

Triggered activity is distinguished from abnormal automaticity in that the spontaneous beats are associated with an initiating stimulus. The underlying mechanism involves the production of afterdepolarizations which may reach threshold to cause extra beats (Cranefield, 1977; Cranefield and Aronson, 1974). Digitalis toxicity produces such afterdepolarizations, and sustained triggered activity can be induced in isolated tissues exposed to digitalis agents (Cranefield and Aronson, 1974). In addition, it has been reported that tissues removed from canine ventricle 24 h following coronary occlusion can exhibit triggered activity (El-Sherif et al., 1981). Other preparations in which triggered activity has been reported are the simian mitral valve leaflet (Wit and Cranefield, 1976), canine coronary sinus (Wit and Cranefield, 1977), and in dilated atria removed from cats with spontaneous cardiomyopathy (Boyden et al., 1977). The arrhythmia-induced aconitine toxicity also appears to be due to early afterdepolarizations (Rosen and Reder, 1981).

Recent studies in pig hearts which have undergone acute coronary occlusion suggest that at the ischemic border between depolarized cells and normal cells, ectopic impulses may occur due to the flow of injury current (Janse et al., 1980). The injured cells which remain electrically coupled to normal tissue for a time during the acute stage may provide sufficient current to cause focal reexcitation of normal cells at the ischemic border. Currently, this phenomenon has not been analyzed sufficiently to provide a reliable model to test the effects of antiarrhythmic agents on focal reexcitation.

Models of Slow Conduction and Block

One determinant of the velocity of impulse conduction is the magnitude of the inward current associated with depolarization of the action potential. In tissues that have been depolarized by increased extracellular potassium or exposed to barium ions, the fast inward sodium current is inactivated. In such tissues, the rate of depolarization due to the slow inward current is usually less than 2 V/s (Aronson and Cranefield, 1973; Cranefield, 1975). The velocity with which these impulses conduct is very slow (below 0.01 m/s). The atrioventricular and sinoatrial nodes normally exhibit slow response-type action potentials and their normal conduction velocities are appropriately slow (Allessie and Bonke, 1979; Billette et al., 1976). In contrast, cardiac fibers exhibiting normal fast inward currents have rates of depolarization between 100 and 800 V/s and conduction velocities between 0.3 and 1 m/s (Hoffman and Cranefield, 1960). These models are sensitive to agents which antagonize the slow inward current.

Cardiac tissues which are depolarized partially at resting potentials greater than −55 mv still maintain the fast inward sodium current although the channels responsible for carrying this current are inactivated partially (Brennan et al., 1978; Lazarra and Scherlag, 1980). Partial depolarization is usually accomplished by increasing the concentration of potassium in the superfusate; however, the magnitude of the fast inward current can also be decreased by decreasing the driving force on the sodium ion by reducing the concentration of sodium in the extracellular fluid (Weidmann, 1955).

The conduction velocity of impulses traversing such tissues is reduced in part due to the depressed inward depolarizing current. Class I antiarrhythmic agents which influence the fast inward current tend to depress depolarization further in such tissues so that areas of slow conduction may be converted to areas of complete block (El-Sherif et al., 1977).

It has been demonstrated recently that, during the acute phase of coronary occlusion (Akiyama, 1980) and also in the infarcted region weeks following coronary occlusion (Spear et al., 1983), reduced cellular electrical coupling can occur. This mechanism decreases the effectiveness of cell-to-cell activation and may be responsible for slowing of conduction and local conduction block. There is relatively little information available concerning the effect of standard antiarrhythmic agents on this parameter of impulse conduction and the importance of affecting cellular coupling in antiarrhythmic action is yet to be elucidated. A suitable model for evaluating the influence of cell-to-cell electrical continuity on impulse conduction involves strands of cardiac tissue which have been partitioned in a tissue bath so that a central segment can be made inexcitable (Antzelevitch et al., 1980). The external path for current flowing between proximal and distal segments can be controlled by a shunt resistor. This system can therefore be used to study the effects of agents on intracellular current flow between cells. Synthetically grown strands of cardiac tissue also exhibit varying degrees of cellular uncoupling and have controllable geometries to study effects of agents on parameters responsible for determining cell coupling (Lieberman et al., 1973).

Membrane excitability has been shown to be important in determining the velocity of impulse conduction (Peon et al., 1978; Arnsdorf and Bigger, 1975). Agents which increase or decrease the threshold for excitation may increase or decrease conduction velocity. Evaluation of the direct effects of an antiarrhythmic agent on excitability can be made in isolated tissues using a microelectrode to inject threshold depolarizing current (Moore et al., 1978).

Conclusion

While it is unlikely that a single animal model will ever be able to determine whether an unknown chemical will be an effective and safe antiarrhythmic drug, electrophysiologic evaluation of agents using a spectrum of experimental models can indicate whether an agent is likely to have antiarrhythmic properties and can determine the specific membrane parameters which are involved in its mode of action. The ultimate objective is to elucidate effects on ionic mechanisms responsible for irregularities in impulse generation and disturbances in impulse conduction. Any given antiarrhythmic agent is not equally effective for all cardiac arrhythmias. Therefore, in evaluating an antiarrhythmic agent, choices must be made about appropriate in vivo or in vitro models to use. The choice of models will be determined by such factors as whether the arrhythmias of interest are of supraventricular or ventricular origin and whether they are associated with specific pathologic conditions or arrhythmogenic settings. As antiarrhythmic agents with increasing pharmacologic diversity become introduced, animal models will become increasingly important in evaluating efficacy and mechanism of antiarrhythmic action.

References

Akiyama, T. 1980. Electrical uncoupling across the ischemic border of in situ porcine hearts. Circulation 62:III-344 (abstr).

Allessie, M.A., and Bonke, F.I.M. 1979. Direct demonstration of sinus node reentry in the rabbit heart. Circ Res 44:557–568.

Allessie, M.A., Bonke, F.I.M., and Schopman, F.J.G. 1977. Circus movement in rabbit atrial muscle as a mechanism of tachycardia. III. The "leading circle" concept: A new model of circus movement in cardiac tissue without the involvement of an anatomical obstacle. Circ Res 41:9–18.

Antzelevitch, C., Jalife, J., and Moe, G.K. 1980. Characteristics of reflection as a mechanism of reentrant arrhythmias and its relationship to parasystole. Circulation 61:182–191.

Arnsdorf, M.F., and Bigger, J.T. 1975. The effect of lidocaine on components of excitability in long mammalian cardiac Purkinje fibers. J Pharmacol Exp Ther 195:206.

Aronson, R.S., and Cranefield, P.F. 1973. The electrical activity of canine cardiac Purkinje fibers in sodium-free, calcium-rich solutions. J Gen Physiol 61:786–808.

Billette, J., Janse, M.J., VanCappelle, F.J.L., Anderson, J.F., Anderson, R.H., Touboul, P., and Durrer, D. 1976. Cycle-length-dependent properties of AV nodal activation in rabbit hearts. Am J Physiol 231:1129–1139.

Boineau, J.P., and Cox, J.R. 1973. Slow ventricular activation in acute myocardial infarction: A source of reentrant premature ventricular contractions. Circulation 48:702–713.

Boyden, P.A., Tilley, L.P., Liu, S.K., and Wit, A.L. 1977. Effects of atrial dilatation on atrial cellular electrophysiology: Studies on cats with spontaneous cardiomyopathy. Circulation 56(4):48.

Brennan, F.J., Cranefield, P.F., and Wit, A.L. 1978. Effects of lidocaine on slow response and depressed fast response action potentials of canine cardiac Purkinje fibers. J Pharmacol Exp Ther 204:312.

Corgalan, R., Verrier, R.L., and Lown, B. 1974. Psychologic stress and ventricular arrhythmia during myocardial infarction in the conscious dog. Am J Cardiol 34:692.

Cranefield, P.F. 1975. The Conduction of the Cardiac Impulse: The Slow Response and Cardiac Arrhythmias. New York:Futura.

Cranefield, P.F. 1977. Action potentials, afterpotentials and arrhythmias. Circ Res 41:415–423.

Cranefield, P.F., and Aronson, R.S. 1974. Initiation of sustained rhythmic activity by single propagated action potentials in canine cardiac Purkinje fibers exposed to sodium-free solution or to ouabain. Circ Res 34:477–481.

Dangman, K.H., and Hoffman, B.F. 1980. Effects of nifedipine on electrical activity of cardiac cells. Am J Cardiol 46:1059–1967.

El-Sherif, N., Gough, W.B., Zeiler, R., and Mehra, R. 1981. Endocardial mapping of triggered automaticity in canine ischemic Purkinje fibers. Am J Cardiol 47:489.

El-Sherif, N., Scherlag, B.J., Lazzara, R., and Hope, R.R. 1977. Reentrant ventricular arrhythmias in the late myocardial infarction period. Mechanism of action of lidocaine. Circulation 56:395–404.

Euler, D.E., and Moore, E.N. 1980. Continuous fractionated electrical activity after stimulation of the ventricles during the vulnerable period: Evidence for local reentry. Am J Cardiol 46: 783–791.

Friedman, P.L., Steward, J.F., Fenoglio, J.J., and With, A.L. 1973. Survival of subendocardial Purkinje fibers after extensive myocardial infarction. Circ Res 33:722.

Garan, H.J., Fallon, J.T., and Ruskin, J.N. 1980. Sustained ventricular tachycardia in recent canine myocardial infarction. Circulation 62:980.

Gupta, R.S., Karma, N.K., and Madan, B.R. 1973. Propranolol/bunolol and phencarbamide in chloroform-induced ventricular fibrillation in mice. Arch Int Pharmacodyn 203:265.

Harris, A.S. 1950. Delayed development of ventricular ectopic rhythms following experimental coronary occlusion. Circulation 1:1318.

Harris, A.S., and Rojas, A.G. 1943. Initiation of ventricular fibrillation due to coronary occlusion. Exp Med Surg (1)1–105–122.

Harry, J.D., Kappagoda, C.T., Linden, R.J., and Snow, H.M. 1971. Effects of beta-adrenoceptor blocking drugs on the chronotropic and inotropic actions of isoprenaline on the acutely denervated dog heart. Br Pharmacol Soc 41(2):387P.

Hasimoto, K., Hauswirth, O., Wehner, H.D., and Ziskoven, R. 1979. The relation between the current underlying pacemaker activity and beta-adrenoceptors in cardiac Purkinje fibres: A study using adrenaline, procaine, Atenolol and Penbutolol. Naunyn-Schmied Arch Pharmacol 307:9–19.

Hiraoka, M., Ikeda, K., and Sano, T. 1980. The mechanism of barium-induced automaticity in ventricular muscle fibers. In: M. Tajuddin, P. Kadas, M. Tariq, N.S. Dhalla, eds. Advances in Myocardiology. University Park Press: Baltimore, 1980.

Hoffman, B.F., and Cranefield, P.F. 1960. Electrophysiology of the Heart. New York: McGraw-Hill.

Horowitz, L.N., Spear, J.F., and Moore, E.N. 1975. Subendocardial origin of ventricular arrhythmias in 24-hour-old experimental myocardial infarction. Circulation 53:56–62.

Janse, M.J., VanCappelle, F.J.L., Morsinke, H, Kleber, A.G., WilmsSchopman, F., Cardinal, R., D'Alnoncourt, N., and Durrer, D. 1980. Flow of "injury" current and patterns of excitation during early ventricular arrhythmias in acute regional myocardial ischemia in isolated porcine and canine hearts. Circ Res 47(2):151–165.

Karagueuzian, H.S., Fenoglio, J.J., Weiss, M.B., and Wit, A.L. 1979. Protracted ventricular tachycardia induced by premature stimulation of the canine heart after coronary artery occlusion and reperfusion. Circ Res 44:833–846.

Kastor, J.A., Spear, J.F., and Moore, E.N. 1972. Localization of ventricular irritability by epicardial mapping. Origin of digitalis-induced unifocal tachycardia from left ventricular Purkinje tissue. Circulation 45:952.

Katzung, B.G. 1975. Effects of extracellular calcium and sodium on depolarization-induced automaticity in guinea pig papillary muscle. Circ Res 37:118–127.

Katzung, B.J., Hondeghem, L.M., and Grant, A.O. 1975. Cardiac ventricular automaticity induced by current of injury. Pfluegers Arch Ges Physiol 360:193–197.

Lawson, J.W. 1968. Antiarrhythmic activity of some isoquinoline derivatives determined by a rapid screening procedure in the mouse. J Pharmacol Exp Ther 160:22.

Lazzara, R., and Scherlag, B.J. 1980. Role of the slow current in the generation of arrhythmias in ischemic myocardium. In: D.P. Zipes, J.C. Bailey, and V. Elharrar, eds. The Slow Inward Current and Cardiac Arrhythmias. The Hague: Martinus Nijhoff.

Lieberman, M., Kootsey, J.M., Johnson, E.A., and T. Sawanobori 1973. Slow conduction in cardiac muscle: a biophysical model. Biophys J 13:37.

Lucchesi, B.R., and Hodgeman, R.J. 1971. Effect of 4-(2-hydroxy-3-isopropylaminopropoxy) acetanilide (AY 21,011) on the myocardial and coronary vascular response to adrenergic stimulation. J Pharmacol Exp Ther 176 (1):200.

Michelson, E.L., Spear, J.F., and Moore, E.N. 1980. Electrophysiologic and anatomic correlates of sustained ventricular tachyarrhythmias in a model of chronic myocardial infarction. Am J Cardiol 45:583–590.

Moore, E.N., and Spear, J.F. 1975. Ventricular fibrillation threshold. Arch Intern Med 135:446–453.

Moore, E.N., Spear, J.F., Horowitz, L.N. et al. 1978. Electrophysiological properties of a new antiarrhythmic drug, tocainide. Am J Cardiol 41:703.

Peon, J., Ferrier, G.R., and Moe G.K. 1978. The relationship of excitability to conduction velocity in canine Purkinje tissue. Circ Res 43:125.

Podzuweit, T. 1980. Catecholamine-cyclec-AMP-Ca^{2+}-induced ventricular tachycardia in the intact pig heart. Basic Res Cardiol 75: 772–779.

Rosen, M.R., and Reder, R.F. 1981. Does triggered activity have a role in the genesis of cardiac arrhythmias. Ann Intern Med 94: 794–801.

Sano, T., Takayama, N., and Shimamoto, T. 1959. Directional difference of conduction velocity in the cardiac ventricular syncytium studied by microelectrodes. Circ Res 7: 262–267.

Schmitt, F.O., and Erlanger, J. 1928. Directional differences in the conduction of the impulse through heart muscle and their possible relation to extrasystolic and fibrillatory contractions. Am J Physiol 87:326–347.

Schwartz, P.J., Brown, A.M., Malliani, A., and Zanchetti, A. 1978. Neural Mechanisms in Cardiac Arrhythmias. New York:Raven Press.

Skinner, J.F., Lie, J.T., and Entman, M.E. 1975. Modification of ventricular fibrillation latency following coronary artery occlusion in the conscious pig: The effect of psychological stress and beta adrenergic blockade. Circulation 51:656.

Spear, J.F., Michelson, E.L., and Moore, E.N. 1983. Reduced space constant in slowly conducting regions of chronically infarcted canine myocardium. Circ Res 53:176–185.

Vassalle, M., and Bhattacharyya, M. 1981. Interactions of norepinephrine and strophanthidin in cardiac Purkinje fibers. Int J Cardiol 1:179–194.

Vassalle, M., and Musso, 1976. On the mechanisms underlying digitalis toxicity in cardiac Purkinje fibers. In: P.E. Roy and N.S. Dhalla, eds. Recent Advances in Studies on Cardiac Structure and Metabolism. 9:355–376. Baltimore: University Press.

Weidmann, S. 1955. The effect of the cardiac membrane potential on the rapid availability of the sodium carrying system. J Physiol 127:213.

Wiggers, C.J., and Wegria, R. 1940. Ventricular fibrillation due to single localized induction and condenser shock applied during the vulnerable phase of ventricular systole. Am J Physiol 128:500–505.

Wit, A.L., and Cranefield, P.F. 1976. Triggered activity in cardiac muscle fibers of the simian mitral valve. Circ Res 38:85–98.

Wit, A.L., and Cranefield, P.F. 1977. Triggered and automatic activity in the canine coronary sinus. Circ Res 41:435–445.

Chapter 7

The Evaluation of Antiarrhythmic Drug Efficacy

J. Thomas Bigger, Jr., and Linda M. Rolnitzky

Introduction

The task of evaluating antiarrhythmic drug efficacy is a challenge. The most elemental aspect of this problem is to determine whether an antiarrhythmic drug significantly changes the frequency of ventricular premature depolarizations (VPD) or of repetitive VPD. This task is complicated by the substantial spontaneous variability in VPD rates. Various statistical techniques have been used to develop rules to determine when drug-induced changes in VPD rate are significantly more than spontaneous variability. These techniques provide lower limits for determining drug efficacy, but do not fully address the problem of designing an effective, nontoxic dosing regimen. Dose-ranging protocols are required to determine effective dose levels. Another consideration when evaluating antiarrhythmic drug efficacy is whether a statistically significant reduction in VPD rate, or rate of occurrence of repetitive VPD, will reduce arrhythmic death rates significantly. A patient with a low rate of ventricular ectopic events by virtue of taking an antiarrhythmic drug may be at a different risk than a patient with the same ventricular ectopic event rate without drug treatment. The fact that a drug reduces VPD frequency does not necessarily insure that the drug will reduce mortality when taken over a sustained period of time. Large scale, controlled drug trials are needed to determine whether significant, even marked, VPD reduction by drug treatment will reduce mortality significantly.

Current Methods for Assessing Spontaneous Variability of VPD

Over the last 5 years, a number of investigators have attempted to define the spontaneous variability in occurrence of VPD in ambulatory ECG recordings. This was done in order to determine the magnitude of reduction in occurrence of VPD, or repetitive VPD, that must be attained to be certain that a drug effect is more marked than that due to random variation.

Heuristic, Nonparametric Approach

To evaluate the utility of acute drug testing, Winkle studied spontaneous variability of VPD frequency in simulated drug tests in 20 patients who had at least 60 VPD/h (Winkle, 1978). Winkle analyzed 5½ continuous hours of ambulatory records in half-hour intervals, calculating the percentage of variability in VPD rate from interval to interval. Winkle determined that the effect of an antiarrhythmic drug can be considered significant if there is a 100% suppression of VPD for a half-hour period or a 90% reduction of VPD in two or three consecutive half-hour periods following drug administration. He defined the limits of spontaneous variability in VPD rate from interval to interval as the maximum variability achieved by 19 out of the 20 patients. This, in effect, established a method with an α level of 0.05. That is, assuming that his patients are representative of patients with high VPD rates, Winkle's criteria for drug efficacy would indicate incorrectly that there is a significant drug effect 5% of the time.

Winkle examined the criteria proposed for acute drug tests in the light of his findings. Gaughan et al. (1976) used as criteria for significant drug effect a 50% reduction in VPD rate or abolition of repetitive VPD in a 30-min period within 1–3 h after administration of a test drug, as compared to a 30-min control period. Winkle observed that, if these criterion were to be applied to his data, 14 of the 20 patients would be classified as responders due solely to spontaneous variability of ventricular ectopic events. Even if an 80% reduction criterion were used, 7 out of the 20 patients would be classified as responders. Winkle concluded that the criteria used by Gaughan et al. (1976) were not stringent enough to distinguish between drug response and spontaneous variability. His paper made the important contribution of alerting researchers to the need to use carefully developed criteria when dealing with events in which there is considerable spontaneous variability.

Winkle's direct, heuristic approach has the appeal of a nonparametric statistic: no assumptions need be made about the underlying distribution of VPD rates. However, the inclusion of only 20 patients in this study seems less than adequate: if only one patient had demonstrated a different pattern in the occurrence of VPD, Winkle's criteria might have been different.

Analysis of Variance Approach

Morganroth et al. (1978) studied 15 patients selected for an antiarrhythmic drug study who had a VPD rate of 30/h or more on an initial 24-h ECG recording. Thirty VPD per h is commonly used as an arbitrary criterion for antiarrhythmic drug therapy. Three 24-h ECG recordings were made on successive days and analyzed for each patient. Morganroth et al. (1978) used classical analysis of variance procedures to evaluate efficacy. They used a logarithmic transformation of their data in order to normalize the distribution and to insure that there was a

Table 7-1 Percentage Reduction in Mean Hourly Frequency of Total VPD, VPD Pairs* and Ventricular Tachycardia (VT) Required to Demonstrate Drug Efficacy.*

Number of Days**		Percentage Reduction		
Control	Test	Total VPD	Pairs	VT
1	1	83	75	65
1	2	79	70	60
1	3	77	68	57
2	1	79	70	60
2	2	72	63	52
3	3	65	55	45
7	7	49	41	33

* After Morganroth et al. (1978) and Michelson and Morganroth (1980).
** Number of 24-h ECG recordings.

homogeneous variance in the subsets of the data used in the analysis. As will be discussed below, the logarithmic transformation does not produce a normal distribution in population studies of VPD frequency. However, restricting the enrollment to patients with a VPD rate of 30 or more/h selects a subset that is far less skewed and is made reasonably normal by logarithmic transformation. In addition, after transformation, the distributions of VPD frequency in all subgroups being analyzed have similar variances. Achieving a reasonably normal distribution and similar variances is essential if analysis of variance techniques are to be successful (Kirk, 1968).

Using a four-way, nested analysis of variance design, Morganroth et al. (1978) computed the minimal per cent VPD reduction values required to prove significant antiarrhythmic drug effect (see Table 7-1). The minimal per cent VPD reduction is a function of the duration of ECG recording and the number of control and test days. The magnitude of VPD reduction required to declare efficacy is greatest, of course, for short durations of recording and few recording periods: for one 8-h control record and one 8-h test record, a 90% reduction is needed. Note that this criterion is similar to Winkle's. The criterion value for one 24-h control record and one 24-h test record is 83% reduction in VPD frequency.

Total variation in VPD frequency was partitioned into variation between patients, between daily records for each patient, between 8-h periods within a 24-h recording and between hourly VPD counts within an 8-h period (see Table 7-2). Interestingly, there was as much variability between three daily ECG recordings within patients as between patients. For an individual patient, the hourly variation accounts for 48% of the total variability, attesting to a substantial hour-to-hour variability. One must keep in mind that the components of variance analysis pertains to a population with a high VPD frequency. The population studied by Morganroth et al. (1978) makes up a small percentage of the total population. In a population of 723 patients discharged from Columbia-Presbyterian Medical Center after a confirmed myocardial infarction, fewer than 15% had 30 or more VPD/h on a routine 24-h ECG recording.

Table 7-2 Sources of Variance in Mean Hourly Frequency of Total VPD, VPD Pairs, and Ventricular Tachycardia (VT).*

Source	Percentage Variance from Each Source		
	Total VPD	VPD Pairs	VT
Pooled			
Between patients	66	65	46
Between days	8	4	7
Between 8-h periods	10	8	9
Between hours	16	23	38
Total	100	100	100
Data from individual patients			
Between days	23	12	12
Between 8-h periods	29	24	17
Between hours	48	64	71
Total	100	100	100

* After Morganroth et al. (1978) and Michelson and Morganroth (1980).

Morganroth et al. (1978) analyzed the electrocardiographic records in 8-h units, making the statistical assumption that there was no difference in VPD rate at different times of the day. However, the effect of circadian rhythm on occurrence of VPD and of repetitive VPD has been noted by several investigators (Steinbach et al., 1982; Lown et al., 1973). There is usually a decrease in the incidence of VPD and of repetitive VPD during sleep. Morganroth et al. (1978) noted a tendency toward decreased arrhythmic frequency during sleep. Therefore, the most valid comparisons for drug effect are made using 24-h records. If records shorter than 24 h are used for between day drug comparisons, they certainly should be recorded during the same time interval each day.

Michelson and Morganroth (1980) extended the analysis of variance procedure to examine the spontaneous variability of repetitive VPD. For this analysis, they used 96 h of consecutive ambulatory electrocardiographic records from 21 patients with various cardiac disorders. As before, they related per cent reduction required to declare a significant reduction of repetitive VPD to the duration of recording (see Table 7-1). Surprisingly, the criteria for repetitive VPD were found to be less stringent than for total VPD frequency. The per cent reduction needed to assert that an antiarrhythmic drug exerts a significant effect on paired VPD is 75% using two 24-h tapes, and 86% using two 8-h tapes. For ventricular tachycardia, the corresponding per cent reductions are 65% and 80%. A diurnal decrease in repetitive ventricular arrhythmias was noted during sleep. As with their earlier paper, the group performed a components of variance analysis for paired VPD and ventricular tachycardia (see Table 7-2). In this study, variance between days for mean hourly frequency of repetitive VPD made up a smaller proportion of total variance than daily variance in total VPD frequency. The proportion of intrapatient variability attributable to day-to-day variability is half as great for repetitive VPD (12%) as for nonrepetitive VPD (23%). Hourly variability made up a larger proportion of variability of repetitive VPD than for VPD frequency. It comprises 64% of intrapatient variability for paired VPD and 71% for ventricular tachycardia, compared with 48% for total VPD frequency. It remains to be seen if this finding holds for many different samples.

Regression Methods

Sami et al. (1980) used linear regression to develop criteria for drug efficacy. Twenty-one patients who had an average of 6 or more VPD/h on a 24-h ECG recording were studied. For each patient, an initial 24-h ambulatory ECG recording was obtained. Each patient was put on a placebo regimen for 2 weeks, and then a second 24-h ECG was recorded. Placebo VPD rate was regressed on initial VPD rate, and 95% and 99% confidence intervals were calculated to account for spontaneous variability. Placebo effect as a possible factor causing changes in VPD rate is a worthwhile consideration. Sami et al. (1980) estimated the minimum per cent reduction in VPD frequency required to establish drug efficacy as a function of the initial VPD rate. For rates below 2.2 VPD/h, this regression method cannot be used. For rates from 2.2–3 VPD/h, the critical value is a 90% reduction in VPD rate. For an initial VPD rate of 20 or more VPD/h, the critical value is a 65% reduction in VPD rate.

Sami et al. (1980) examined VPD frequencies far lower than those examined by Morganroth et al. (1978). This raises questions about the ability of the logarithmic transformation of VPD frequency to normalize the distribution and stabilize variance. As is seen in Figure 7-2, transformed data are still very highly skewed for the population with a minimum VPD frequency of 6 VPD/h.

Sami et al. (1980) proposed one-tailed confidence intervals. One-tailed interval estimation is appropriate when one is interested only in detecting a significant decrease in VPD rate caused by antiarrhythmic drug treatment. Since these statistical methods are often used for drugs in a developmental stage, it is unwise to ignore the possibility that any new drug may be proarrhythmic. For a variety of antiarrhythmic drugs, both marketed and unmarketed, Velebit et al. (1982) found an 11% proarrhythmic effect, even when using very stringent criteria. This proportion has held up in over 1,200 antiarrhythmic drug trials (Podrid, P.J., personal communication).

Comparison of the Methods of Morganroth and Sami

There is a considerable difference in the one criterion value that can be compared in the Morganroth and Sami studies, i.e., the minimum per cent reduction in VPD frequency required to prove antiarrhythmic drug efficacy using two 24-h ECG recordings in patients with 30 or more VPD/h in the initial record. Morganroth proposed an 83% reduction for this analysis; Sami proposed a 65% reduction.

Shapiro et al. (1982) applied both Morganroth's and Sami's methods to a much more extensive data set. The data set consisted of three 24-h ambulatory ECG recordings, obtained within a 14-day period, for 162 patients with severe ventricular arrhythmias. Each recording averaged at least 30 VPD/h.

Shapiro obtained very similar results using both Morganroth's analysis of variance approach and Sami's regression method. He obtained separate results for each pairwise comparison of the three records obtained for each patient. Required per cent reduction varied from 74% (record 1 versus record 2) to 83% (record 1 versus record 2) with the analysis of variance approach of Morganroth et al. (1978). With regression techniques, required per cent reduction varied 73% (record 1 versus record 3) to 84% (record 1 versus record 3). The similarity of results is somewhat surprising, since the two models are not equivalent. As an example of the disparity between the two methods, Morganroth's method analyzed ECG data in 8-h units, while Sami used data averaged over a 24-h period. Shapiro more closely aligned the two methods by using a one-tailed nested analysis of variance in his analysis. This differs from Morganroth's two-tailed analyses, and is equivalent to Sami's one-tailed approach. (As mentioned previously, in view of the fact that antiarrhythmic drugs have proarrhythmic potential, we prefer a two-tailed approach.) Shapiro attributed the discrepancy between Sami's results and those of Morganroth and himself to a smaller day-to-day variance of the VPD in the Sami sample.

It is somewhat surprising that Sami's data demonstrated less daily variability than Morganroth's, since Morganroth's data consisted of sets of recordings made on consecutive days, while Sami's recordings were made 2 weeks apart. Also, Sami's second record for each patient included any effect due to placebo. The discrepancy in the two data sets is probably best explained by the fact that they are both very small, too small to be representative of the population of patients with high VPD rates. Shapiro's study points out the need for using data sets large enough to represent adequately the population to which results will be applied.

The Distribution of VPD Frequency and Its Logarithmic Transformation

Winkle's method of assessing the limits of spontaneous variability of the occurrence of VPD is a nonparametric method. A proven nonparametric method for judging treatment effects of VPD would have appeal because it would require no assumptions as to the underlying distribution describing the occurrence of VPD. Both Morganroth and Sami used statistical methods that require that the data to be analyzed be distributed approximately normally. The distribution of hourly VPD frequency is highly skewed to the left, as is common with distributions of counts. In an effort to normalize the data, Morganroth and Sami used a logarithmic transformation of the VPD rate, a commonly used technique. (The value 1 is added to the VPD frequency value before the logarithm is calculated, to enable the transformation to be used with VPD frequencies of zero.)

In order to illustrate the properties of the distribution of hourly VPD frequency and its logarithmic transformation, we used 723 24-h ECG recordings of patients admitted to Columbia-Presbyterian Medical Center with a myocardial infarction over the past 5 years.

Figure 7-1 shows that the distribution of hourly VPD frequency for these 723 patients is highly skewed to the left. Figure 7-2 shows that the distribution of log

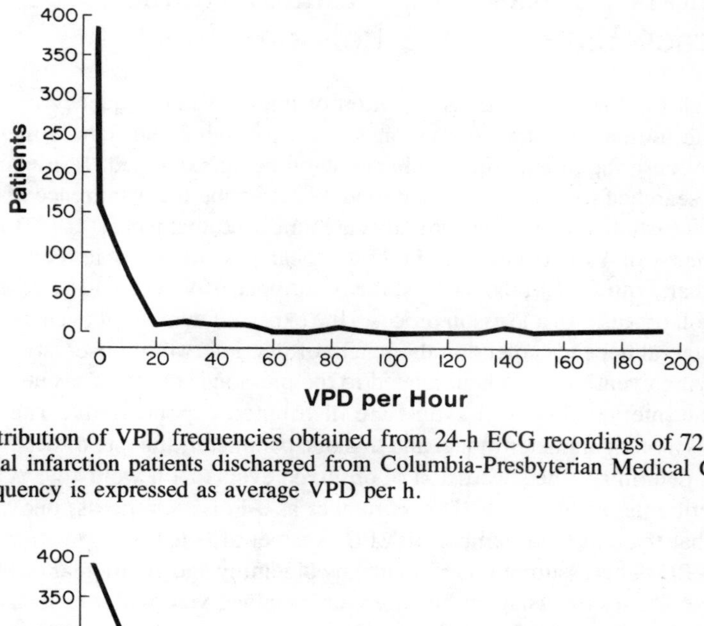

7-1 Distribution of VPD frequencies obtained from 24-h ECG recordings of 723 post-myocardial infarction patients discharged from Columbia-Presbyterian Medical Center. VPD frequency is expressed as average VPD per h.

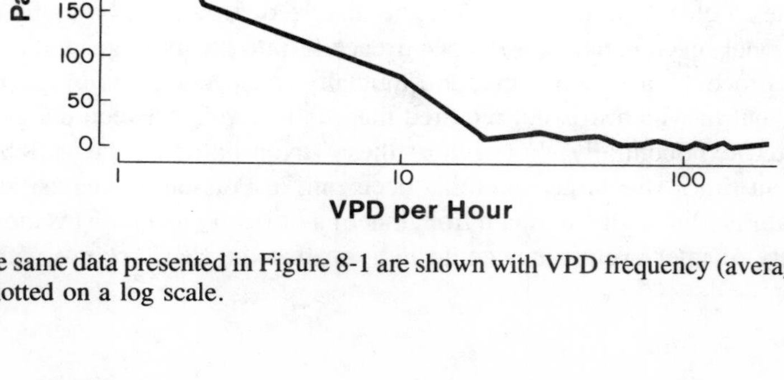

7-2 The same data presented in Figure 8-1 are shown with VPD frequency (average VPD per h) plotted on a log scale.

(VPD frequency + 1) also is highly skewed to the left. However, when we restrict the analysis to patients who have a rate of 30 or more VPD/h, the logarithmic transformation of this truncated sample is reasonably symmetrical. The logarithmic transformation appears to be adequate when applied to populations with high VPD rates. However, even when the data are limited to VPD frequencies of 30 or greater, using the logarithmic transformation is superior to using the raw data, since the effect of outliers, i.e., patients with unusually high VPD frequencies, will be reduced markedly (Tukey, 1977).

Methods for Assessing Antiarrhythmic Drug Efficacy Based on the Poisson Model

Although the logarithmic transformation of hourly VPD frequency provides an adequate normalizing transformation for Morganroth's and Sami's methods, it does not describe or explain the phenomenon being examined. Ruttimann et al. (1972) searched for a mathematical model to describe the occurrence of VPD in 21 patients studied while in a coronary care unit. Ruttimann et al. (1972) analyzed the patterns of VPD occurrence in 21 24-h electrocardiographic recordings and found that, with 51% of the records, the occurrence of VPD could be described as a Poisson process. In a Poisson process, the expected number of events in a given time interval depends solely on the length of that interval of observation and the underlying event rate and is unrelated to the previous pattern of events. In addition, the intervals between events are distributed exponentially. The Poisson model is a one-parameter model and this one parameter, the rate of occurrence of events, determines the succession of observed events. If it were always possible to describe the pattern of VPD occurrences as a Poisson process, one could assume that the expected number of VPD is never affected by the pattern of previous VPD. This assumption is violated by bigeminy and ventricular tachycardia. During episodes of sustained bigeminy or sustained ventricular tachycardia, the expected number of VPD is influenced by the regular VPD pattern that is occurring, violating the Poisson assumptions. However, unless sustained bigeminy or tachycardia are frequent in a record, the Poisson model is adequate.

Ruttimann et al. (1972) found the Poisson model to be appropriate in only 11 out of the 21 electrocardiographic records analyzed. However, he found that for an additional seven patients, VPD occurrence fit into the more general class of a renewal process, in which events are mutually independent, as in the Poisson process, but in which it is not required that the intervals between the events be distributed exponentially. For five of these seven patients, the variability in inter-event times was larger than that occurring in Poisson processes, although the variability did not differ much from that of a Poisson process. This increase in variability of inter-event times could indicate that the ECG records sometimes contain periods with clustering of VPD episodes or that the underlying event rate is not constant.

Ruttimann et al. (1972) developed a computer program for on-line testing of drug efficacy. The program required only that the VPD occur as a renewal process. The program calculated the underlying rate of occurrence of VPD, and tested for a significant change in this rate as an indication of significant drug effect. A program such as Ruttimann's could be used in experimental antiarrhythmic drug studies, but would be limited by poor performance in patients who have very high VPD rates in predrug recordings.

Thomas and Miller (1984) used the Poisson approach to derive a set of criteria that can be used easily in a clinical research setting. They used the variance of a Poisson process to estimate daily variability and combined this with estimates of day-to-day intrapatient variability to derive criteria for assessing antiarrhythmic drug efficacy. Although Ruttimann et al. (1972) found that only half of the ECG records he examined fit the Poisson model, he did find that the variance of intervals between VPD was close to the variance of a Poisson process in four-fifths of the cases. It therefore seems justified to use the Poisson variance in this analysis. Estimates of daily intrapatient variability were obtained from records collected on 20 patients as part of an unpublished drug intervention trial.

Figure 7-3 shows the 95% confidence limits for spontaneous variability of ventricular ectopic events. This figure is to be used to define confidence limits for simple ventricular ectopic episodes as well as for rarer events such as VPD pairs. The range of values of events per day, as shown on the abscissa, does not extend far enough into the low range so that the figure could be used routinely to detect significant changes in even rarer events such as ventricular tachycardia in records made in postinfarction patients. This approach indicates that the per cent reduction required to show significant antiarrhythmic drug efficacy varies with VPD frequency in the predrug ambulatory ECG recording. For initial ECG recordings with 20 or more VPD in 24 h, an 84% reduction in frequency is required to demonstrate antiarrhythmic drug efficacy. This value is essentially identical with Morganroth's value of 83%. For predrug 24-h ECG recordings with less than 20 ventricular events, Thomas and Miller require a 95% reduction to show a significant antiarrhythmic drug effect. They state that this criterion might be used when investigating the effect of an antiarrhythmic drug on relatively rare events such as VPD pairs. For even rarer events such as ventricular tachycardia, the confidence limits would become even wider. Results of Thomas and Miller (1984) concerning VPD pairs differ from those of Michelson and Morganroth (1980). Michelson and Morganroth found that a smaller per cent reduction in frequency of VPD pairs was needed to show a significant drug effect than for VPD frequency. These divergent results were in part due to the fact that Michelson et al. (1980) used different variance estimates for simple and for repetitive ventricular episodes. Michelson's variance estimates for simple ventricular ectopic events were calcu-

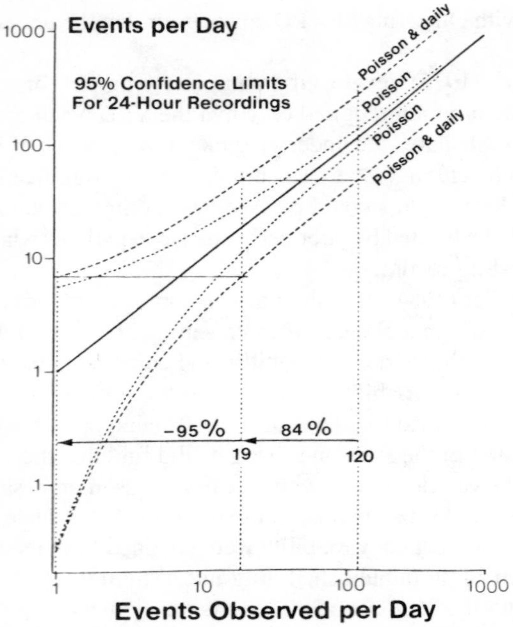

7-3 Ninety-five per cent confidence limits for the number of ventricular premature depolarizations observed in a 24-h recording (on a log-log scale). Confidence limits are shown for Poisson counting statistics alone, as well as for that plus day-to-day variation. Reprinted with permission of the authors and publisher (Thomas and Miller, 1984).

lated from the records of only 15 patients; the variance estimates for repetitive ventricular ectopic events were obtained from the records of 20 patients. Substantiation of variance estimates for paired VPD or ventricular tachycardia with a larger data set is needed to settle the issue of whether or not components of variance differ for simple and repetitive ventricular events.

In view of the fact that Thomas and Miller assume that VPD episodes are Poisson-distributed, and that even when the broader category of a renewal process is used, only four-fifths of the population can be considered, it is surprising that their results are identical with Morganroth et al. (1978) when comparing one 24-h predrug tape with one 24-h tape made after a drug is administered. A possible explanation is that, as is shown in Figure 7-3, as VPD rate increases, the proportion of total variation due to daily variability decreases, and the proportion due to between-day variability predominates. As the VPD rate increases, although the Poisson model may become less adequate, it contributes less and less to the confidence interval used to define the limits of spontaneous variability.

Observations on Computer Simulations Using the Poisson Model

Figures 7-4 and 7-5 show the results of computer simulations performed in our laboratory. Figure 7-4 is an example of the hourly spontaneous VPD variability in 8 h of simulated ECG record assuming that the record has an underlying VPD rate of 200/h, and that the occurrence of VPD is a Poisson process.

Figure 7-5 shows a simulated 8 h of VPD frequency after an 800-mg dose of quinidine is administered. The quinidine blood level over an 8-h period following the administration of a single 800-mg dose of quinidine was calculated using a standard drug kinetics equation (Rowland, 1972). The relation between quinidine blood level and VPD reduction was calculated using a general drug concentration-response equation (Meffin, 1977). The expected VPD rate was then calculated assuming that the drug-free VPD rate for each hour was as shown in Figure 7-4. In this example, it appears that the spontaneous VPD variability does not obscure the effect of quinidine. This is in part due to the dramatic effect of quinidine on VPD frequency; at 4 mg/l, quinidine reduces VPD frequency by 80%. The effect of a less potent drug, or the effect of a potent drug at a low dosage, may be masked by the spontaneous variability in VPD frequency. For example, assume that the initial low level effect of an antiarrhythmic drug used in a dose-ranging experiment on an individual patient should be a 10% reduction in VPD fre-

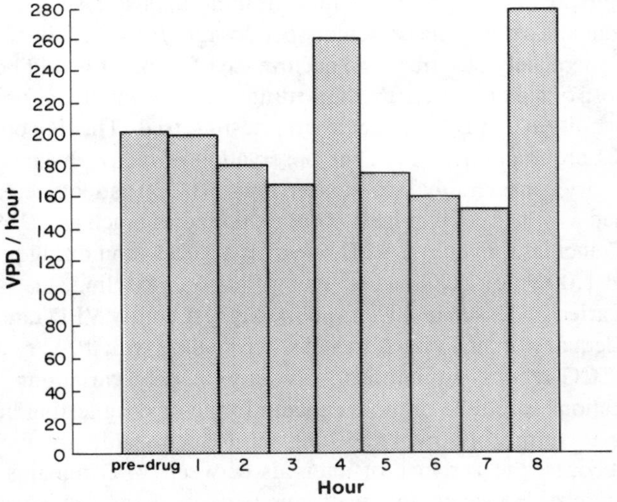

7-4 Results of simulated ECG record of eight consecutive hourly VPD frequencies for a patient with an underlying VPD rate of 200 VPD/h. The VPD events are assumed to occur as a Poisson process.

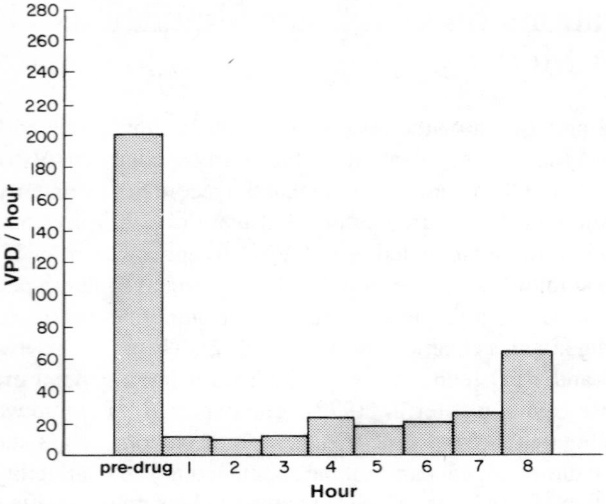

7-5 Results of 8 h of simulated ECG record of a patient with an underlying VPD rate of 200/h who is administered an 800-mg dose of quinidine.

quency. This can be masked easily by a 10% spontaneous variability in VPD rate. At a rate of 200 VPD/h, this will happen about 10% of the time. Therefore, it would be unrealistic to expect to obtain a meaningful dose-response curve using a single patient and a single measurement per dosage. However, if in fact the Poisson model adequately described the occurrence of VPD, it would be rare that an effective dose of a potent antiarrhythmic drug would be totally masked by spontaneous variability of VPD in an acute drug-testing trial. This is counter to Winkle's (1978) observations, and of the observation of many physicians that VPD rates often vary considerably from hour to hour. The 20 patients selected by Winkle, who had a VPD rate of at least 60/h, exhibited as much as a 99% reduction, and a 101% increase, in hourly VPD rate over a $5^1/_2$-h monitoring period. Yet, in a simulated 1,000 h of ECG record, using Poisson modeling, the lowest hourly VPD rate varied by less than 40% from the highest hourly VPD rate. This points out the inadequacy of the Poisson model when dealing with the very real phenomenon that ECG records sometimes show large hourly variations. These large hourly variations would be of more concern for acute drug testing but are of less importance for protocols involving long term electrocardiographic recordings. For 24-h records, the variance of intervals between VPD remains close to the Poisson variance. However, for small time periods, there is evidence of clustering of VPD episodes that can give misleading results in acute drug-testing protocols.

Misapplications of Antiarrhythmic Drug-Testing Techniques in Clinical Practice

It is not simple for clinicians to apply the methods proposed by Winkle, Morganroth, or Sami. In clinical practice, physicians may use these methods in a way that appears valid but which is incorrect. For example, a patient who has symptoms or who is in a high risk group for significant ventricular arrhythmias has a 24-h ECG recording that contains frequent VPD (e.g., >100 VPD/h) and a few paired VPD but no ventricular tachycardia. Physicians may not treat based on these findings because ventricular tachycardia is not present, but instead may obtain another recording because of high VPD frequency. If the second 24-h ECG recording has a similar average VPD frequency but contains nonsustained ventricular tachycardia, physicians often will initiate treatment with moderate doses of an antiarrhythmic drug, i.e., a dose that is likely to be safe and well tolerated, but one that has only a moderate chance of efficacy, e.g., quinidine sulfate, 300 mg, four times a day. Most physicians will repeat a 24-h Holter on treatment but the time that they perform the recording varies significantly. Some physicians will repeat the recording after five assumed drug elimination half-lives elapse. Others will measure plasma drug concentrations and adjust doses until a target concentration is exceeded before repeating the 24-h ECG. If the first postdrug recording shows little or no effect and the plasma concentration of the drug is moderate to high, many doctors will change to another drug before repeating the 24-h ECG recording. If the first 24-h ECG recording on the drug shows a large effect, e.g., greater than 70% reduction in VPD frequency and total suppression, the physician is likely to declare the drug effective without any further assessment of efficacy. If the first 24-h ECG recording on drug shows a moderate effect at a moderate drug level, the usual action is to increase the drug dose and to repeat the 24-h ECG. Such a sequence has the hazard of declaring a drug effective when it is not.

Clinical sequences in antiarrhythmic drug usage can be much more complex than these examples. However, it is apparent that even these sequences depart markedly from the analysis of variance or regression approaches discussed above. By focusing on those 24-h recordings that show what a physician wants or expects to see, an incorrect conclusion may be drawn that a drug is effective or ineffective.

Dose-Ranging Studies

The purpose of dose-ranging studies is 2-fold: 1, to determine whether a drug is significantly effective in reducing VPD frequency and repetitiveness, and 2, to determine an effective but nontoxic dose range. Each subject has one or more base-line 24-h ECG recordings, and then is given increasing doses of the test drug; an additional 24-h ECG recording is made at each dosage level. This approach provides the strongest evidence for a causal relationship between drug dosing and VPD response. Alternatively, patients can be assigned randomly to be tested at only one of several dosage levels. The proportion of patients "responding" at each dosage is calculated, and this proportion is used to produce the standard "dose-response curve." In view of the magnitude of spontaneous variability in VPD frequency, it is clear that the definition of a "response" should not be chosen arbitrarily, but should be based on recommendations such as those of Winkle, Morganroth, Sami, or Thomas.

Dose ranging relates changes in response to changes in plasma drug concentration. The advantage of working with groups of patients is that results will describe the concentration-response relationship as it pertains to the population as a whole. Individual responses to the drug may vary from this pattern to some degree; however, this information gives the clinician a point of reference from which to manage any new patient's dose regimen. In addition, when working with substantial numbers of patients, one can estimate the type and frequency of concentration-related adverse drug effects. This information is essential in deriving effective doses that have a low probability of producing dose-related toxicity.

Figure 7-6 presents a dose-response curve for patient response to imipramine that was obtained in a study by Giardina et al. (1982). This curve contains such pertinent information as the minimum dose that is likely to produce a desirable response, the dose at which virtually every responder will respond, and the dosage level at which one-half of the responders are expected to respond.

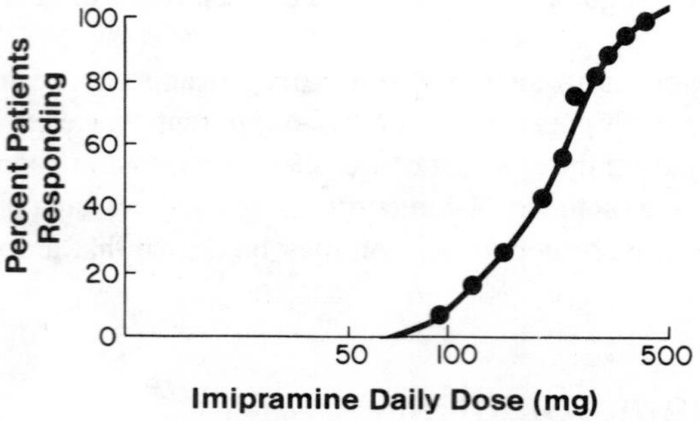

7-6 Dose-response curve for 16 patients who responded to imipramine with at least 80% suppression of ventricular premature complexes. After a figure by Giardina and Bigger (1982), with the permission of the authors and publisher.

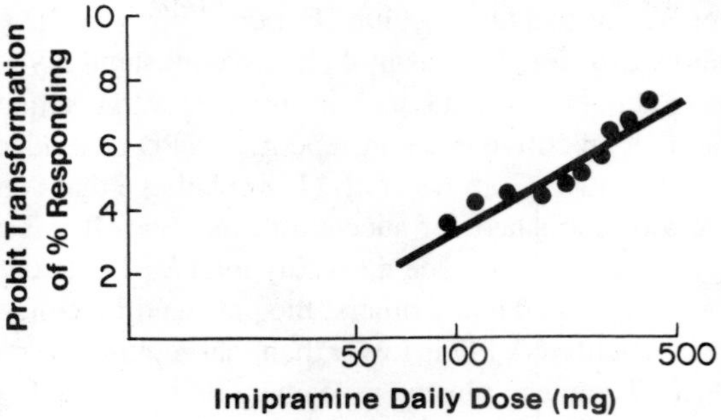

7-7 Probit transformation of dose-response curve in Figure 7-6.

The dose-response relationship can be linearized using transformations. Figure 7-7 shows a probit transformation of the dose-response data in Figure 7-6 (Finney, 1952). Investigators often prefer to work with such linear relationships. Outliers are easy to spot in a linear relationship, and it is easy to interpolate values and to extrapolate, although one must be wary about extrapolation into areas not adequately described by the data.

Antiarrhythmic Drug Therapy and Improvement in Patient Prognosis

Recent epidemiologic studies have sought to quantitate the relation between the VPD frequency and repetitiveness and subsequent cardiac events. In a prospective multicenter study of 866 post-myocardial infarction subjects who participated in the Multicenter Post Infarction Program (MPIP) (1983), Bigger et al. (1984) assessed the relation of ventricular arrhythmias detected in 24-h ECG recordings made about 10 days after myocardial infarction to death during the subsequent 2 years. Death is an S-shaped function of VPD frequency; the risk of death increases considerably for a VPD rate of 3/h or greater. Both VPD frequency and incidence of repetitive VPD are independently associated with mortality in postinfarction patients. This finding suggests that in antiarrhythmic drug testing, it is wise to examine the effect of the drug on the rate of occurrence of both nonrepetitive and repetitive VPD.

There are many questions remaining about treatment of potentially malignant arrhythmias in the years after myocardial infarction. Everyone is asking whether reduction in VPD will cause a corresponding decrease in mortality rate. A number of questions derive from this primary question. Should VPD frequency be reduced by a percentage or to a target value? For example, if VPD frequency must be reduced to below 3/h to reduce arrhythmic risk substantially, this will be almost impossible to achieve for patients with predrug VPD frequency of greater than 100/h. Must both repetitive and non-repetitive VPD be reduced or abolished to reduce risk significantly? Graboys et al. (1982) believe that ventricular tachycardia must be totally abolished for successful outcome. It is easier to abolish ventricular tachycardia than to reduce markedly total VPD frequency. As shown by Myerburg et al. (1981) and many others, the plasma drug concentration that is needed to suppress repetitive VPD is lower than that required to reduce VPD frequency by 70–80%. The mean plasma procainamide level required for complete suppression of ventricular tachycardia (9 μg/ml) was considerably lower than the mean plasma level needed for 85% suppression of VPD (15 μg/ml). The decrease in VPD frequency at the plasma level that effectively suppressed spontaneous ventricular tachycardia was only 36%. So, it is possible that significant protection against sustained ventricular tachycardia and fibrillation can be afforded by doses of antiarrhythmic drugs that do not reach conventional criteria for effective reduction in VPD frequency.

Epidemiologic Drug Trials

Assessment of antiarrhythmic drug efficacy would be incomplete if no account were taken of the effect of the drug on a patient's prognosis. Intervention trials, in which patients are randomly selected for a control or intervention group, are powerful tools to determine the effect of a drug on mortality or symptomatic arrhythmic events. Unless patients are randomly assigned to control or intervention groups, it becomes very difficult to isolate the effect of the drug on outcome. If it is desirable that patients with certain characteristics appear in both the control and intervention groups, then stratified random sampling should be used. This allows for the numbers of patients in various subgroups of the control and intervention groups to be planned, enabling the use of statistical designs with maximum power.

It is also highly desirable that antiarrhythmic drug trials be double-blind. One often finds that physicians opt for conventional therapy rather than enroll the sicker patients. Thus, the death rates in the placebo groups are often lower than expected.

The difficulty in isolating the drug effect in a nonrandomized, nonblinded study is apparent in the ongoing debate about the effect of digitalis on patients following a myocardial infarction. Three retrospective studies show a lack of agreement. Moss et al. (1981) found a significant adverse digitalis effect on 4-month mortality in that subgroup of 812 post-myocardial infarction population with congestive heart failure and repetitive VPD on a predischarge ambulatory electrocardiographic recording. Bigger et al. (1981) found a significant adverse digitalis effect in a population of 490 postmyocardial infarction patients after adjusting for previous myocardial infarction, left ventricular failure in the CCU, enlarged heart on discharge chest X-ray, frequent ventricular arrhythmias and other risk factors. However, the Coronary Artery Surgery Study of 1,592 postmyocardial infarction patients with chest pain syndromes concluded that digitalis did not have an independent effect on mortality in the $4^1/_2$ years following their infarcts (Ryan et al., 1983). A randomized controlled trial is the best way to address controversial issues arising from retrospective studies such as these.

Six major long term trials that have been conducted to assess the effect of antiarrhythmic drugs on mortality in postinfarction patients are discussed by May et al. (1982). The study populations cited ranged in size from 112–568. Study designs were simple, with patients randomly allocated to control or intervention group. Five of the six studies were double-blind. There was no attempt in these studies to relate drug use to suppression of arrhythmias; mortality was the only endpoint examined. In all six studies, there was no significant effect of antiarrhythmic drugs on mortality.

This result is not surprising given the design and sample size of these studies. Some did not even select patients with arrhythmias to treat. None of these studies required dosing to a predetermined standard of efficacy. Most important, all of the studies were thousands of patients short of the number needed for a trial in order to have an 80% chance of detecting a 25% reduction in mortality. A significant effect of antiarrhythmic drugs on survival of patients with malignant ventricular arrhythmia who respond to antiarrhythmic therapy was reported by Graboys et al. (1982). They followed 123 patients with malignant ventricular arrhythmias over an average follow-up period of 30 months. The death rate due to sudden death (defined as death occurring within 1 h of onset of symptoms) was 11%. A breakdown of that death rate indicated that the annual death rate for drug responders (defined as patients with abolition of repetitive VPD and R on T VPD) was 3%, contrasted with a 41% annual death rate for nonresponders. This study is most encouraging to physicians who have patients with malignant ventricular arrhythmias who are responding favorably to antiarrhythmic drug therapy. However, the design of the study limits conclusions that may be drawn. There is no control group in this study because the authors considered it unethical. With such a design, it is possible that the response to the drug may select patients who will survive, i.e., the drugs may not be responsible for the increased survival.

Summary

In patients with coronary heart disease, VPD has a peculiar, unusually skewed distribution and substantial spontaneous variability in frequency of occurrence. The factors responsible for these characteristics are largely unknown at the present time and represent significant obstacles to be overcome in the evaluation of antiarrhythmic drug efficacy. Techniques for judging efficacy have been developed but these are not simple to apply in clinical practice. Whether arrhythmia control translates into improved quality and length of life overall is yet to be determined. Some recent studies in malignant arrhythmias are encouraging in this regard.

Acknowledgments

We wish to thank Dr. Elsa Giardina for providing dose-response data on patients treated for ventricular arrhythmias with imipramine. We thank Professors Joseph L. Fleiss and Bruce Levin for discussions of the statistical issues addressed in this manuscript.

Supported in part by National Institutes of Health grants HL-22982, HL-12736, and HL-70204 from the National Heart, Lung and Blood Institute, Bethesda, MD; by grant RR-00645 from the Research Resources Administration, Bethesda, MD; by funds from Merck, Sharp and Dohme Research Laboratories, West Point, PA; and by the Winthrop and Chernow Foundations, New York, NY.

References

Bigger, J.T., Fleiss, J.L., Kleiger, R., Miller, J.P., Rolnitzky, L.M., and the Multicenter Post-Infarction Research Group. 1984. The relationship between ventricular arrhythmias, left ventricular dysfunction and mortality in the two years after myocardial infarction. Circulation 69:250–258.

Bigger, J.T., Weld, F.M., Rolnitzky, L.M., and Ferrick, K.J. 1981. Is digitalis treatment harmful in the year after acute myocardial infarction? Circulation 64(IV):83.

Finney, D.J. 1952. Probit Analysis. Cambridge, England: University Press.

Gaughin, C.E., Lown, B., Lanigan, J., Voukydis, P., and Beser, H. 1976. Acute oral drug testing for determining antiarrhythmic drug efficacy. 1. Quinidine. Am J Cardiol 38: 677–684.

Giardina, E.V.G., and Bigger, J.T. 1982. Antiarrhythmic effect of imipramine hydrochloride in patients with ventricular premature complexes without psychological depression. Am J Cardiol 50:172–179.

Graboys, T.B., Lown, B., Podrid, P.J., and DeSilva, R. 1982. Long-term survival of patients with malignant ventricular arrhythmia treated with anitarrhythmic drugs. Am J Cardiol 50: 437–443.

Kirk, R.E. 1968. Experimental Design: Procedures for the Behavioral Sciences. pp. 60–67. California; Brooks/Cole Publishing Co.

Lown, B., Tykocinski, A., Garfein, M., and Brooks, P. 1973. Sleep and ventricular premature beats. Circulation 48:691–701.

May, G.S., Eberlein, K.A., Furberg, C.D., Passamani, E.R., and DeMets, D.L. 1982. Secondary prevention after myocardial infarction: a review of long-term trials. Progr Cardiovasc Dis 24:331–352.

Meffin, P.J., Winkle, R.A., Blaschke, T.F., Fitzgerald, J., Harrison, D.C., Harapat, S.R., and Bell, P.A. 1977. Response optimization of drug dosage: Antiarrhythmic studies with tocainide. J Clin Pharmacol Ther 22:42–47.

Michelson, E.L., and Morganroth, J. 1980. Spontaneous variability of complex ventricular arrhythmias detected by long-term electrocardiographic recording. Circulation 61: 690–695.

Morganroth, J., Michelson, E.L., Horowitz, L.N., Josephson, M.E., Pearlman, A.S., and Dunkman, W.B. 1978. Limitations of routine long-term monitoring to assess ventricular ectopic frequency. Circulation 58:408–414.

Moss, A.J., Davis, H.T., Conard, D.L., DeCamilla, J.J.,and Odoroff, C.L. 1981. Digitalis-associated cardiac mortality after myocardial infarction. Circulation 64:1150–1156.

Myerburg, R.J., Kessler, K.M., Kiem, I., Pefkaros, K.C., Conde, C.A., Cooper, D., and Castellanos, A. 1981. Relationship between plasma levels of procainamide, suppression of premature ventricular complexes and prevention of recurrent ventricular tachycardia. Circulation 64:280–290.

Rowland, M. 1972. Drug administration and regimens. In: K.L. Melmon and H.F. Morrelli, eds. Clinical Pharmacology: Basic Principles in Therapeutics. pp. 21–90. New York: MacMillan Co.

Ruttman, U.E., Bassir, R., and Yamamoto, W.S. 1972. A statistical description of the occurrence of premature ventricular contractions based on the Poisson process. Computers Biomed Engr 10:431–442.

Ryan, T.J., Bailey, K.R., McCabe, C.H., Luk, S., Fisher, L.D., Mock, M.B., and Killip, T. 1983. The effects of digitalis on survival in high-risk patients with coronary artery disease. Circulation 67:735–742.

Sami, M., Kraemer, H., Harrison, D.C., Houston, N., Chimasaki, S., and DeBusk, R.F. 1980. A new method for evaluating antiarrhythmic drug efficacy. Circulation 62:1172–1179.

Shapiro, W., Canada, W.B., Lee, G., DeMaria, A.N., Low, R.I., Mason, D.T., and Laddu, A. 1982. Comparison of two methods of analyzing frequency of ventricular arrhythmias. Am Heart J 104:874–875.

Steinbach, K., Golgar, D., Weber, H., Joskowicz, G., and Kaindl, F. 1982. Frequency and variability of ventricular premature contractions—the influence of heart rate and circadian rhythms. PACE 5:38–51.

The Multicenter Postinfarction Research Group. 1983. Risk stratification and survival after myocardial infarction. N Engl J Med 309: 331–336.

Thomas, L.J., and Miller, J.P. Long-term ambulatory ECG recording in the determination of antidysrhythmic drug efficacy. In: B.R. Lucchesi, J.V. Dingell, and R.P. Schwartz, eds. Clinical Pharmacology of Antiarrhythmic Therapy. pp. 249–265. New York: Raven Press.

Tukey, J.W. 1977. Exploratory Data Analysis. pp.83–85. Philippines: Addison-Wesley Publishing Co.

Velebit, V., Podrid, P., Lown, B., Cohen, B.H., and Graboys, T.B. 1982. Aggravation and provocation of ventricular arrhythmias by antiarrhythmic drugs. Circulation 65:886–894.

Winkle, R.A. 1978. Antiarrhythmic drug effect mimicked by spontaneous variability of ventricular ectopy. Circulation 57:1116–1121.

Chapter 8

Indices of Antiarrhythmic Drug Efficacy Using Invasive Techniques

Leonard N. Horowitz

Introduction

Sudden cardiac death accounts for approximately 500,000 deaths yearly in the United States. The majority of these deaths are caused by ventricular tachyarrhythmias. Since the recognition of this major public health crisis, many modalities for identifying patients at risk for these life-threatening arrhythmias and for selecting therapy to prevent them have been proposed. Noninvasive means of identifying risk and selecting therapy are discussed elsewhere in this symposium. We will present invasive clinical cardiac electrophysiologic techniques for the identification and selection of treatment for patients with life-threatening ventricular tachyarrhythmias.

Programmed electrical stimulation in the human heart has been used to assess vulnerability to ventricular arrhythmias and to assess the suppressant effect of antiarrhythmic treatment. Programmed electrical stimulation is performed with electrode catheters which are typically introduced percutaneously and positioned in various cardiac chambers under fluoroscopic guidance. Stimulation protocols vary between laboratories, but they generally include the introduction of ventricular extrastimuli during sinus rhythm and ventricular pacing at several rates. The amplitude of the stimuli is generally twice the late diastolic threshold. Our stimulation protocol is outlined in Table 8-1. It is critical to emphasize that observations using programmed electrical stimulation should be reproducible, particularly when these are used for selection of antiarrhythmic therapy.

Table 8-1 Stimulation Protocol for Ventricular Arrhythmias.

1. Single, double, and triple extrastimuli delivered during sinus rhythm and ventricular pacing at several cycle lengths.
2. Bursts (5–15 complexes) of ventricular pacing at increasing rates.

Responses of Programmed Electrical Stimulation

Programmed electrical stimulation of the ventricle can produce repetitive ventricular responses or a ventricular tachyarrhythmia (ventricular tachycardia and ventricular fibrillation). Repetitive ventricular responses are single or multiple extra ventricular complexes which are produced by ventricular extrastimuli (Farshidi et al., 1980). Two types of repetitive ventricular responses have been identified (Fig. 8-1). Bundle branch reentry is recognized by the occurrence of an extra ventricular response following the stimulated premature complex which is dependent upon retrograde His-Purkinje conduction delay. Bundle branch reentry, as its name implies, is thought to result from reentry within the normal conduction system. Bundle branch reentrant repetitive ventricular responses are preceded by a His bundle deflection. On the other hand, intraventricular repetitive responses to

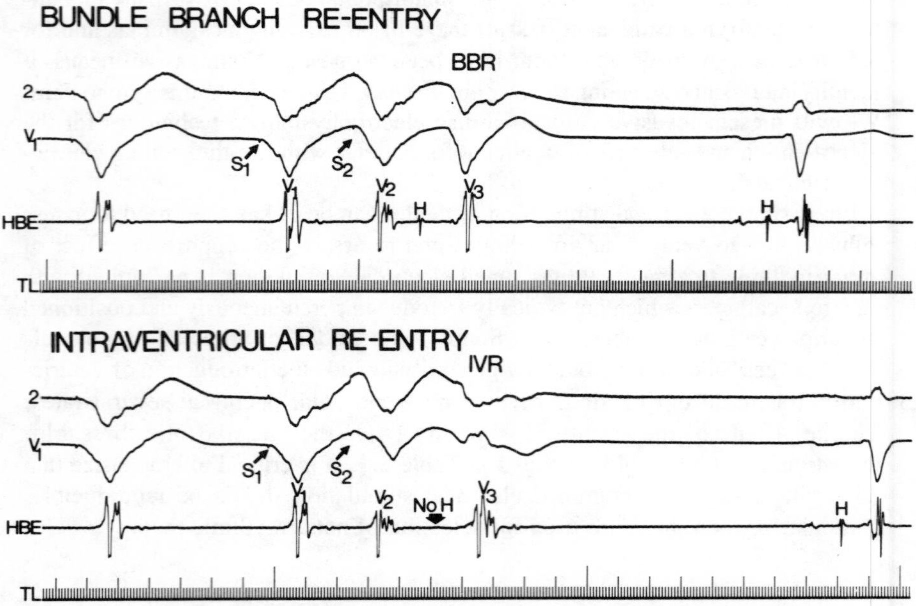

8-1 Examples of bundle branch and intraventricular reentry. In both panels, ECG leads 2 and V_1 are shown with a His bundle electrogram (HBE) and 10-ms time lines. In the upper panel, following the ventricular premature stimulus (S_2), an additional complex is noted (BBR). Note that a His bundle deflection precedes the extra response which is similar in morphology to the paced complexes. In the bottom panel, following the premature extrastimulus (S_2), an additional complex is noted. This one, however, is not preceded by a His bundle deflection and is different in QRS morphology. This latter complex is an intraventricular reentrant response.

extrastimuli are independent of retrograde His-Purkinje delay and are not necessarily preceded by His bundle depolarizations. The site of reentry for this type of response is not known, but it is thought to be an area of pathologic change in the ventricle.

The predictive value of repetitive ventricular responses in identifying patients at risk for ventricular arrhythmias has been investigated extensively (Farshidi et al., 1980; Greene et al., 1978; Troup et al., 1978; Mason, 1980). The bundle branch reentrant response is considered by most investigators to be a normal physiologic occurrence. It occurs in more than 50% of individuals undergoing programmed ventricular stimulation whether or not heart disease is present. It has not been associated with an increased risk of cardiovascular mortality or documented ventricular tachyarrhythmias. Intraventricular responses, on the other hand, are observed in less than 10% of normal subjects undergoing electrophysiologic studies and are considered a pathologic response. The intraventricular response is noted more commonly in patients who have had a documented clinical episode of ventricular tachycardia or ventricular fibrillation.

In one study of 424 consecutive patients undergoing programmed ventricular stimulation, the clinical relevance of repetitive responses was evaluated (Farshidi et al., 1980). Intraventricular reentrant responses occurred in 78/119 patients with clinically documented ventricular tachycardia/fibrillation, whereas no intraventricular responses occurred in 253/305 patients without ventricular tachyarrhythmias. This relationship was statistically significant; however, the clinical usefulness of this measurement was minimal. One-third of patients with known ventricular arrhythmias fail to manifest the intraventricular reentrant response, and thus, the test has low sensitivity for prospectively identifying patients at risk for life-threatening arrhythmias. Others have presented divergent conclusions (Greene et al., 1978), but these generally have not been confirmed (Troup et al., 1978; Mason, 1980).

The other potential response to programmed ventricular stimulation is induction of a ventricular tachyarrhythmia. These arrhythmias include ventricular tachycardia, either sustained or nonsustained, or ventricular fibrillation. The use of programmed electrical stimulation to determine vulnerability to these arrhythmias is based on the assumption that an arrhythmia can be initiated only in susceptible patients and that the arrhythmia initiated by programmed stimulation is similar to the clinical rhythm disturbance to which the patient is prone. This assumption is supported by many studies, although most are retrospective analyses. In one report of patients undergoing electrophysiologic study with a standard stimulation protocol, ventricular tachycardia was initiated by programmed stimulation in 48/57 (84%) with previously documented ventricular tachycardia (Horowitz et al., 1982). Whereas, in a group of 112 patients without documented clinical ventricular tachyarrhythmia, ventricular tachycardia was initiated in only 3 (3%). Similar results have been reported by other groups (Spielman et al., 1978; Mason and Winkle, 1978).

Hamer and co-workers (1982), studying patients who had survived acute myocardial infarction, found that programmed electrical stimulation prospectively could identify patients at risk to develop life-threatening arrhythmias. They found that sudden death occurred in 4/12 (33%) of patients in whom ventricular tachycardia could be induced by programmed stimulation, whereas sudden death occurred in only 1/25 (4%) of patients in whom no arrhythmia was inducible. In a similar prospective study, the sensitivity of inducible ventricular tachycardia or fibrillation as a predictor of subsequent sudden death or spontaneous ventricular tachycardia was 86% and the specificity was 83% (Richards et al., 1983). Conversely, the inability to induce a ventricular tachyarrhythmia had a predictive accuracy of 98% for the absence of subsequent sudden death. Thus, ventricular tachyarrhythmias are rarely induced by programmed ventricular stimulation in patients without clinical ventricular tachyarrhythmias or vulnerability to them, and conversely, in most patients who have ventricular tachyarrhythmias clinically, these arrhythmias can be induced in the electrophysiology laboratory.

Methods for Selecting Antiarrhythmic Regimens

Antiarrhythmic regimens can be selected by several methods. The empiric method in which agents and their doses are selected without objective data is the easiest but least effective. Successful suppression of ventricular tachyarrhythmias is uncommon (less than 20%). It is difficult if not impossible to determine drug efficacy because the arrhythmia-free interval between recurrences is unpredictable. Furthermore, selection of effective doses based on "therapeutic ranges" developed from grouped data from large populations is not effective.

Other methods of selecting antiarrhythmic regimens use objective testing to assess drug efficacy. Noninvasive techniques are discussed elsewhere in the symposium. In general, these techniques rely on data obtained by electrocardiographic monitoring during drug administration to assess suppression of ventricular premature complexes (Graboys et al., 1982). Selection of therapy for sustained arrhythmias by this means is flawed by reliance upon a drug's effect on ventricular premature complexes which may not necessarily predict the drug's effect on sustained tachyarrhythmias. Of particular importance in this regard are the reports of a disparate effect of drugs on these parameters (Herling et al., 1980; Myerburg et al., 1981). Myerburg and co-workers (1981) have shown, for example, that the elimination of premature ventricular complexes with procainamide occurs at different plasma concentrations than does suppression of sustained ventricular tachyarrhythmias.

Invasive electrophysiologic testing, on the other hand, is a provocative technique in which drug efficacy against the sustained arrhythmias is tested. In the procedure by which pharmacologic regimens are devised using electrophysio-

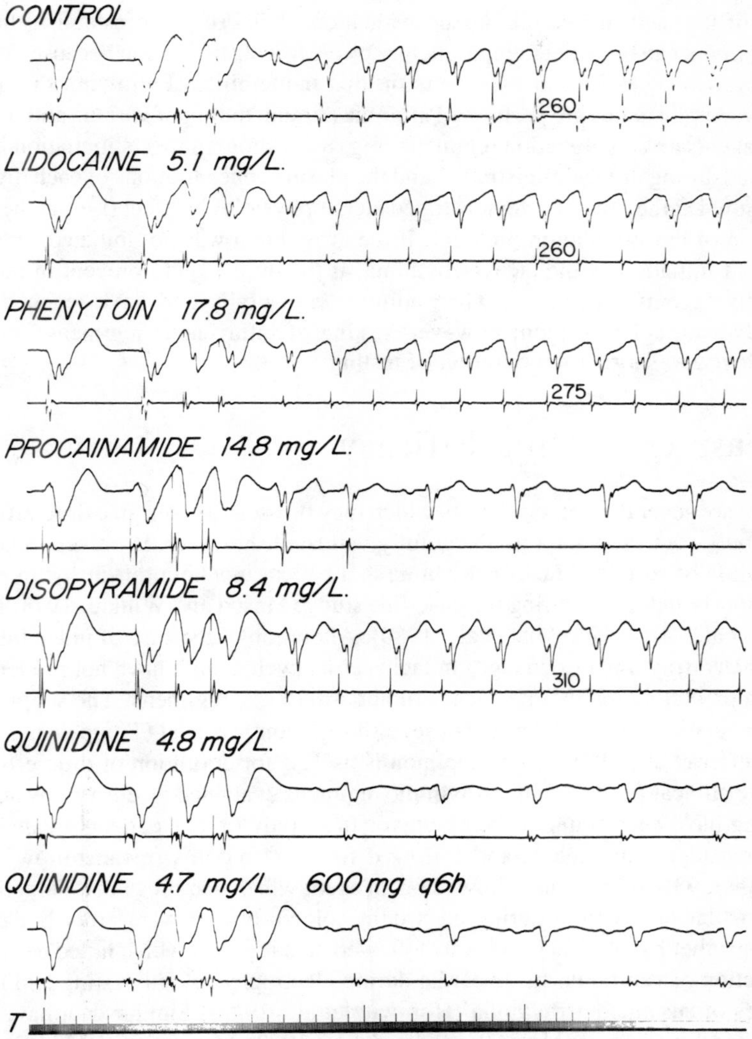

8-2 Serial electrophysiologic study for ventricular tachycardia. In each panel, a V_1 rhythm strip is shown with an intracardiac electrogram recorded at the right ventricular apex. The drug and drug level at the time of electrophysiologic study are shown. The number written to the right is the cycle length of the induced ventricular tachycardia. Note that, in this patient, lidocaine, phenytoin, and disopyramide failed to prevent ventricular tachycardia. Procainamide and quinidine prevented the induction of ventricular tachycardia. Quinidine, in an oral regimen which produced a blood level comparable to that obtained during electrophysiologic testing, also prevented induction of ventricular tachycardia.

logic techniques, a base-line study is performed to document reproducible initiation of the tachyarrhythmia under evaluation. It is critical to establish that the arrhythmia can be initiated reproducibly by electrical stimulation because drug efficacy will be evaluated by effects on this inducibility. Following this initial study, serial studies are performed after the administration of various antiarrhythmic agents and combination regimens (Fig. 8-2). Programmed stimulation is performed during drug administration and the plasma concentrations of each drug are measured at the time of a demonstrated electrophysiologic effect (i.e., at the completion of the stimulation protocol, if the arrhythmia was not initiated, or at the time of initiation of the tachyarrhythmia, if the drug fails to prevent initiation). Ideally, agents are studied when administered orally and have reached their steady-state concentration; however, testing of intravenous regimens has been employed to shorten the duration of testing.

Measures of Drug Efficacy

There are several potential indices which may be used to determine drug efficacy. The only measure which has been fully validated, however, is prevention of the initiation of sustained tachyarrhythmia in a patient in whom this arrhythmia was previously inducible during the base-line study (Mason and Winkle, 1978; Horowitz et al., 1978; Horowitz et al., 1980). Alteration of the ease of inducibility of the tachyarrhythmia or changes in tachycardia cycle length have not proven useful in predicting long term efficacy of antiarrhythmic regimens. The suppression of the repetitive ventricular response, although controversial (Troup et al., 1978; Schaeffer et al., 1978), in my opinion is useless for definition of drug efficacy.

The clinical results of antiarrhythmic regimens evaluated by electrophysiologic testing have been found to be effective. In a study of 111 patients treated with noninvestigational agents and followed for 9–54 months (mean follow-up 18 months), 93% of patients followed on an agent which had prevented induction of ventricular tachycardia during electrophysiologic testing were arrhythmia-free. On the other hand, 90% of patients followed on a regimen which failed to prevent induction of ventricular tachycardia during electrophysiologic testing had recurrences of sustained arrhythmia (Horowitz et al., 1982). Similar data have been reported by many authors (Horowitz et al., 1982; Mason and Winkle, 1978; Horowitz et al., 1978; Fisher et al., 1977; Mason and Winkle, 1980; Ruskin and Garan, 1979). Similar results have been reported in those patients who have been evaluated by electrophysiologic testing following resuscitation from out-of-hospital cardiac arrest (Ruskin et al., 1980; Morady et al., 1983). Ruskin et al. (1980) reported the results of selecting antiarrhythmic therapy using electrophysiologic testing in 31 patients who had survived out-of-hospital cardiac arrest. In 19 of 19 patients in whom a previously inducible arrhythmia was suppressed by an antiarrhythmic regimen, no symptomatic arrhythmias occurred during follow-up, whereas in patients who remained inducible, sudden death occurred in 50%. In several studies, the prevention of induction of ventricular tachyarrhythmias has correlated with 80–90% long term efficacy rates using this approach.

Data collected using a variety of antiarrhythmic drugs has shown that the results of electrophysiologic testing have been highly predictive of subsequent clinical course. The usefulness of electrophysiologic testing has been controversial, however, when applied to amiodarone. Some have presented data which indicate that electrophysiologic testing is unhelpful in selecting the clinical course of patients treated with amiodarone (Waxman, 1983; Hamer et al., 1981), while others have suggested that the contrary is true and that electrophysiologic testing is very helpful (Horowitz et al., 1983; McGovern and Ruskin, 1983). There is general agreement that the inability to induce ventricular tachyarrhythmia following initiation of amiodarone therapy predicts long term success in the suppression of the ventricular tachyarrhythmia. Recurrence rates in patients in whom ventricular tachyarrhythmias remain inducible during amiodarone treatment, however, are lower than with other agents. Whether longer follow-up is needed to assess this difference is not known. Also, electrophysiologic testing can predict the severity of a recurrence which may occur on amiodarone therapy and can be useful for deciding whether adjunctive therapy is advisable (Horowitz et al., 1983).

Investigational antiarrhythmic agents can be assessed in a manner similar to that used for routinely available agents. Excluding the experience with amiodarone most investigational agents currently available appear similar in their responses to electrophysiologic selection techniques.

Risk Benefit Considerations

The invasive electrophysiologic technique for selecting therapy for ventricular tachyarrhythmias is applicable only to those patients in whom programmed electrical stimulation is able to initiate a ventricular tachyarrhythmia. Although this includes 80–90% of patients with recurrent ventricular tachyarrhythmias, there are some patients in whom the arrhythmia is noninducible, and thus for these patients this technique is not applicable. In many patients, these life-threatening arrhythmias cannot be terminated by programmed stimulation and cardioversion is necessary. This, of course, is a liability. These patients, however, represent a group which is at highest risk for sudden cardiac death because of hemodynamic deterioration or rapid degeneration to ventricular fibrillation, and the benefits of electrophysiologic testing would be expected to be most appreciable.

Provocative tests of this sort carry some risk of morbidity and potential mortality. Even in a setting in which frequent studies are performed by experienced physicians, serious complications may occur. The reported incidence of these complications is low; however, it must be acknowledged. The risk/benefit ratio considering these known risks and reported results, however, continue to favor the use of provocative electrophysiologic testing in patients with potentially lethal ventricular arrhythmias.

References

Farshidi, A., Michelson, E.L., Greenspan, A.M., Spielman, S.R., Horowitz, L.N., and Josephson, M.E. 1980. Repetitive responses to ventricular extrastimuli: Incidence, mechanism and significance. Am Heart J 199:59–68.

Fisher, J.D., Cohen, H.L., Mehra, R., Altschuler, H., Escher, D.J.W., and Furman, S. 1977. Cardiac pacing and pacemakers. II. Serial electrophysiologic pharmacologic testing for control of recurrent tachyarrhythmias. Am Heart J 93:658–668.

Graboys, T.B., Lown, B., Podrid, P.J., and DeSilva, R. 1982. Long-term survival of patients with malignant ventricular arrhythmia treated with anti-arrhythmic drugs. Am J Cardiol 50:437–443.

Greene, H.L., Reid, P.R., and Schaeffer, A.H. 1978. The repetitive ventricular response in man: A predictor of sudden death. N Engl J Med 299:729–736.

Hamer, A.W., Finerman, W.B., Peter, T., and Mandel, W.J. 1981. Disparity between the clinical and electrophysiologic effects of amiodarone in the treatment of recurrent ventricular tachyarrhythmias. Am Heart J 102: 992–1000.

Hamer, A., Vohra, J., Hunt, D., and Sloman, G. 1982. Prediction of sudden death by electrophysiological studies in high risk patients surviving acute myocardial infarction. Am J Cardiol 50:223–229.

Herling, I.M., Horowitz, L.N., and Josephson, M.E. 1980. Ventricular ectopic activity following medical and surgical treatment of recurrent sustained ventricular tachycardia. Am J Cardiol 45:633–639.

Horowitz, L.N., Josephson, M.E., Farshidi, A., Spielman, S.R., Michelson, E.L., and Greenspan, A.M. 1978. Recurrent sustained ventricular tachycardia. 3. Role of the electrophysiologic study in selection of antiarrhythmic regimens. Circulation 58:986–997.

Horowitz, L.N., Josephson, M.E., and Kastor, J.A. 1980. Intracardiac electrophysiologic studies as a method for the optimization of drug therapy in chronic ventricular arrhythmia. Progr Cardiovasc Dis 23:81–98.

Horowitz, L.N., Spielman, S.R., Greenspan, A.M., and Josephson, M.E. 1982. Role of programmed stimulation in assessing vulnerability to ventricular arrhythmias. Am Heart J 103:604–608.

Horowitz, L.N., Spielman, S.R., Greenspan, A.M., Webb, C.R., and Kay, H.R. 1983. Ventricular arrhythmias—Use of electrophysiologic studies. Am Heart J 106:881–886.

Mason, J.W. 1980. Repetitive heating after single ventricular extrastimuli: Incidence and prognostic significance in patients with ventricular tachycardia. Am J Cardiol 45:407 (abstr).

Mason, J.W., and Winkle, R.A., 1978. Electrode catheter arrhythmia induction in the selection and assessment of antiarrhythmic drug therapy for recurrent ventricular tachycardia. Circulation 58:971–985.

Mason, J.W., and Winkle, R.A. 1980. Accuracy of the ventricular tachycardia-induction study for predicting long-term efficacy and inefficacy of antiarrhythmic drugs. N Engl J Med 303:1073–1077.

McGovern, B., and Ruskin, J.N. 1983. The efficacy of amiodarone for ventricular arrhythmias can be predicted with clinical electrophysiologic studies. Int J Cardiol 3:71–76.

Morady, F., Scheinman, M.M., Hess, D.S., Sung, R.J., Shen, E., and Shapiro, W. 1983. Electrophysiologic testing in the management of survivors of out-of-hospital cardiac arrest. Am J Cardiol 51:85–89.

Myerburg, R.J., Kessler, K.M., Kiem, I., Pefkaros, K.C., Conde, C.A., Cooper, D., and Castellanos, A. 1981. Relationship between plasma levels of procainamide suppression of premature ventricular complexes and prevention of recurrent ventricular tachycardia. Circulation 64:280–290.

Richards, D.A., Cody, D.V., Denniss, A.R., Russell, P.A., Young, A.A., and Uther, J.B. 1983. Ventricular electrical instability: A predictor of death after myocardial infarction. Am J Cardiol 51:75–80.

Ruskin, J.N., DiMarco, J.P., and Garan, H. 1980. Out-of-hospital cardiac arrest: Electrophysiologic observations and selection of long-term antiarrhythmic therapy. N Engl J Med 303:607–613.

Ruskin, J.N., and Garan, H. 1979. Chronic electrophysiologic testing in patients with recurrent sustained ventricular tachycardia. Am J Cardiol 43:400 (abstr).

Schaeffer, A.H., Greene, H.L., and Reid, P.R. 1978. Suppression of the repetitive ventricular response: An index of long-term antiarrhythmic effectiveness of aprindine for ventricular tachycardia in man. Am J Cardiol 42:1007–1012.

Spielman, S.R., Farshidi, A., Horowitz, L.N., and Josephson, M.E. 1978. Ventricular fibrillation during programmed ventricular stimulation: Incidence and clinical implications. Am J Cardiol 42:913–918.

Troup, P.J., Pederson, D.N., and Zipes, D.P. 1978. Effects of premature ventricular stimulation in patients with ventricular tachycardia. Circulation 58:II-154 (abstr).

Waxman, H.L. 1983. The efficacy of amiodarone for ventricular arrhythmias cannot be predicted with clinical electrophysiologic studies. Int J Cardiol 3:76–80.

EDITOR'S NOTES

Indices of Antiarrhythmic Drug Efficacy

The indices of antiarrhythmic drug efficacy are not readily defined at present nor uniformly accepted. Drs. Spear and Moore present the concept that animal models for evaluating drug effects and efficacy must be selected for the precise application of the data being collected. Thus animal models that are employed to assess efficacy of antiarrhythmic drugs in man must, by definition, be complex and mimic the clinical situation to the greatest extent possible. In this regard, some of the larger animal models (e.g., dog and pig), may mimic the clinical situation to a greater extent based on their electrophysiologic responsiveness and coronary anatomy. An initial consideration is the question of whether an animal model is sought for the purpose of establishing drug efficacy or for the purpose of more specifically understanding the drug mechanism. Animal models developed primarily for elucidating mechanistic information of both arrhythmias and antiarrhythmic drug action tend to be simpler, with fewer, noncontrolled variables. Also, such models only rarely tend to mimic the clinical situation. Alternatively, some of the more complex efficacy-oriented models must employ techniques and approaches that encompass the diversity of clinical parameters realized in the patient setting. An example utilizing this latter approach relates to the induction of myocardial infarction in larger animal models. Historically, the induction of myocardial infarction has generally been carried out by a permanent occlusion of a major epicardial artery, resulting mostly in transmural and rather homogeneous infarct development. In contrast, to better reflect a larger clinical population, newer techniques induce infarction by occluding and reperfusing a coronary artery, resulting in a more "mottled" type of infarct. Indeed, such an infarct results in a higher degree of electrical instability, as evidenced by the relative ease with which one can induce ventricular tachycardia or fibrillation. Alternatively, since it is not yet possible to fully predict antiarrhythmic efficacy or toxicity in man from data generated by individual animal models, it is important to consider a spectrum of animal models in assessing antiarrhythmic drugs. Although such an approach seems rational, its major pitfall lies in the interpretation of the diverse drug responses obtained, both qualitatively and quantitatively, in various animal models of several animal species. Furthermore, whether such animal models are in vitro or in vivo, anesthetized or conscious, adds another pitfall to interpretation of data generated from these models. Ultimately, the appropriate balance of in vitro versus in vivo and anesthetized versus conscious models in animal species physiologically more similar to man may be a more important consideration than utilizing many different animal species. However, this viewpoint remains to be proven.

Regarding evaluation of antiarrhythmic drug efficacy both clinically and by noninvasive techniques in man, the level of agreement is no better than that for defining comparable problems at the animal level. Significant questions and uncertainties in the statistical evaluation of the effect of antiarrhythmic drugs on ambient ventricular arrhythmias are highlighted in the chapter by Bigger and Rolnitzky. The nonparametric nature of ambient ventricular arrhythmias has caused considerable debate about the appropriate statistical means for evaluating modulation by antiarrhythmic drugs. Furthermore, even the most simple of these statistical techniques cannot be easily applied to individual patients in the typical clinical situation in which antiarrhythmic drugs are used. In addition, the question of greatest significant clinical impact, whether drug treatment will ultimately reduce mortality, is difficult, if not impossible, to assess from the current spectrum of clinical studies. An additional point of contention emphasized in Dr. Bigger's chapter also relates to the misapplications of antiarrhythmic drug testing techniques in clinical practice. In this regard, the impact of a preconceived notion by a physician can often lead to or be the basis of drawing an incorrect conclusion as to whether a drug is efficacious or not. Due to the skewed distribution and substantial variability of VPD's, it may be that only large-scale, multicenter, long-term, placebo-controlled drug trials will effectively determine the appropriate drug efficacy of a new agent.

Alternate and newer concepts in the evaluation of drug efficacy were discussed by Dr. Horowitz. His chapter details current techniques used in invasive electrophysiologic studies assessing the efficacy of antiarrhythmic drugs. Basic assumptions underlying the use of invasive electrophysiologic technique include: 1) it is applicable to life-threatening arrhythmias; 2) it is reproducible; 3) evoked arrhythmias are safely abolished; and 4) related drug testing facilitiates therapy. In view of the technique's current status, one is left with the conclusion that not all of these assumptions have been fully met and that methodologic uniformity among various investigators continues to be lacking. However, based upon evolving studies of long-term results of therapy evaluated in this way, the data suggest that this technique is both safe and promising. A major question relates to timing the use of invasive electrophysiologic testing in the course of patient therapy. At this point, it is unclear whether such techniques should be employed in the patient with assumed non-life-threatening arrhythmias. On the other hand, the utility and application of invasive (PES) electrophysiologic testing in patients with life-threatening ventricular arrhythmias appears rational and necessary.

It is interesting to note that a dichotomy continues to exist between the evaluation of noninvasive and invasive techniques for assessing antiarrhythmic efficacy. In noninvasive evaluations, studies have concentrated on the statistical approach to antiarrhythmic drug response. Therefore, considerable research has been devoted to understanding and providing the statistical soundness of observed antiarrhythmic efficacy. However, as noted by Bigger and Rolnitzky, little work has been done on the clinical impact of the arrhythmia reduction determined by this technique. On the other hand, in studies employing invasive techniques in the evaluation of antiarrhythmic efficacy, considerable evidence has been brought to bear that the prediction of efficacy made by invasive techniques is valid in the long-term management of patients; however, little statistical analysis has been devoted to the specific indices of antiarrhythmic drug responses.

Thus major issues regarding indices of drug efficacy relate to statistical, methodologic, and invasive-versus-noninvasive approaches. Despite the presence of various controversies, it seems apparent that a need exists for newer approaches to allow more effective drug efficacy evaluation. Although noninvasive approaches are likely to maintain an important role in the future, more invasive techniques, when clinically justifiable, may provide an important adjunct to the evaluation of arrhythmias and antiarrhythmic drugs which may prove to be of significant benefit in particular to patients with life-threatening arrhythmias.

Part II

Basic and Clinical Effects of Antiarrhythmic Drugs: Classification of Drug Effects

The Classification of Antiarrhythmic Drugs Reviewed After a Decade

E. M. Vaughan Williams

Introduction

More than a decade has passed since I suggested a classification of antiarrhythmic drugs (Vaughan Williams, 1970) originally based on three major actions, which was increased a few years later to four in collaboration with Bramah Singh (Singh and Vaughan Williams, 1972), who was working for a doctorate in my laboratory at that time. Several of the drugs studied had more than one of the four actions, so that it deserves emphasis that the classification did not so much categorize drugs, in accordance with chemical structure or physical properties, but it described four ways in which the compounds could prevent or correct abnormal cardiac rhythm. More than 20 new antiarrhythmic drugs have been introduced since 1970, several of which were synthesized for quite different roles, but which were discovered by screening experiments to be cardioactive. It is of considerable interest, therefore, that all but one of them has been found to possess one or more of the actions originally proposed as responsible for the antiarrhythmic effects. Much work has been done in the meantime on the older compounds in analyzing their mode of action, as well as on the newer drugs.

Historically, the first class of action was that exerted by quinidine and a number of other remedies (Szekeres and Vaughan Williams, 1962), which incidentally, at 10–100 times their antiarrhythmic concentrations, behaved as local anesthetics in nerves. These compounds, although differing in other respects, had in common the property of ''interfering specifically with the process by which depolarizing charge is transferred across the membrane'' (Szekeres and Vaughan Williams, 1962) (i.e., by fast inward depolarizing current carried by sodium ions). The effect was revealed as a depression of the maximum rate of depolarization, unless the interstimulus interval was so long that it permitted full recovery between beats. Sodium channels are inactivated rapidly after depolarization, and remain in the inactivated state until repolarization proceeds to voltages more negative than about −55 mv. It was suggested that the (class I) antiarrhythmic drugs interfered with the process in which Na^+ channels were ''reactivated in response to repolarization,'' and that in consequence, they ''extended the effective refractory period to a point long after the time at which repolarization was already complete'' (Szekeres and Vaughan Williams, 1962).

The above explanation was not universally accepted. Davis and Temte, discussing the effects of lidocaine and diphenylhydantoin (DPH), concluded that ''a reduction in rising velocity is not a necessary feature for antiarrhythmic activity'' (Davis and Temte, 1969). On the contrary, they concluded that ''the most significant effect of lidocaine with regard to its antiarrhythmic action is the prevention of decremental conduction in Purkinje fibers.'' They considered that diphenylhydantoin and propranolol acted in the same way as lidocaine. Bassett and Hoffman (1971) also took the view that ''DPH and lidocaine may abolish a reentrant rhythm by improving conduction. DPH either increases or does not substantially alter membrane responsiveness and conduction velocity.'' There are two reasons why it might be concluded that therapeutic concentrations of lidocaine would be insufficient to reduce the rate of depolarization ($\dot{V}_{max}$). The first is that if the extracellular potassium concentration is low, the resting potential will be hyperpolarized, and the depressant effect on $\dot{V}_{max}$ will be nullified (Singh and Vaughan Williams, 1971). The second is that lidocaine delays recovery from inactivation, but for a brief period only, so that if the interval between action potentials is long, no effect on $\dot{V}_{max}$ will be seen (Vaughan Williams, 1980). Both these points are of clinical significance, because lidocaine may be ineffective in patients in whom, perhaps as a result of diuretic therapy, serum potassium has fallen. Secondly, even when no effect on H-V conduction time or QRS is apparent in sinus rhythm, the class I effect of lidocaine could nevertheless be responsible for depressing or eliminating the conduction of premature ventricular beats, or for slowing a ventricular tachycardia. Recently, El-Sherif and Lazzara studied experimentally induced reentrant ventricular arrhythmias in the late myocardial infarction period in dogs, and found that, at the time at which lidocaine (El-Sherif et al., 1977) and DPH (El-Sherif and Lazzara, 1978) exerted an antiarrhythmic action, the effect of both drugs was to slow conduction. They concluded that ''there is currently no basis to substantiate the concept that both DPH and lidocaine can abolish reentrant rhythms by improving conduction in the reentrant pathway.''

Another complicating factor is that some drugs, notably lidocaine and mexiletine, shorten action potential duration (APD) in the ventricular conduction pathway, especially in the preterminal Purkinje fibers, in which APD is normally much longer than in the His bundle or ventricular muscle. This led Wittig and his colleagues (1973) to suggest that the shortening of APD could constitute an antiarrhythmic action, permitting premature action potentials to conduct slowly before the drug because they ''took off'' from partially depolarized tissue, and to conduct more rapidly after the drug, because they would, as a result of the shortening of APD, be initiated from fully repolarized cells.

There are several reasons for not accepting this hypothesis: 1, Even in isolated tissues, it is difficult to select proximally an interstimulus interval which will ensure that the second action potential takes off from distal partially repolarized cells. The repolarizing limb of the Purkinje fiber action potential is so steep that if the second stimulus arrives a few milliseconds too late, the membrane is already repolarized; if a little too early, the cell is refractory and there is no second potential. 2, Because the second potential conducts more slowly, it will lag behind the first, so that it will again take off from a fully repolarized membrane, and will then conduct as rapidly as the first. 3, There is no evidence that premature action potentials occurring in man, rather than from preparations artificially stimulated with paired stimuli, behave in this way. 4, There is abundant evidence in animals (Vaughan Williams, 1980) and man (Olsson et al., 1971) that shortening of APD is an arrhythmogenic factor. 5, The class I action of lidocaine provides a sufficient explanation for its antiarrhythmic effects. Thus, in my view, lidocaine is antiarrhythmic in spite of, rather than because of, the shortening of APD.

Nevertheless, shortening of APD in the ventricular conduction pathway is a fact which must have some explanation, and it was concluded from voltage clamp experiments on sheep Purkinje fibers by Arnsdorff and Bigger (1972) that lidocaine, at a concentration (2.14×10^{-5} M) "considered equivalent to clinical plasma antiarrhythmic levels," . . . "increased chord conductance for the potassium ion (g_k)." In contrast, Carmeliet and Saikawa (1982), who also studied sheep Purkinje fibers under voltage clamp, while observing that in the presence of lidocaine $1.85–3.7 \times 10^{-5}$ M "steady-state currents were shifted outward," they found that the "outward shift of current at the plateau level by lidocaine was not observed in the presence of tetrodotoxin (TTX): in Na-free medium the effect of lidocaine was totally suppressed." They concluded that "local anesthetics do not increase the K inward-rectifier current, and have no effect on background current at potentials negative to -60 mV." It would appear, therefore, that in Purkinje fibers, sodium channels are not fully inactivated at the potential of the plateau. Coraboeuf and Deroubaix (1978), in a study of canine Purkinje fibers, came to a similar conclusion, finding that TTX shortened APD, and stating that "the effect is probably due to the fact that in Purkinje fibers the TTX-sensitive steady-state sodium current flows in a larger potential range than in the myocardium."

All this recent work confirms that the actions of lidocaine and other class I drugs can be attributed to interference with recovery from inactivation of sodium channels, without involving other effects. Thus, the differences in clinical behavior of various class I compounds can be explained partly by the duration of their attachment to the channel, a topic to be discussed later (Vaughan Williams, 1984a), or to incidental other properties, such as anticholinergic action (quinidine, disopyramide), effects on the central nervous system (diphenylhydantoin, lorcainide, lidocaine, mexiletine), or differences in distribution and rate of removal.

Turning to the class II antiarrhythmic agents, the most exciting development in the past decade is the evidence, now, in spite of some criticism (Mitchell, 1981), indisputable after so many careful trials, that prolonged treatment of postinfarction patients with β-blockers can protect a significant number of them against reinfarction and sudden death (Wilhelmsson et al., 1974; Multicentre International Study, 1977; The Norwegian Multicenter Study Group, 1981; Beta-Blocker Heart Attack Trial Research Group, 1982). The reasons for the protection are unclear. It has been found in animals (Raine and Vaughan Williams, 1978; Raine and Vaughan Williams, 1981) and in man (Edvardsson and Olsson, 1981; Vaughan Williams et al., 1980), that long term β-blockade induces a significant prolongation of action potential duration and Q-T interval, greater than can be accounted for by any concomitant bradycardia, and since the phenomenon is observed uniformly throughout the myocardium, it could constitute a prophylactic (class III) antiarrhythmic action. The reason for the protection against reinfarction is equally unclear, but it has been found in animals that prolonged β-blockade induces increased capillarity of the ventricular myocardium, especially in the midwall (Tasgal and Vaughan Williams, 1981).

Whether or not prolongation of action potential duration is truly responsible for an antiarrhythmic effect has been doubted, because of a long known association between a prolonged Q-T interval and susceptibility to serious ventricular arrhythmias (Vaughan Williams, 1980). The topic will be discussed in greater detail later (Vaughan Williams, 1984b), but it is a fact that amiodarone, the initial class III agent, has proved to be spectacularly successful as an antiarrhythmic drug, especially for the treatment of atrial arrhythmias and for reentrant arrhythmias of the Wolff-Parkinson-White type (Rosenbaum et al., 1976). More recently, some other compounds which prolong action potential duration in a uniform manner, melperone (Millar and Vaughan Williams, 1982) and sotalol (Singh and Vaughan Williams, 1970), have also proved effective as antiarrhythmic agents in the clinic.

Finally, with regard to drugs with a class IV action, restricting slow inward current, some of the newer compounds have proved disappointing as antiarrhythmic remedies. The so-called "calcium antagonists" comprise a group of drugs which are widely different in chemical structure and tissue selectivity. Nifedipine, for example, acts primarily on smooth muscle, especially vascular smooth muscle, and its cardiac effects are less pronounced than those of verapamil. It has been suggested that although all cardiac tissues, apart from cells in and around the sino-atrial and atrio-ventricular nodes, are normally depolarized by fast inward (sodium) current, in ischemia or in other situations causing partial diastolic depolarization and inactivation of fast current, slow inward current may "take over," as it were, permitting the activation of slowly conducting action potentials to initiate reentry. The antiarrhythmic action of calcium antagonists is thus attributed to abolition of these abnormal slow depolarizations.

There are several reasons for doubting this hypothesis. 1, If it were true, verapamil should be especially effective in ventricular arrhythmias associated with ischemia. In practice, this is not so; the class I agents are more effective in these conditions. 2, Verapamil is most effective in controlling supraventricular arrhythmias involving the nodes, which are normally depolarized by slow inward current. 3, Arrhythmias induced by experimental ischemia originate in the border zone outside the ischemic region, and although the action potentials are of short duration, they are initiated by fast inward current.

Nevertheless, verapamil has been reported to be effective occasionally in ventricular arrhythmias associated with ischemia, and if the effect is not directly due to block of slow action potentials, what is the explanation? Cell-to-cell conduction is mediated through gap junctions, which provide a low resistance pathway for intracellular current. Recent evidence has indicated that these junctions may be closed or narrowed when the intracellular calcium concentration $[Ca]_i$ rises (Dahl and Isenberg, 1980). If the changes in $[Ca]_i$ which normally are associated with the activation of contraction are sufficient to affect gap-junction resistance, then a concentration of verapamil causing a negative inotropic effect by reducing $[Ca]_i$ should also decrease intercellular resistance. A secondary consequence should be an increase in conduction velocity. In our original paper on the electrophysiologic effects of verapamil, Singh and I had noted a dose-related increase in conduction velocity (Table 1), which we had found difficult to explain, although we did consider the possibility of reduced cell-to-cell resistance. "The core resistance includes the specialized contacts at the intercalated discs, which could be

Table 1 Effects of Verapamil on Spontaneous Rate, Maximum Drive Frequency, Electrical Threshold, Conduction Velocity, and Contraction Amplitude in Isolated Rabbit Atria.

Concentration of Verapamil	Spontaneous Rate	Maximum Drive Frequency	Electrical Threshold	Conduction Velocity	Contraction Amplitude
mg/l (μM)					
0.075 (0.152)	0	0	0	0	−32.8 (4.9)
0.15 (0.304)	0	0	0	0	−56.7 (4.3)
0.30 (0.608)	−8.6 (2.2)	+2.1 (1.3)	−3.9 (1.2)	+6.7 (1.9)	−67.4 (5.9)
1.0 (2.03)	−21.5 (3.1)	+3.9 (1.7)	−10.4 (2.8)	+16.8 (3.3)	−78.7 (8.2)
3.0 (6.08)	*	+14.1 (2.8)	−12.8 (3.1)	+19.7 (4.2)	−90.3 (9.4)

Each value indicated is a mean percentage change (± S.E.M.) from controls from three experiments. The observations were made after a steady-state was achieved at 60 min of exposure to drug.

*Spontaneous pacemaker frequency ceased in two preparations (at 30 min in one and at 42 min in the other); the atria could still be driven electrically.

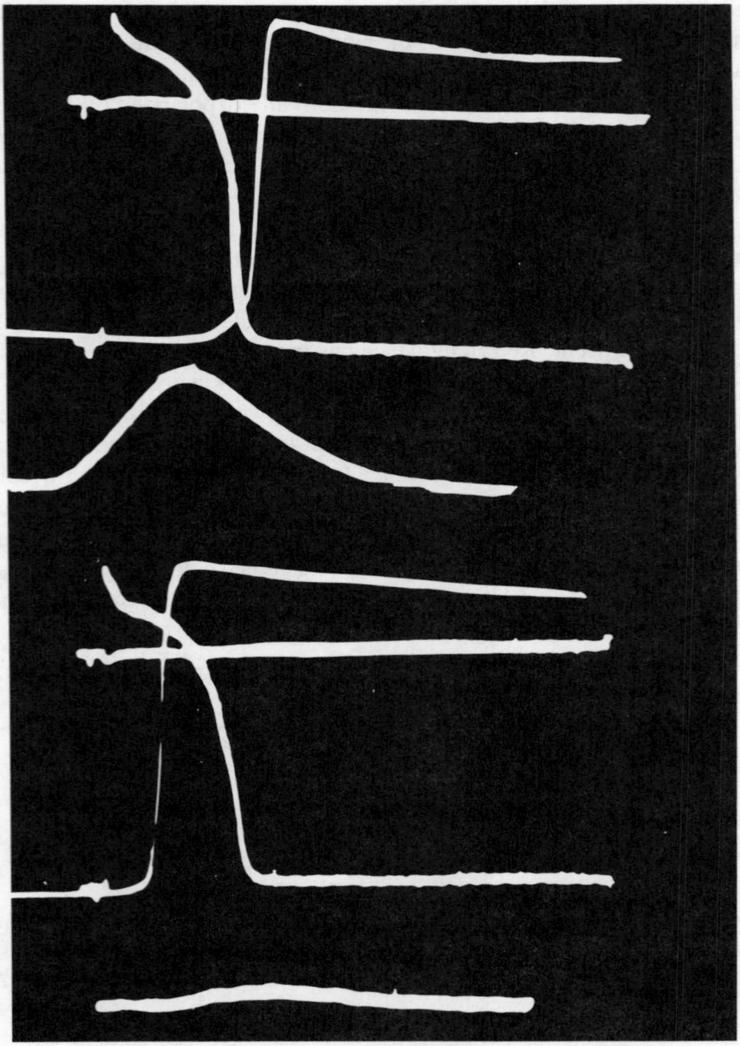

1 Effect of verapamil on intracellular potentials and contractions of rabbit ventricular muscle, paced at 1 Hz. In each panel, horizontal trace: zero potential with the microelectrode in the bath; middle traces: intracellularly recorded potentials at slow and fast sweep speeds; lowest trace: contraction at the slower sweep speed. Upper panel: control records. Vertical calibration: 1 g. Lower panel: in the presence of verapamil 2 μmol l^{-1}. Vertical calibration: 100 mv. Horizontal calibration 200 or 20 ms.

affected by drugs." We did not know then, of course, that gap junctions could be controlled by $[Ca]_i$. Another consequence of opening up gap junctions should be a smaller "foot" to the action potential, since the passive discharge of the membrane capacity into an approaching active region would have a shorter time constant. I therefore reviewed some original records and, to my surprise, noted that the foot of the ventricular action potential was greatly attenuated (Fig. 1).

I would like to suggest, therefore, that although the main antiarrhythmic effect of class IV drugs is on transitional cells in and around the nodes, which are normally depolarized by slow inward current, they may exert an indirect action in Purkinje cells and myocardial cells normally depolarized by fast inward current. The primary effect is still on slow inward current, of course, but because $[Ca]_i$ falls, gap junctions open up and conduction is improved. The effect is thus similar to that which lidocaine was once supposed to have, as already described. Considerable support has been given to this hypothesis in a recent paper by El-Sherif and Lazzara (1979), who found that, at the time at which experimental reentrant arrhythmias in the late myocardial infarction period were attenuated by verapamil and D600, although sinus rate and A-V conduction were slowed as expected, ventricular conduction was improved, and the dispersion of abnormal activity reduced. Both these findings would be consistent with improved intercellular coupling.

Summary

The past decade has seen the introduction of many new class I drugs, which restrict fast inward current. Furthermore, the action of lidocaine and diphenylhydantoin as class I agents which primarily depress conduction has been confirmed. The original class III drug, amiodarone, is increasingly in use as an antiarrhythmic of first choice for Wolff-Parkinson-White-type arrhythmias and for arrhythmias associated with hypertrophic myopathy, and as a reserve drug in resistant arrhythmias of other types. Other compounds delaying repolarization have been proven to be clinically effective as antiarrhythmics. Recent research suggests that inhibition of slow inward current may lead, as a secondary consequence of lowered $[Ca]_i$, to improved cell-to-cell conduction. Finally, all but one of the new antiarrhythmic drugs, none of which existed in 1972, have turned out to possess one or more of the four classes of action originally described. The single exception, alinidine, a selective bradycardic agent, may restrict anionic currents (Millar and Williams, 1981), which would constitute a fifth class of action, but this is far from proven.

References

Arnsdorf, M.F., and Bigger, J.T. 1972. Effect of lidocaine hydrochloride on membrane conductance in mammalian cardiac Purkinje fibers. J Clin Invest 51:2252–2263.

Bassett, A.L., and Hoffman, B.F. 1971. Antiarrhythmic drugs: electrophysiological actions. Annu Rev Pharmacol 11:143–170.

β-Blocker Heart Attack Trial Research Group. 1982. A randomized trial of propranolol in patients with acute myocardial infarction. JAMA 247:707–1714.

Carmeliet, E., and Saikawa, T. 1982. Shortening of the action potential and reduction of pacemaker activity by lidocaine, quinidine and procainamide in sheep cardiac Purkinje fibers. Circ Res 50:257–272.

Coraboeuf, E., and Deroubaix, E. 1978. Shortening effect of tetrodotoxin on action potentials of the conducting system in the dog heart. J Physiol 280:24P.

Dahl, G., and Isenberg, G. 1980. Decoupling of heart muscle cells: correlations with increased cytoplasmic calcium activity and with changes of nexus ultrastructure. J Membr Biol 53:63–75.

Davis, L.D., and Temte, J.V. 1969. Electrophysiological actions of lidocaine on canine ventricular muscle and Purkinje fibres. Circ Res 24:639–655.

Edvardsson, N., and Olsson, S.B. 1981. Effects of acute and chronic beta-receptor blockade on ventricular repolarization in man. Br Heart J 45:628–636.

El-Sherif, N., Scherlag, B.J., Lazzara, R., and Hope, R.F. 1977. Re-entrant ventricular arrhythmias in the late myocardial infarction period. 4. Mechanism of action of lidocaine. Circulation 56:395.

El-Sherif, N., and Lazzara, R. 1978. Re-entrant ventricular arrhythmias in the late myocardial infarction period. 5. Mechanism of action of diphenylhydantoin. Circulation 57:465–472.

El-Sherif, N., and Lazzara, R. 1979. Re-entrant ventricular arrhythmias in the late myocardial infarction period. 7. Effect of verapamil and D-600, and the role of the "slow inward current." Circulation 60:605–615.

Millar, J.S., and Vaughan Williams, E.M. 1981. Pacemaker selectivity. Influence on rabbit atria of ionic environment and of alinidine, a possible anion antagonist. Cardiovasc Res 15:335–350.

Millar, J.S., and Vaughan Williams, E.M. 1982. Differential actions on rabbit nodal, atrial, Purkinje cell and ventricular potentials of melperone, a bradycardic agent delaying repolarization: effects of hypoxia. Br J Pharmacol 75:109–121.

Mitchell, R.A. 1981. Timolol after myocardial infarction: an answer or a new set of questions? Br Med J 282:1565.

Multicentre International Study. 1977. Reduction in mortality after myocardial infarction with long-term beta-adrenoceptor blockade. Br Med J 2:419–421.

The Norwegian Multicenter Study Group. 1981. Timolol-induced reduction in mortality and reinfarction in patients surviving acute myocardial infarction. N Engl J Med 304: 801–807.

Olsson, S.B., Cotoi, S., and Varnauskas, E. 1971. Monophasic action potential and sinus rhythm stability after conversion of atrial fibrillation. Acta Med Scand 190:381–388.

Raine, A.E.G., and Vaughan Williams, E.M. 1978. Electrophysiological basis for the contrasting prophylactic efficacy of acute and prolonged beta-blockade. Br Heart J 40(Suppl):71–77.

Raine, A.E.G., and Vaughan Williams, E.M. 1981. Adaptation to prolonged beta-blockade of rabbit atrial, Purkinje, and ventricular potentials, and of papillary muscle contraction. Time-course of development of, and recovery from, adaptation. Circ Res 48:804–812.

Rosenbaum, M.B., Chiale, P.A., Halpern, M.S., Nau, G., Przybylski, J., Levi, R.J., Lazzari, J.O., and Elizari, M.W. 1976. Clinical efficacy of amiodarone as an antiarrhythmic agent. Am J Cardiol 38:934–944.

Singh, B.N., and Vaughan Williams, E.M. 1970. A third class of antiarrhythmic action. Effects on atrial and ventricular intracellular potentials, and other pharmacological actions on cardiac muscle, of MJ 1999 and AH 3474. Br J Pharmacol 39:675–687.

Singh, B.N., and Vaughan Williams, E.M. 1971. The effect of altering potassium concentration on the action of lidocaine and diphenylhydantoin on rabbit atrial and ventricular muscle. Circ Res 29:286–296.

Singh, B.N., and Vaughan Williams, E.M. 1972. A fourth class of antiarrhythmic action? Effect of verapamil on ouabain toxicity, on atrial and ventricular intracellular potentials, and on other features of cardiac function. Cardiovasc Res 6:109–119.

Szekeres, L., and Vaughan Williams, E.M. 1962. Antifibrillatory action. J Physiol 160: 470–482.

Tasgal, J., and Vaughan Williams, E.M. 1981. Stereological identification of capillary density gradients in the left ventricles of young rabbits, and effect of prolonged treatment with propranolol. J Physiol 315:353–367.

Vaughan Williams, E.M. 1970. Classification of antiarrhythmic drugs. In: E. Sandoe, E. Flensted-Jensen, and K.H. Olesen, eds. Symposium on Cardiac Arrhythmias. pp. 449–472. Sodertalje, Sweden: AB Astra.

Vaughan Williams, E.M. 1980. Antiarrhythmic Action. London: Academic Press.

Vaughan Williams, E.M. 1984a. Sub-divisions of class I drugs. In: H.J. Reiser and L.N. Horowitz, eds. Mechanisms and Treatment of Cardiac Arrhythmias: Relevance of Basic Studies to Clinical Management. Baltimore: Urban and Schwarzenberg.

Vaughan Williams, E.M. 1984b. Class III antiarrhythmic action and long Q-T interval. In: H.J. Reiser and L.N. Horowitz, eds. Mechanisms and Treatment of Cardiac Arrhythmias: Relevance of Basic Studies to Clinical Management. Baltimore: Urban and Schwarzenberg.

Vaughan Williams, E.M., Hassan, M.O., Floras, J.S., Sleight, P., and Jones, J.V. 1980. Adaptation of hypertensives to treatment with cardio-selective and non-selective beta-blockers. Absence of correlation between bradycardia and blood-pressure control, and reduction in the slope of the Q-T/R-R relation. Br Heart J 44:473–487.

Watanabe, Y., Dreifus, L.S., and Likoff, W. 1963. Electrophysiological antagonism and synergism of potassium and antiarrhythmic agents. Am J Cardiol 12:702–710.

Wilhelmsson, C., Vedin, J.A., and Wilhelmsen, L. 1974. Reduction of sudden deaths after myocardial infarction by treatment with alprenolol: preliminary results. Lancet (2): 1157–1160.

Wittig, J.H., Harrison, L.A., and Wallace, A.G. 1973. Electro-physiological effects of lidocaine on distal Purkinje fibres of canine heart. Am Heart J 86:69–78.

A. Antiarrhythmic Effects of Conduction-Slowing Agents (Class I)

Chapter 9

Subdivisions of Class I Drugs

E.M. Vaughan Williams

Antiarrhythmic drugs such as quinidine, lidocaine, and disopyramide appear so different from each other in clinical use, that many physicians have been reluctant to accept that they could have a fundamentally similar mode of antiarrhythmic action. Nevertheless, there are now good grounds for believing that all class I drugs do owe their antiarrhythmic property to a capacity to delay recovery from inactivation of sodium channels, so that fewer channels are available to depolarize cells at risk of premature excitation. The remedies differ from each other clinically, therefore, for a variety of other reasons, the most important of which are the following:

1. Some class I drugs are anticholinergic, the most potent in this respect being quinidine and disopyramide. Apart from the noncardiac complications of antimuscarinic actions, there are several cardiac consequences. In a patient with substantial background vagal activity, sinus tachycardia may supervene; or, more seriously, an atrial fibrillation or supraventricular tachycardia which was previously innocuous because impulses were blocked at the A-V node, may develop into ventricular tachycardia when A-V conduction is improved by the blockade of vagal tone. Secondly, the fact that the drugs depress A-V conduction by reason of their class I action may be masked by the simultaneous improvement in conduction caused by the anticholinergic effect, and the result may be no change in A-V conduction time.

In a patient with little vagal background, however, and with depressed A-V conduction, the full class I depression by quinidine or disopyramide will be revealed, and serious A-V block may occur (Birkhead and Vaughan Williams, 1977).

2. Distribution into the CNS varies considerably between class I drugs, and more information is required concerning the extent to which this is influenced by fat solubility, pK_a, and molecular size (Table 9-1). Certainly, dizziness and other CNS effects, even convulsions, limit the use of several class I drugs, including lidocaine, mexiletine, and lorcainide in high dosage, and quinidine also presents CNS problems in addition to its other side effects.

Table 9-1 Physiological Properties and Rates of Onset of Rate-Dependent Block for 11 Antiarrhythmic Drugs.

Drug	Fat Solubility log P	pk_a	Concentration μM	% Rate $\dot{V}_{max}$	Block Onset Rate (AP^{-1})	Recovery Time Constant(s)	Mol Wt
Lidocaine	2.76	7.8	200	40.4	(>0.6)		234
Mexiletine	1.3	9.3	20	49.2	(>0.6)	0.47	179
Tocainide	0.8	7.8	300	45.2	0.277		190
Disopyramide	1.8	8.4	100	50.9	0.113	12.2	339
ORG 6001	3.93	8.0	30	57.7	0.079	4.6	305
Quinidine	3.6	8.8	20	52.5	0.068		324
Procainamide	0.8	9.2	180	41.0	0.055		236
Flecainide	1.15	9.3	5	50.7	0.029	15.5	408
Encainide	0.91	10.2	3	50.0	0.025	20.3	358
Lorcainide	4.16	9.4	2	45.0	0.022	13.2	371
CCI 22277	7.19	9.5	2	68.0	0.014	80.4	463

Ventricular muscle paced at an interstimulus interval (ISI) of 300 ms. Figures are means (±S.E.M.). (AP = action potential. Block onset rate calculated as AP^{-1}).

Table 9-2 Elimination Half-Lives and Volumes of Distribution.

Drug	Elimination Half-life (h)	Volume of Distribution (l/kg)
Lidocaine	1.8	1.6
Mexiletine	13.0	6.6
Tocainide	13.0	2.8
Disopyramide	7.0	0.5
Quinidine	6.3	2.5
Procainamide	3.0	2.9
Flecainide	14.0	
Lorcainide	7.7	7.9
Aprindine	50.0	4.0

3. Metabolism and rates of excretion may vary enormously between drugs. Elimination half-life depends on both factors, and the rapid metabolism of lidocaine makes its oral use impracticable, since its half-life may be as short as 30 min in some patients. At the other extreme, aprindine has an elimination half-life of 2 1/2 days. The half-lives and volumes of distribution of nine class I drugs are given in Table 9-2 (Ronfeld, 1980).

4. There are wide variations in the rapidity with which the drugs become attached to and released from the sodium channels.

On the basis of early microelectrode studies it was long ago suggested that the antiarrhythmic action of the drugs examined at that time was due to their "interfering with the process by which (sodium) carrier is reactivated in response to repolarization" (Szekeres and Vaughan Williams, 1962). This interference might be accounted for if the drugs actually eliminated a proportion of the channels in some way, as tetrodotoxin is believed to do in nerves (Fig. 9-1C, left). The maximum rate of depolarization (MRD or $\dot{V}_{max}$) would thus be reduced, but the rate of recovery from inactivation of the remaining unblocked channels need not be affected, in which case there would be no change in refractory period, if it were measured as the shortest distance between a basal driving stimulus, S_1, and an interpolated premature stimulus, S_2, which could elicit a second response (Fig. 9-1, A and B, "programmed stimulation"). Alternatively, no channels need be permanently eliminated, but, instead, the recovery of sodium channels from inactivation could be delayed "until long after the time at which repolarization was already complete" (Szekeres and Vaughan Williams, 1962) (Fig. 9-1C, right).

At this point it is necessary to clarify the terms "effective and absolute refractory periods." Historically, the term "effective RP" was coined by Lewis (Lewis and Drury, 1926) in order to explain why quinidine might still reduce the frequency at which cardiac muscle could follow pacing stimuli, in spite of the fact that it had been shown by Love (1926) (Fig. 9-1A) that quinidine did not alter the "absolute refractory period" defined as the interval between S_1 and a third stimulus, S_3, which would abolish the response to S_2, even though S_2 was well outside the refractory period for S_1-S_2 alone.

S_3 did not evoke any response measurable at that time (Lewis and Drury, 1926) (Fig. 9-1A). With hindsight, it can be seen (Fig. 9-1B) that, if S_3 arrives just before the point at which sufficient sodium channels have recovered from inactivation to sustain propagation, there may, nevertheless, be enough recovered channels to induce a small depolarization, thus reversing the process of recovery and ensuring that the response to S_2 is now insufficient for propagation.

It was known from early studies (Vaughan Williams, 1958; Johnson and McKinnon, 1957) that the effect of quinidine in depressing the rate of depolarization was greater if the myocardium was paced at higher frequency. A drug which caused only a brief delay in the recovery from inactivation (e.g., lidocaine), might have no apparent effect on MRD at sinus rhythm, because diastole would be long enough to allow full recovery before the next beat (Vaughan Williams, 1980). A premature stimulus applied very early in diastole, however, would elicit a response with a depressed MRD, since it would arrive soon enough for recovery from inactivation to be still incomplete. Class I drugs might thus be subdivided on the basis of the varying extents to which they delayed recovery from inactivation after repolarization.

This problem has been investigated recently by T.J. Campbell, as part of his doctorate study program (Campbell and Vaughan Williams, 1982; Campbell, 1983). The effects of a number of class I drugs were examined on the maximum rate of depolarization in guinea pig ventricular muscle. After control responses to trains of stimulus had been recorded, the drugs were applied in the absence of stimulation. If the rate of depolarization in response to the first stimulus after a period of exposure to the drug was slower than that observed before the drug application, the effect, expressed as a percentage reduction from control, was termed "resting block."

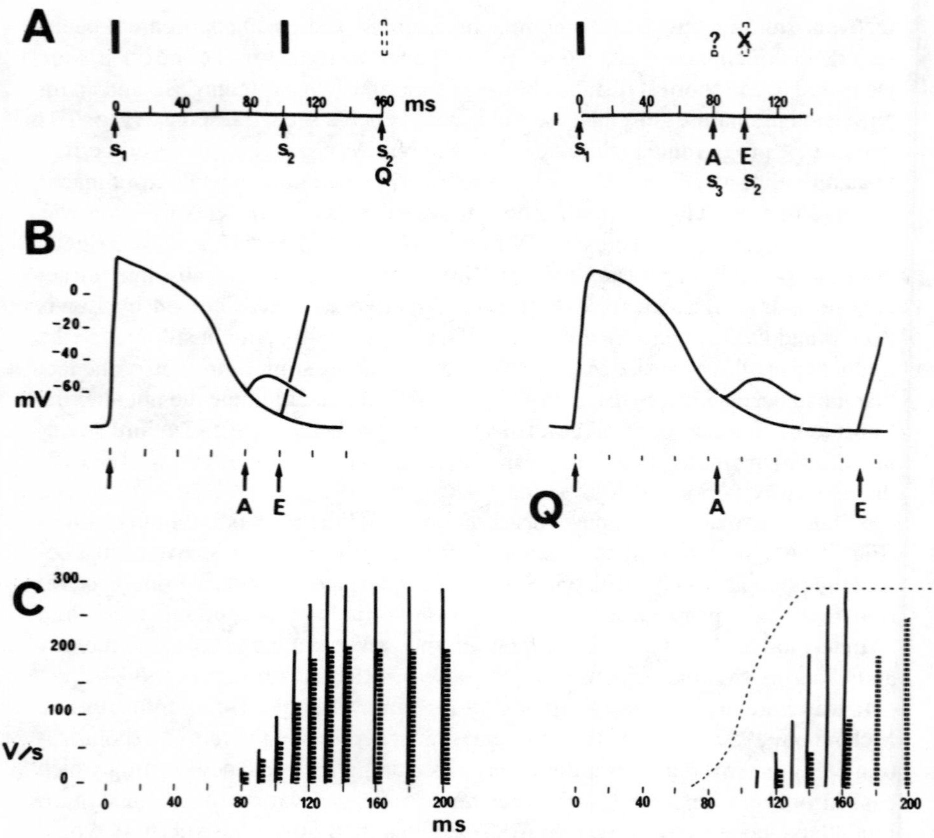

9-1 Time dependence of disappearance of inactivation of fast inward current in contracting muscle (from reference: Vaughan Williams, 1980). A, left, Lewis measured refractory period as the shortest interval between a stimulus (S_1) causing a recordable response, and a second stimulus (S_2) causing another recordable response. Quinidine lengthened refractory period, thus defined. Right, Love (1926) measured refractory period as the shortest interval between S_1 and an interpolated stimulus S_3 which would abolish a previously observed response to S_2. This interval (S_1-S_3) was called the "absolute" refractory period (A) by Lewis, and the S_1-S_2 interval above was renamed the "effective" refractory period (E). The query above S_3 indicates that this stimulus must have had some effect, which abolished the response to S_2, although it produced no recordable response itself. B, the action potential recorded before (left) and after (right) exposure to quinidine. Stimulation at the absolute refractory period (A) causes a local response, which delays further the disappearance of inactivation of fast inward channels (thus explaining Love's results). Quinidine increases this delay, so that the return of excitability is dissociated from repolarization, and the effective refractory period is postponed until long after repolarization is complete. C, MRD (V/s) in response to stimuli at various times in the wake of an action potential with the same duration as that depicted in B above. Left, solid lines, controls; interrupted lines, MRD on the assumption that 40% of channels were eliminated, but that no additional de-

The tissue was then stimulated by further trains of stimuli, at various frequencies similar to those applied before the drug, until the depression of MRD had settled to a stable level. The latter, expressed as a percentage reduction from the MRD of the first response in the train, may be termed "frequency-dependent" or "rate-dependent" block. It was found that with some drugs, the new steady-state level was not achieved until after a long series of stimuli, i.e., the frequency-dependent block was slow in onset. With others, on the other hand, the new steady-state was achieved within one or two beats. The results of experiments on 11 class I agents are presented in Table 9-3, the concentrations having been chosen (from many dose-response curves) as those which produced approximately a 50% steady-state reduction in MRD.

The drugs have been arranged in order of rapidity of onset of frequency-dependent block (expressed as the fraction of the ultimate block per beat), and fall into the three distinct groups. Lidocaine, mexiletine, and tocainide had a very rapid onset (one or two beats only for full effect); flecainide, encainide, lorcainide and CCI 22277 (a new antiarrhythmic with a steroid structure) were of very slow onset; and the remainder required 10–20 beats to reach the steady-state at the stimulation frequency chosen (3.3 Hz). The drugs in the slow onset group were far more potent than the others. In the fast group, mexiletine was 10 times

Table 9-3 Rates of Onset of Rate-Dependent Block for 11 Antiarrhythmic Drugs.

Drug	Concentration μM	% Rate-dependent Depression of $\dot{V}_{max}$	Rate of Onset of Block (AP^{-1})	Time Constant of Recovery (s)
Lidocaine	200	40.4 (2.1)	Very fast	
Mexiletine	20	49.2 (7.7)	Very fast	0.471 (0.036)
Tocainide	300	45.2 (3.6)	0.277 (0.029)	
Disopyramide	100	50.9 (2.1)	0.113 (0.007)	12.2 (1.0)
ORG 6001	30	57.7 (1.9)	0.079 (0.004)	4.6 (0.5)
Quinidine	20	52.5 (2.3)	0.068 (0.005)	
Procainamide	180	41.0 (2.2)	0.055 (0.003)	
Flecainide	5	50.7 (5.0)	0.029 (0.002)	15.5 (0.5)
Encainide	3	50.0 (3.5)	0.025 (0.006)	20.3 (0.9)
Lorcainide	2	45.0 (4.1)	0.022 (0.004)	13.2 (1.3)
CCI 22277	2	68.0 (3.6)	0.014 (0.001)	80.4 (7.4)

Ventricular muscle paced at an interstimulus interval (ISI) of 300 ms. Figures are means (± S.E.M.). (AP = action potential).

(9-1 *continued*)
lay was introduced between repolarization and the disappearance of inactivation of the surviving channels. Right, the dotted line represents the peaks of the control MRD measurements depicted on the left. The vertical lines depict MRD on the assumption that no fast channels were eliminated, but that a moderate (solid lines) or substantial (interrupted lines) additional delay was introduced between repolarization and the disappearance of inactivation. The first case resembles the effect of lidocaine, and shows that no effect on MRD would be observed unless the frequency of stimulation reduced the interstimulus interval to less than 160 ms.

more potent than lidocaine, and 15 times more potent than tocainide, but was about equipotent with quinidine and ORG 6001 (another steroid) in the intermediate group.

When MRD had reached its steady-state value in a train, stimulation was arrested, and a single stimulus applied at varying times after the end of the train. When the rate of depolarization in response to this single stimulus became as fast as that in response to the first stimulus in the train, recovery was considered to be complete. It was found that, for all drugs, the rate of recovery followed a single exponential time course, and was independent of drug concentration. The time constants for recovery (τ_{re}) of seven of the drugs studied have also been presented in Table 9-3, and fall into exactly the same groups as for rates of onset, drugs with the fastest onset recovering most rapidly.

More than a decade ago it was suggested that class I drugs "have a variety of chemical structures, but are mostly lipophilic" and "are taken up into the primary membrane, from where they press their attack on the sodium channels." Class I action by the local anesthetic type of drug may involve restriction of the freedom of charged elements controlling the ion gates to move in response to changes of voltage across the membrane (Vaughan Williams, 1972). Others have preferred a model in which local anesthetics gain access to the sodium channel from the inside of the cell and are attached to it in ionized form. Since, however, to gain access to the cell interior, the drugs probably traverse the membrane in uncharged form, the pK_a is of interest as well as the fat solubility (expressed as log P, the octanol-water partition coefficient). These values, and the molecular weights of the drugs studied, are presented in Table 9-1. It is clear that there was a correlation ($r = 0.94$) between molecular weight and the time constant of recovery, and these two parameters have been plotted in Figure 9-2. The conclusion to be drawn from this very close correlation is that, although fat solubility and dissociation constant may influence access to the sodium channels, once the agent has become attached, the main determinant of the strength of binding is molecular size, implying attachment by short range Van der Waal's forces rather than by electrostatic forces.

From the clinical point of view, the main interest of the above subdivision of class I drugs into fast, intermediate, and slowly dissociating groups is that the intermediate group corresponds to the original class I agents (A), which caused some prolongation of refractory period and slowing of conduction, even in sinus rhythm. Some other class I drugs introduced later (lidocaine, mexiletine, tocainide) formed a second subgroup (B) which had little effect on conduction at normal heart rates, but which prolonged refractory period as measured by programmed stimulation. The slowest group (C) includes some very recently studied drugs, such as encainide (Harrison et al., 1980), which depress conduction and widen QRS even at slow heart rates, but which have little effect on the refractory period measured by interpolated stimuli.

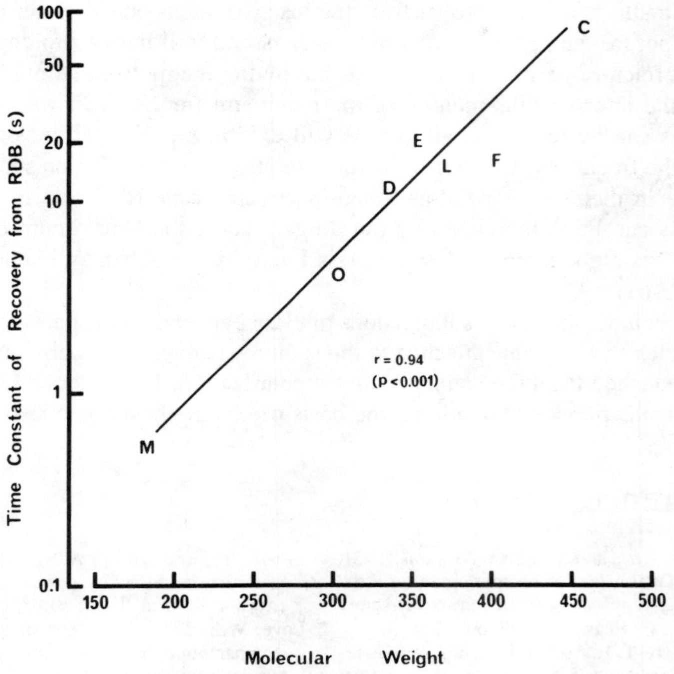

9-2 Positive correlation between the log of the time constant of recovery from rate-dependent block (RDB) (τ_{re}), M = mexiletine, 10 μM; O = ORG 6001, 60 μM; D = disopyramide, 20 μM; E = encainide, 6 μM; L = lorcainide, 2 μM; F = flecainide, 5 μM; C = CCI 22277, 4 μM.

With lidocaine and the other "fast-on, fast-off" drugs, very high concentrations are required to block a substantial number of sodium channels. Class I drugs are attached to the channel in its inactivated form. If a drug is rapidly detached during diastole, many more channels are inactivated at the beginning of diastole than at the end. Thus, MRD may be depressed detectably only if a test stimulus is applied during the first 50–100 ms after repolarization. Refractory period is prolonged if it is measured by a premature stimulus interpolated on a slow basal frequency (Fig. 9-1C, right). With the third group of class I drugs, attachment to the sodium channel is so strong that virtually the same number of channels is inactivated at the end as at the beginning of diastole. Consequently, there is no change in refractory period measured by an interpolated stimulus, but the threshold will be augmented, and MRD will be slower, because the total number of available channels is reduced (Fig. 9-1C, left). The remaining channels, however, without any drug attached, will recover from the inactivation as quickly after repolarization as before, and programmed refractory period will not be prolonged.

If "refractory period" is measured, not by the interpolated stimulus method, but as the interstimulus interval of the maximum frequency at which a pacing stimulus can be followed, all groups will exhibit a prolongation, because the higher the frequency, the longer the total duration of time in which sodium channels are in their depolarized-and-then-inactivated state (the state in which the channels can be immobilized by the drugs). Thus, the "maximum driven frequency" is a good general test for class I activity (Vaughan Williams and Szekeres, 1961).

To conclude, the above subdivisions of class I agents, on the basis of the speed with which they become attached to the sodium channels after activation and become detached from the channels after repolarization, fits remarkably well with subdivisions previously made on the basis of electrophysiologic tests in man.

References

Birkhead, J.S., and Vaughan Williams, E.M. 1977. Dual effect of disopyramide on atrial and atrio-ventricular conduction and refractory periods. Br Heart J 33:657–660.

Campbell, T.J. 1983. Resting and rate-dependent depression of maximum rate of depolarization ($\dot{V}_{max}$) in guinea-pig ventricular action potentials by mexiletine, disopyramide and encainide. J Cardiovasc Pharmacol 5:291–296.

Campbell, T.J., and Vaughan Williams, E.M. 1982. Electrophysiological and other effects in rabbit hearts of CCI 22277, a new steroidal antiarrhythmic drug. Br J Pharmacol 76:337–345.

Harrison, D.C., Winkle, R., Sami, M., and Mason, J. 1980. Encainide: a new and potent antiarrhythmic agent. Am Heart J 100:1046–1054.

Johnson, E.A., and McKinnon, M.G. 1957. The differential effect of quinidine and pyrilamine on the myocardial action potential at various rates of stimulation. J Pharmacol Exp Ther 120:460–468.

Lewis, T., and Drury, A.N. 1926. Revised views of the refractory period, in relation to circus movement. Heart 13:95–100.

Love, W.S. 1926. The effect of quinidine and strophanthin upon the refractory period of the tortoise ventricle. Heart 13:87–93.

Ronfeld, R.A. 1980. Comparative pharmacokinetics of new antiarrhythmic drugs. Am Heart J 100:978–983.

Szekeres, L., and Vaughan Williams, E.M. 1962. Antifibrillatory action. J Physiol 160: 470–482.

Vaughan Williams, E.M. 1958. The mode of action of quinidine on isolated rabbit atria interpreted from intracellular potential records. Br J Pharmacol 13:276–287.

Vaughan Williams, E.M. 1972. Biophysical background to beta-blockade. In: New Perspectives in Beta-Blockade. Horsham: CIBA.

Vaughan Williams, E.M. 1980. Antiarrhythmic Action. London: Academic Press.

Vaughan Williams, E.M., and Szekeres, L. 1961. A comparison of tests for antifibrillatory action. Br J Pharmacol 17:424–432.

Chapter 10

Class I Antiarrhythmic Agents: Diversity of Action

Jeffrey L. Hill

Introduction

Since the original proposition of Vaughan Williams to classify antiarrhythmic agents according to their effect on action potential characteristics (Vaughan Williams, 1970), many schemes have been devised to group agents according to their basic electrophysiologic properties (Gettes, 1979). In most cases, the comparisons are made using normal tissues under relatively normal conditions. An understanding of the mechanism(s) of antiarrhythmic action of class I agents requires consideration of a variety of properties in addition to the basic electrophysiologic actions of reducing action potential upstroke and conduction slowing. Class I agents have been subclassified into three groups according to the effect on action potential duration of normal isolated cardiac tissue. It is important to consider these additional electrophysiologic effects in order to appreciate the antiarrhythmic activity of a class I agent. Although class I antiarrhythmic agents share the electrophysiologic property of slowing conduction in cardiac tissues, the extent of conduction slowing at a given extracellular concentration of the agent depends on several factors. These same factors often influence other electrophysiologic actions of the agent, such as the effect on action potential duration. The intent of this chapter is to review some of these factors which provide for diversity of antiarrhythmic action among the class I agents. Indeed, not all agents are influenced by these factors in the same way or to the same degree. Basic electrophysiologic considerations (Rosen and Danilo, 1984; Wit, 1984) and current viewpoints of classification of antiarrhythmic agents (Vaughan Williams, 1984) are presented elsewhere in this book.

Subclassification of Class I Agents

Class I antiarrhythmic agents have been subclassified into three groups according to their effects on action potential duration in isolated cardiac tissue (usually Purkinje fibers). Table 10-1 illustrates these groups and includes many of the

Table 10-1 Subclassification of Class I Antiarrhythmic Agents.

A Prolong APD	B Shorten APD	C No Effect on APD
Quinidine	Lidocaine	Encainide
Procainamide	Diphenylhydantoin	Lorcainide
Disopyramide	Aprindine	Flecainide
Ajmaline	Ethmozin	Propafenone
Tricyclics	Mexiletine	
Pirmenol	Tocainide	
Prajmalium		
ORG 6001		
Cibenzoline		

APD = Action potential duration.

agents currently studied. The importance of the additional ability of a class I agent to prolong, shorten, or to have no effect on action potential duration in the manifestation of the antiarrhythmic effect is not well understood. However, the shortening of action potential duration has been considered to be an important factor in the arrhythmogenesis associated with some of the agents in this group (Olsson et al., 1971).

The above subclassification has been compared to that obtained by grouping the agents according to the effect of stimulation rate on the degree of slowing of the action potential upstroke (Vaughan Williams, 1984; Campbell, 1983). A detailed discussion of this relationship and a consideration of the physical-chemical properties of these agents in regard to the rate of interaction of the agent with the membrane channel is provided in another chapter.

Factors to Consider

Several factors important to consider in the diversity of antiarrhythmic activity among class I agents are shown in Table 10-2. Class I agents affect automaticity, conduction, and refractoriness by varying degrees, both quantitatively and qualitatively. Specific examples regarding automaticity have been described in Chapter 4 (Rosen and Danilo, 1984). The relationship between changes in conduction relative to refractoriness for a given agent and the extent to which prolongation of action potential duration is of additional benefit for antiarrhythmic activity is not yet apparent. For example, in a reentrant ventricular tachycardia, a delicate balance exists between conduction and refractoriness to perpetuate the arrhythmia. Interruption of the reentry pathway could be affected by changes in conduction or refractoriness, or both. The impact of prolonged refractoriness due to lengthening of action potential duration and the combination of this effect with slowed conduction has not been characterized.

An evaluation of the electrophysiologic basis for an agent to produce antiarrhythmic effects must also consider the fiber type. In many cases, class I agents have qualitatively as well as quantitatively different effects on Purkinje fibers com-

Table 10-2 Diversity of Class I Antiarrhythmic Drug Activity: Factors to Consider.

Automaticity vs conduction vs refractoriness
Fiber type
Disease state (normal vs ischemic/infarcted)
Rate (use) dependency
Normal vs premature beat
Tissue distribution
Ca^{2+} antagonism
Actions on/by the autonomic nervous system
Actions on/by the central nervous system
Cardiac Depression
Side effects
Duration of action

pared to ventricular muscle fibers. These differences are particularly evident in the effects on action potential duration (Millar and Vaughan Williams, 1981).

A factor readily identified but not yet fully appreciated in the diversity of response among class I agents is the electrophysiologic action of the agent in normal versus ischemic or infarcted myocardial tissues. One example of this phenomenon is the well known effect of lidocaine on conduction in ischemic tissue (Allen et al., 1978; Kupersmith et al., 1975). Lidocaine slows conduction and prolongs refractoriness in the ischemic zone without affecting conduction in the nonischemic tissue. This type of effect is not limited to drug-induced changes in conduction. Recent studies have shown the effects of class I agents on action potential duration (APD) to vary between ischemic or infarcted and normal zones, and also in the margin between these zones. Figure 10-1 illustrates an example of the variation in the effect of encainide on APD of isolated rabbit ventricular muscle fibers recorded in normal and ischemic tissues (Wong et al., 1982). Low concentrations of encainide, a class IC agent, had little effect on APD of normal cells, but lengthened APD of cells that were ischemic for 30 min. The APD had been shortened, relative to nonischemic cells; thus encainide reduced the disparity of APD between these two regions. The authors consider the potential for this effect to be part of the mechanism of antiarrhythmic action for encainide.

Similar studies conducted with procainamide, a class IA agent, indicate procainamide to have significantly different actions on APD of cat ventricular muscle cells located in the zone of acute infarction (90–120 min) than in cells located in a zone of healed infarction, 2–4 months following infarction (Myerburg et al., 1982). Procainamide prolonged the APD of the muscle cells in the acutely infarcted zone, while it had little effect on APD recorded from cells in the healed infarct zone (Fig. 10-2). APD of the cells in the normal zone was always prolonged by procainamide. In both cases, the disparity between APD was reduced. However, the mechanism for this increase in homogeneity was different in these two situations employing the same antiarrhythmic agent. The authors were able to rule out differences in tissue distribution of procainamide as a possible explanation for these effects.

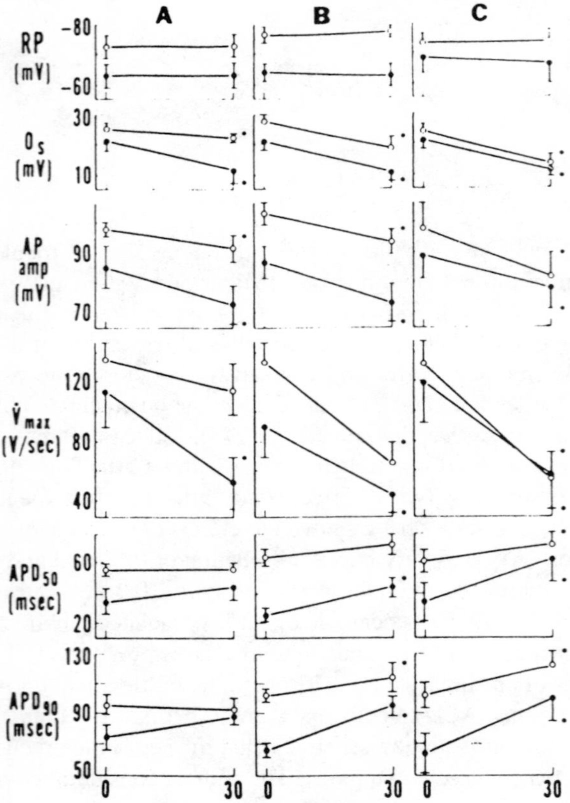

10-1 The effects of encainide on the action potential characteristics of stimulated ventricular muscle cells from the ischemic zone and the normal tissues surrounding the ischemic region. For each concentration of encainide: 10^{-6} M (A), 5×10^{-6} M (B), and 10^{-5} M (C), changes in resting potential (RP), overshoot (OS), AP amplitude (AP amp), $\dot{V}_{max}$, APD_{50}, and APD_{90} at 30-min exposure are shown. The open circles show data from normal cells, while the filled circles show data from depressed cells in the ischemic zone. *$p < 0.05$. (Figure and legend reproduced with permission from Wong et al.: European Journal of Pharmacology, Elsevier Press, 1982.)

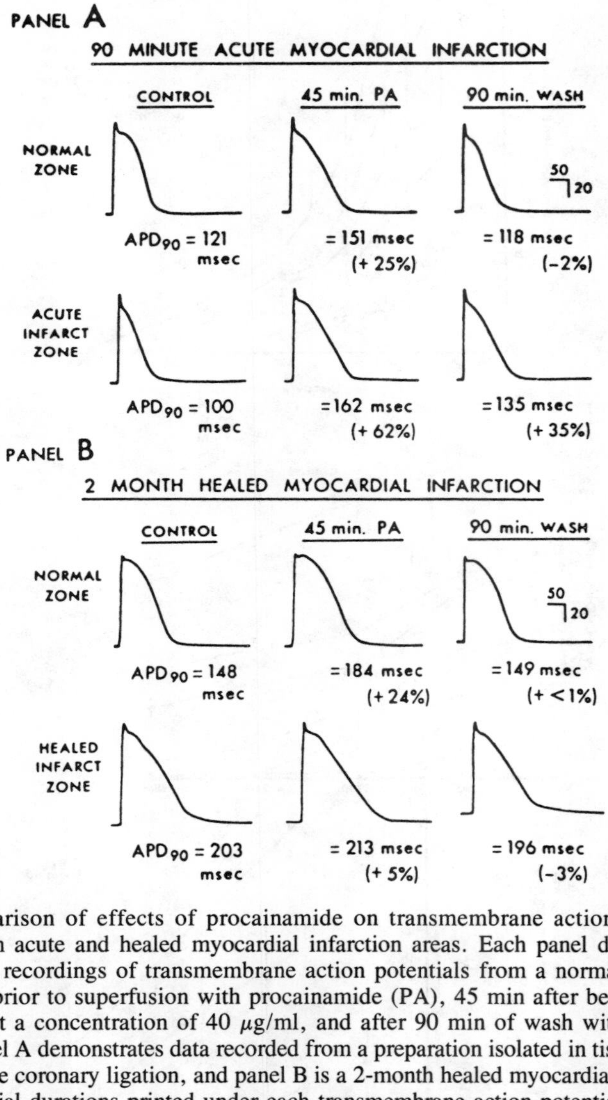

10-2 Comparison of effects of procainamide on transmembrane action potentials recorded from acute and healed myocardial infarction areas. Each panel demonstrates simultaneous recordings of transmembrane action potentials from a normal zone and infarct zone prior to superfusion with procainamide (PA), 45 min after beginning PA superfusion at a concentration of 40 μg/ml, and after 90 min of wash with Tyrode's solution. Panel A demonstrates data recorded from a preparation isolated in tissue bath 90 min after acute coronary ligation, and panel B is a 2-month healed myocardial infarction. Action potential durations printed under each transmembrane action potential recording were measured at 90% repolarization (APD_{90}) and the percentages in parentheses under APD_{90}'s compare APD_{90} during and after PA superfusion to control for each recording. Horizontal calibration = 50 ms, vertical calibration = 20 mv. (Reproduced with permission from Myerberg et al.: Circulation Research, American Heart Association, 1982.)

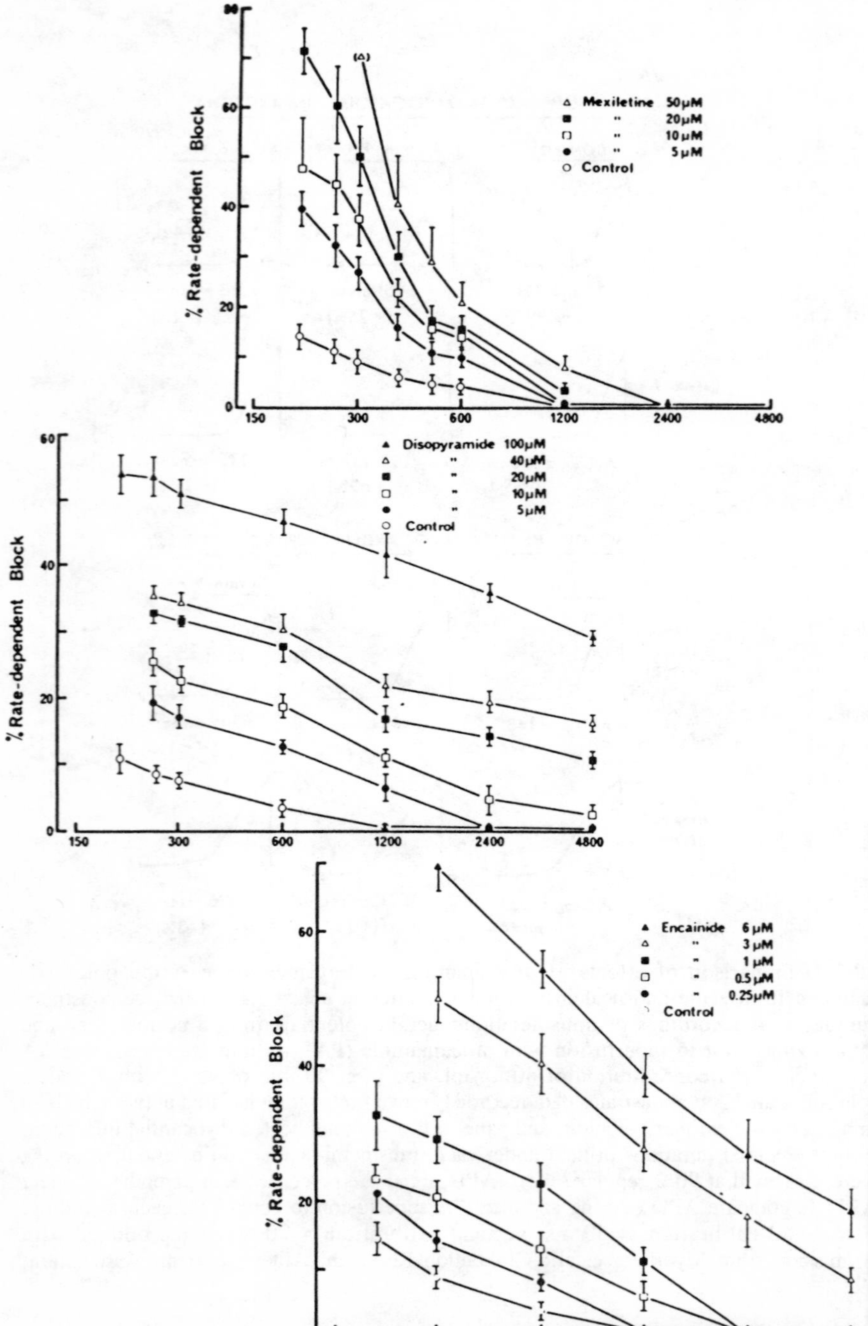
Mexiletine 50μM
" 20μM
" 10μM
" 5μM
Control
% Rate-dependent Block
Disopyramide 100μM
" 40μM
" 20μM
" 10μM
" 5μM
Control
Encainide 6μM
" 3μM
" 1μM
" 0.5μM
" 0.25μM
Control
150
300
600
1200
2400
4800
Inter-stimulus Interval (ms)

A factor described earlier and discussed in more detail by Vaughan Williams (Vaughan Williams, 1984) is the effect of interstimulus interval and stimulation rate on the drug-induced conduction block. Disopyramide (IA), mexiletine (IB), and encainide (IC) have been shown to produce rate-dependent (or use-dependent) block in guinea pig ventricular muscle fibers (Campbell, 1983). The onset and recovery from the rate-dependent block varied among the three agents (Fig. 10-3). Mexiletine exhibited the fastest response to a sudden change in stimulation frequency; disopyramide was the slowest, while encainide was intermediate. Some of the differences in the antiarrhythmic effects observed in vivo may be explained by the kinetic differences observed in studies such as this.

Another factor to consider in the diversity of a class I agent in regard to its potential for antiarrhythmic activity, is the effect of the agent on the premature action potential. This concept is not new to the study of action potential upstroke and intramyocardial conduction. However, only limited information exists concerning the diversity of class I effects on action potential duration of the premature beat. In fact, most class I agents shorten the premature APD. Figure 10-4 illustrates an example of prolongation of APD of premature beats delivered at early intervals in man following the administration of mexiletine (Harper et al., 1979). Mexiletine prolonged the monophasic APD recorded at the right ventricular outflow tract without significantly affecting the nonpremature APD. The authors suggest that this effect is potentially important in the antiarrhythmic activity of this drug. Further investigation into this concept may yield yet another method for the classification or subclassification of antiarrhythmic agents based on APD effects of the premature beat.

One other electrophysiologic effect to consider in the diversity of class I antiarrhythmic agents is the property of calcium antagonism. Agents such as quinidine (Grant and Katzung, 1976) and a newer agent, cibenzoline (Millar and Vaughan Williams, 1982) have been shown to have some component of calcium antagonist activity (class IV) in addition to their primary effect to slow sodium-dependent action potential upstroke and conduction. Other agents, propafenone, for example, may have β-adrenergic blocking (class II) activity in addition to the class I effect.

There are several nonelectrophysiologic parameters that are important in the diversity of antiarrhythmic action of agents in this class. The distribution of an antiarrhythmic agent between normal and abnormal tissues plays an important role in

10-3 Relationships between rate, expressed as the log of the interstimulus interval (ISI), and the per cent of rate-dependent reduction in $\dot{V}_{max}$ at various concentrations of mexiletine (top panel), disopyramide (middle), and encainide (bottom). The points are means +/−S.E. (n = 5 in each case). The highest concentration of mexiletine produced inexcitability at ISI of 300 ms in three of five preparations, and the average of the remaining two experiments is plotted in brackets. (Note that the scale on the vertical axis is different for mexiletine from that used for the other two drugs.) (Reproduced with permission from Campbell, Terence J.: J. Cardiovasc Pharmacol:5, Raven Press, 1983.)

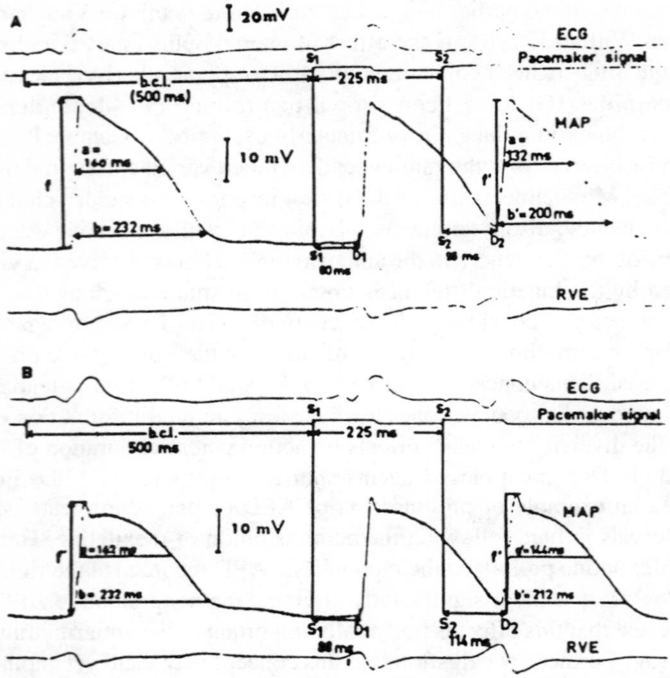

10-4 Monophasic action potential (MAP) recordings from subject No. 6 demonstrating the effect of mexiletine on an early induced ectopic beat. Panel A, control recording. Panel B, recording after mexiletine. Note that the MAP durations of the basic paced beats are very similar. The MAP durations of the induced ectopic beat, however, are longer after mexiletine. In addition, mexiletine has increased both the S_1-D_1 interval and the S_2-D_2 interval. The voltage calibration of the MAP signal is 4 times that of the ECG and RVE. (Reproduced from Harper et al., (1979), with permission.)

the homogeneity of electrophysiologic effect in the ischemic heart. The physical-chemical nature of the compound, the time of administration of the compound relative to ischemic injury, and the biochemical environment presented to the compound upon its delivery to the affected myocardium, may influence tissue concentrations and thus electrophysiologic actions at various sites within the myocardium. Zipes et al. (1982) have shown the myocardial distribution of aprindine to be widely variable depending on time of administration relative to the induction of the ischemic episode. Furthermore, weak bases such as quinidine and lidocaine distribute between extracellular and intracellular compartments according to the pH gradient. The pH of the ischemic myocardium varies markedly in different regions in the ischemic heart (Hill et al., 1981), and thus, weak bases will distribute preferentially to areas of lower pH (assuming some degree of perfusion is maintained).

Other nonelectrophysiologic effects important in the diversity of action of the class I agents include: direct or indirect actions involving the central and autonomic nervous systems, cardiac depression, cardiac and non-cardiac side effects, and duration of action. The involvement of each of these factors varies in scope and intensity among the different agents. In some cases, the agent may influence one or more of these factors; while in other cases such as autonomic tone, the factor may influence the electrophysiologic action of the antiarrhythmic agent. These factors have been extensively reviewed by others (Vaughan Williams, 1984) and are important upon considering the activity and clinical utility of any antiarrhythmic agent.

Summary and Conclusions

The extent to which a class I antiarrhythmic agent slows conduction, prolongs refractoriness, and shortens or lengthens action potential duration depends on a variety of factors. These factors, which may be present to varying degrees, must be considered alone and in combination before an understanding of the mechanism of antiarrhythmic action can be appreciated. It is often difficult to predict whether the antiarrhythmic agent or subgroup of agents will prove efficacious in the treatment of a presented cardiac arrhythmia. Electrophysiologic actions of the agent, in addition to those seen routinely in isolated normal tissues, are often altered to a varying degree in the diseased heart. Discrepencies between effects on normal and ischemic or infarcted tissues are well established. Uncertainty of the actual mechanism of antiarrhythmic action often arises when the basic electrophysiologic actions of an agent are considered in normal versus abnormal tissue. This uncertainty is more readily apparent and, potentially, more serious as one moves from animal studies to man. As new experimental techniques develop and as a better understanding of the mechanisms for arrhythmogenesis is achieved, our approach to the effective and safe treatment of cardiac arrhythmias (or, at least, an understanding of our limitations) will improve. The factors considered in the diversity of action of class I agents that have been provided in this chapter may, of course, be extrapolated to other classes of antiarrhythmic agents.

References

Allen, J.D., Brennan, F.J., and Wit, A.L. 1978. Actions of lidocaine on transmembrane potentials of subendocardial Purkinje fibers surviving infarcted canine hearts. Circ Res 43:470–481.

Campbell, T.J. 1983. Resting and rate-dependent depression of maximum rate of depolarisation ($\dot{V}_{max}$) in guinea pig ventricular action potentials by mexiletine, disopyramide, and encainide. J Cardiovasc Pharmacol 5: 291–296.

Gettes, L.S. 1979. On the classification of antiarrhythmic drugs. Mod Concepts Cardiovasc Dis 48:13–18.

Grant, A.O., and Katzung, B.G. 1976. Effect of quinidine and verapamil on electrically induced automaticity in the ventricular myocardium of guinea pig. J Pharmacol Exp Ther 196:407–419.

Harper, R.W., Bertil Olsson, S., and Varnauskas, E. 1979. Effect of mexiletine on monophasic action potentials recorded from the right ventricle in man. Cardiovasc Res 13(6):303–310.

Hill, J.L., McCown, P.M., and Gettes, L.S. 1981. Relationship between changes in extracellular pH and K^+ during acute myocardial ischemia. Circulation (suppl).

Kupersmith, J., Antman, E.M., and Hoffman, B.F. 1975. In vivo electrophysiological effects of lidocaine in canine acute myocardial infarction. Circ Res 36:84–91.

Millar, J.S., and Vaughan Williams, E.M. 1981. Pharmacological mapping in the rabbit heart. Br J Pharmacol 74:827P.

Millar, J.S., and Vaughan Williams, E.M. 1982. Effects on rabbit nodal, atrial, ventricular and Purkinje cell potentials of a new antiarrhythmic drug, cibenzoline, which protects against action potential shortening in hypoxia. Br J Pharmacol 75:469–478.

Myerburg, R.J., Bassett, A.L., Epstein, K., Gaide, M.S., Kozlovskis, P., Wong, S.S., Castellanos, A., and Gelband, H. 1982. Electrophysiological effects of procainamide in acute and healed experimental ischemic injury of cat myocardium. Circ Res 50:386–393.

Olsson, S.B., Cotoi, S., and Varnauskas, E. 1971. Monophasic action potential and sinus rhythm stability after conversion of atrial fibrillation. Acta Med Scand 190:381–388.

Rosen, M.R., and Danilo, P., Jr. 1984. In: H.J. Reiser and L.N. Horowitz, eds. Mechanisms and Treatment of Cardiac Arrhythmias: Relevance of Basic Studies to Clinical Management. Baltimore: Urban and Schwarzenberg.

Vaughan Williams, E.M. 1970. Classification of antiarrhythmic drugs. In: E. Sandøe, E. Flensted-Jensen, K.H. Olsen, eds. Symposium on Cardiac Arrhythmias. pp. 449–472. Sodertalje, Sweden:AB Astra.

Vaughan Williams, E.M. 1984. In: H.J. Reiser and L.N. Horowitz, eds. Mechanisms and Treatment of Cardiac Arrhythmias: Relevance of Basic Studies to Clinical Management. Baltimore: Urban and Schwarzenberg.

Wit, A.L. 1984. In: H.J. Reiser and L.N. Horowitz, eds. Mechanisms and Treatment of Cardiac Arrhythmias: Relevance of Basic Studies to Clinical Management. Baltimore: Urban and Schwarzenberg.

Wong, S.S., Myerburg, R.J., Ezrin, A.M., Gelband, H., and Bassett, A.L. 1982. Electrophysiologic effects of encainide on acutely ischemic rabbit myocardial cells. Eur J Pharmacol 80:323–329.

Zipes, D.P., Prystowsky, E.N., and Heger, J.J. 1982. Electrophysiologic testing of antiarrhythmic agents. Am Heart J 103:610–615.

Chapter 11

Class I Antiarrhythmic Agents: Classification, Electrophysiologic Considerations, and Clinical Effects

N. A. Mark Estes, III, Hasan Garan, Brian McGovern, and Jeremy N. Ruskin

Introduction

In the past 15 years, multiple classification schemes for antiarrhythmic agents have been proposed, categorizing drugs according to their influences on isolated cardiac tissues (Vaughan Williams, 1970; Hoffman and Bigger, 1971; Singh and Vaughan Williams, 1971; Singh and Hauswirth, 1974; Vaughan Williams, 1975; Rosen et al., 1975; Gettes, 1979; Hauswirth and Singh, 1979; Singh et al., 1980). Although once the subject of considerable controversy, there is increasing uniformity of thought about classification of antiarrhythmic drugs. Of the many proposed systems, that of Vaughan Williams in 1970 is the most widely used. In this classification system, antiarrhythmic drugs are placed into four classes based primarily on their cellular electrophysiologic effects (Table 11-1). Drugs which alter the transmembrane action potential and particularly the maximal rate of rise of depolarization ($\dot{V}_{max}$) are included in class I. Class II drugs are those with antisympathetic or sympatholytic effects. Agents which prolong action potential duration without significantly altering $\dot{V}_{max}$ are classified as class III. Finally, a separate category, class IV, exists for agents that block the slow inward calcium channel currents (Singh and Vaughan Williams, 1971).

Table 11-1 Vaughan Williams Classification of Antiarrhythmic Agents.

Class	Effect	Prototype
I	Local anesthetic action	Quinidine
II	β-adrenergic blockade	Propranolol
III	Prolong action potential repolarization	Amiodarone
IV	Calcium channel blockade	Verapamil

Limitations of this and other classification systems have become increasingly apparent as antiarrhythmic agents with greater pharmacologic diversity are introduced and as the mechanisms of actions of drugs are better defined with the use of more clinically appropriate and relevant experimental models (Singh and Vaughan Williams, 1971; Singh and Hauswirth, 1974; Rosen et al., 1975; Spear and Moore, 1982). Current classification systems tend to obscure similarities among drugs in different classes and, more importantly, differences among drugs in the same class. This is particularly true for the broad category of class I drugs which now include agents with a wide spectrum of basic and clinical electrophysiologic effects. To illustrate, lidocaine and quinidine are both categorized as class I drugs with local anesthetic properties. Both block the rapid inward sodium current in vitro. The effect of lidocaine is strongly voltage-dependent and far greater in partially depolarized tissues such as ischemic myocardium than in normal fibers (Kupersmith et al., 1975). Lidocaine causes a dose-dependent decrease in the steady-state $\dot{V}_{max}$ that becomes much more pronounced when resting potential is made less negative. By contrast, quinidine depresses $\dot{V}_{max}$ equally in normally and partially depolarized fibers at all levels of resting potential, and its effect is strongly rate-dependent (Gettes, 1981).

A classification system based on the electrophysiologic effects of antiarrhythmic drugs promotes a more rational basis for therapeutic decisions in the treatment of clinical arrhythmias. To that end, three subcategories of class I agents recently have been proposed, based on the distinct electrophysiologic properties of the drugs in each category (Harrison, 1981). It is the purpose of this chapter to explore further this new classification scheme for class I drugs. Although it is not the authors' intent to review the basic electrophysiologic effects of these agents, certain fundamental electrophysiologic properties that are relevant to clinical observations will be noted. Finally, the current advantages and limitations of this proposed division of class I agents will be reviewed.

Definition of Class I Agents

Class I drugs can be divided into three distinct subgroups as presented in Table 11-2. Class IA drugs are those that depress phase 0 of the action potential, prolong conduction, and slow repolarization, and include quinidine, procainamide, and disopyramide (Sekiya and Vaughan Williams, 1963). Lidocaine and the lidocaine-like drugs, mexiletine, and tocainide constitute class IB (Roos et al., 1976; Winkle et al., 1976). Electrophysiologic characteristics of these agents include the shortening of repolarization, and increase in fibrillation thresholds with little effect on phase 0 of the action potential in normal myocardium. Finally, agents that depress phase 0 markedly, affect repolarization minimally, and result in a profound slowing of conduction are categorized as class IC. Encainide, fle-

Table 11-2 Modified Class I Based on Cellular Electrophysiologic and Clinical Profiles.

Class	Action
IA	Depress phase 0 Slow conduction Prolong repolarization
IB	Little effect on phase 0 in normal tissue Depress phase 0 in abnormal fibers Shorten repolarization
IC	Markedly depress phase 0 Profound slowing of conduction Slight effect on repolarization

cainide, lorcainide, and propafenone are included in this group (Hodess et al., 1979).

Electrophysiologic Considerations

Through detailed studies of the cellular electrophysiologic effects of antiarrhythmic agents, it is possible to predict some of the action of antiarrhythmic drugs on specific cardiac tissues and their effects on clinical arrhythmias (Bassett and Hoffman, 1971; Gettes, 1981; Hoffman, 1981). The effect of class IA, IB, and IC drugs on such basic parameters as conduction velocity, length of refractory periods, action potential amplitude and duration, maximal rate of depolarization ($\dot{V}_{max}$), maximum diastolic potential, phase 4 automaticity, and membrane responsiveness are well characterized and are summarized in Table 11-3 (Bassett and Hoffman, 1971; Singh et al., 1980; Gettes, 1981; Campbell, 1983).

All class I agents can act on the fast inward sodium current and can diminish $\dot{V}_{max}$ in a dose-dependent fashion through a number of mechanisms (Bigger, 1980). Partial block of the fast inward channel has a number of predictable effects on electrical activity such as slowing conduction velocity and prolonging the time of recovery from inactivation (Luckstead and Tarr, 1972; Ducouret, 1975). By contrast, only in very high concentrations does lidocaine (class IB) reduce gNa, slow conduction, or prolong repolarization in normal myocardium (Bigger and Mandel, 1970; Davis and Temte, 1969). Class IC drugs tend to cause marked slowing of conduction relative to class IA or IB drugs as a result of their more profound effects on the fast inward channel and $\dot{V}_{max}$ (Kesteloot and Stoobandt, 1977; Hodess et al., 1979; Duff et al., 1981; Hellestrand et al., 1982; Keefe et al., 1982; Abitol et al., 1983). The action potential amplitude is decreased by both IA and IC agents.

Table 11-3 Basic Electrophysiologic Effects of Class I Drugs in Normal Cardiac Tissue.

Class	Cond Vel	ERP	APA	APD	$\dot{V}_{max}$	Onset of RDB	MDP	V_{th}	Phase 4	Memb Resp
IA	↓	↑↑	↓	↑	↓	Inter	↓	↑	↓	↓
IB	↓	0	0	↓	↓	Fast	0	0	↓	↓
IC	↓↓	↑	↑	0	↓↓	Slow	↓	↑	↓	↓

Cond Vel = conduction velocity; ERP = effective refractory period; APA = action potential amplitude; APD = action potential duration; $\dot{V}_{max}$ = maximal rate of rise of upstroke (phase 0) of action potential; RDB = rate-dependent block; MDP = maximum diastolic potential; V_{th} = threshold voltage for fiber activation; Memb Resp = membrane responsiveness.

Key: ↑ = increase; ↓ = decrease; ↑↑ = marked increase; ↓↓ = marked decrease; 0 = no change; Inter = intermediate.

Quinidine and other class I drugs shorten the plateau phase of the action potential but prolong the repolarization phase (Weld et al., 1982). The magnitude of increase in the effective refractory period (ERP) caused by class IA drugs is greater than the increase in the action potential duration (APD) in normal cardiac tissue. Class IB drugs shorten the effective refractory period less than they shorten the action potential duration (Kupersmith et al., 1975). Drugs in both classes prolong the effective refractory period relative to the action potential duration. However, it is evident that quinidine- and lidocaine-like drugs affect the ERP to APD relationship through different mechanisms. Class IA drugs do so by decreasing the membrane responsiveness, as defined by the $\dot{V}_{max}$ to V_m relationship, so that the maximal rate of phase 0 depolarization and conduction velocity is decreased at any given transmembrane voltage. Class IB drugs cause a dose-dependent decrease in the steady-state $\dot{V}_{max}$ that becomes much more pronounced when the resting potential (V_m) becomes less negative in abnormal fibers (Chen et al., 1975). Thus, conduction is slowed at any given resting membrane potential with more pronounced results at less negative potentials (Singh and Vaughan Williams, 1971). Lidocaine-like drugs reduce membrane responsiveness to stimuli delivered at low transmembrane voltages and shift the curve on its voltage axis in a direction opposite to that seen with class IA drugs (Gettes, 1981). Lidocaine slows the recovery kinetics of $\dot{V}_{max}$, which is the other determinant of refractoriness besides action potential duration. Accordingly, it will cause $\dot{V}_{max}$ and conduction of a premature response to be slower than would be anticipated from the membrane potential from which the response originates. Lidocaine's slowing of conduction with partially depolarized myocardium or with premature impulses may contribute to its antiarrhythmic effects. By contrast, quinidine does not significantly alter recovery kinetics of $\dot{V}_{max}$ after premature beats.

Recent observations regarding the kinetics of onset of rate-dependent depression of $\dot{V}_{max}$ by various class I drugs provide an attractive theoretical explanation for the clinical electrophysiologic effects of class IA, IB, and IC agents. Using standard microelectrode techniques, class I agents were found by Campbell to fall into three well demarcated subgroups with fast (lidocaine, mexiletine, tocainide), intermediate (quinidine, disopyramide, procainamide), or slow (flecainide, encainide, lorcainide) onset of rate-dependent depression of $\dot{V}_{max}$ (Campbell, 1983). All class I drugs demonstrate progressive enhancement of their depressant effects on $\dot{V}_{max}$ with increasing frequency of stimulation (rate-dependent block). However, the rate at which $\dot{V}_{max}$ declines to a new plateau following a sudden increase in frequency shows marked differences among the class I agents. When considered in terms of the onset of rate-dependent block, the class I drugs fall into three distinct subgroups with fast, intermediate, and slow kinetics corresponding to the subgroups IB, IA, and IC, respectively. The lidocaine-like drugs were found to prolong the effective refractory period relative to the action potential duration. The "slow" drugs (class IC) had only minor effects on this parameter. The quinidine-like drugs produced small to moderate increases in the effective refractory period relative to action potential duration. The class IB agents significantly prolonged the action potential duration which was shortened by the "fast" drugs. The differences observed between drugs in their onset kinetics and prolongation of effective refractory period relative to action potential duration is a consequence of their differing abilities to prolong recovery of the sodium channel from inactivation (Campbell, 1983).

The speed with which a class I drug responds to a sudden increase in pacing rate by further depressing $\dot{V}_{max}$ seems to be a factor in determining the ability of that drug to prolong the effective refractory period relative to the action potential duration (Campbell, 1983). Consideration of the kinetics of interaction of class I antiarrhythmic agents with the sodium channel in vitro allows insights into a number of clinical observations with these drugs. Of the "fast" kinetics group, Campbell found that only mexiletine significantly increases the effective refractory period in therapeutic concentrations (Campbell, 1983). The class IB agents combine the effect of decreasing the action potential duration and increasing the ratio of effective refractory period to action potential duration. This is consistent with the clinical reports showing little change in the ventricular effective refractory period, except in toxic doses (Josephson et al., 1972; McComish et al., 1977). The class IC drugs which have a marked effect on cardiac conduction and the slowest onset of rate-dependent block have the least effect on the ratio of effective refractory period to action potential duration, and prolong the effective refractory period only moderately as suggested by clinical reports (Hellestrand et al., 1982; Campbell, 1983).

The broad category of class I drugs is thus extremely diverse electrophysiologically when one examines the basic electrophysiologic effects of the individual antiarrhythmic agents. Categorization of the antiarrhythmic agents into subgroups based on these considerations promotes a clearer understanding of both their electrophysiologic and antiarrhythmic actions. For example, the mechanisms by which class IA, IB, and IC agents affect automatic arrhythmias due to enhanced phase 4 depolarization vary. A property common to all of the class I drugs is the suppression of phase 4 depolarization (Bigger, 1972). Inhibition of diastolic depolarization by decreasing the slope of phase 4 depolarization frequently abolishes clinical arrhythmias due to enhanced automaticity. Class IA and IC drugs have the unique effects of decreasing the maximal diastolic potential and increasing the threshold voltage. These properties are not shared by the class IB drugs. A decrease in the maximum diastolic potential and an increase in the threshold for fiber activation caused by class IA and IC drugs will extend the cycle length of an automatic arrhythmia that is not terminated by these agents.

Clinical Effects of Class IA, IB, and IC Antiarrhythmic Agents

The clinical electrophysiologic effects of class IA, IB, and IC drugs are summarized in Table 11-4. Whereas both class IA and IC agents depress sinus node function, those in class IB are generally without significant effects on the sinus node (Lippestad and Forfang, 1971; Seipel and Breithardt, 1976; Horowitz et al.,

Table 11-4 Electrophysiologic Effects of Class I Drugs on Various Cardiac Tissues.

Cardiac Tissue	Parameter	IA	IB	IC
Sinus node	Sinus node recovery time	↑	0	↑
Atrium	Conduction	↑	0	↑↑
	ERP	↑↑	0	↑
A-V node	Conduction	0	0	0
	ERP			
	Normal	0	0	0
	Antegrade fast pathway	—	—	0
	Retrograde fast pathway	↑	—	↑↑
His-Purkinje system	Conduction	↑	0	↑↑
	ERP			
	Antegrade	↑	↓	—
	Retrograde	↑	—	—
Ventricle	Conduction	↑	0	↑↑
	ERP	↑	0	↑
Accessory A-V pathway	Conduction			
	Antegrade	↑	0	↑↑
	Retrograde	↑	0	↑↑
	ERP			
	Antegrade	↑	↑	↑↑
	Retrograde	↑	0	↑↑

ERP = effective refractory period.

Key: ↑ = increase; ↓ = decrease; ↑↓ = increase or decrease; 0 = no change; ↑↑ = marked increase; — = sufficient data not available.

1978; Bigger and Reiffel, 1979; Kasper et al., 1979). The direct effect of quinidine is to depress sinus node automaticity, but its indirect effects tend to increase the resting heart rate because of its α-blocking and vagolytic effects (Schmid et al., 1974; Hoffman et al., 1975). In the denervated human heart, quinidine slows the sinus rate minimally, whereas in the presence of an intact autonomic nervous system, quinidine may cause an increase in the sinus rate by cholinergic blockade or a reflex increase in sympathetic activity (Mason et al., 1977). Depression of sinus node activity in humans by lidocaine or other class IB drugs is unusual but can occur in subjects with preexisting sinus node dysfunction (Cheng and Wadhwa, 1983; Bigger and Reiffel, 1979). Mexiletine has not shown any consistent effect on the sinus node automaticity in man (Roos et al., 1976; McComish et al., 1977). Flecainide has been shown to decrease the rate of sinus node discharge in animal models (Campbell et al., 1981; Vik-mo et al., 1982). In patients with no preexisting abnormalities of sinus node function, flecainide is reported to have no significant effect on the basic sinus rate (Somani, 1980; Granrud et al., 1981; Hodges et al., 1982). However, two recent clinical studies have shown prolongation of sinus node recovery time after flecainide administration (Anderson et al., 1981; Vik-mo et al., 1982). Lorcainide results in a slight increase in the heart rate with a prolongation of the sinus node recovery time (Keefe et al., 1982). In general, class I drugs exert no clinically significant effects on the normal sinus node. However, both class IA and IC drugs may have profound depressant effects in patients with preexisting sinus node dysfunction.

Conduction via specialized atrial fibers and the effective refractory period of atrial myocardium is unaffected by class IB agents. This would be expected as lidocaine-like drugs cause no significant change in the action potential duration of either ordinary or specialized atrial fibers (Mandel and Bigger, 1971). By contrast, class IA agents increase the effective refractory period in the atrium and depress intra-atrial conduction (Singh et al., 1980). These differences may account for the clinical observation that these agents have a salutary effect in suppressing atrial flutter and fibrillation.

Lidocaine causes substantial decreases in the action potential duration of Purkinje fibers and ventricular muscle (Bigger and Mandel, 1970); the greatest changes are seen in those regions of the His-Purkinje system in which the action potential duration is longest (Wittig et al., 1973). Clinically, prolongation of conduction through the normal His-Purkinje system is not seen with class IB drugs. With ischemia, low $[K_o]$, or partial depolarization by stretch, significant increases in the H-V interval have been reported with lidocaine (Bigger and Mandel, 1970; Kupersmith et al., 1975; Bigger, 1980; Rosen et al., 1976). The effective refractory period of the His-Purkinje system decreases after lidocaine (Arnsdorf and Bigger, 1972). These electrophysiologic effects are representative of those caused by other class IB agents such as tocainide and mexiletine (Anderson et al., 1978; Horowitz et al., 1978; Swedberg et al., 1978).

Both class IA and IC agents slow the rate at which an excitatory stimulus is propagated through the His-Purkinje system and myocardium. Class IC drugs have a particularly marked effect on the conduction velocity on the His-Purkinje system (Cocco and Strazzi, 1976; Kasper et al., 1979; Sami et al., 1979a; Sami et al., 1979b; Somani, 1980; Olsson and Edvardsson, 1981; Hellestrand et al., 1982; Vik-mo et al., 1982). Both these classes of drugs increase the duration of the effective refractory period of the ventricular specialized conduction system. Generally, this increase is substantially greater with class IA than IC agents. Drugs from both classes shift the threshold potential (V_{th}) to more positive values and excitability is thereby reduced. Block of the fast inward sodium channel modifies the action potential and its propagation. Action potential amplitude and $\dot{V}_{max}$ decrease and the impulse propagates less rapidly and becomes a less effective stimulus for adjacent fibers. This decrease in excitability accounts for the ability of antiarrhythmic agents to prevent or interrupt a reentrant circuit (Hoffman, 1981). It will be recalled that reentry, which is the mechanism responsible for many tachyarrhythmias, has as prerequisites two functional pathways with block of impulse conduction over one and slowed conduction over the other (Moe, 1975). In theory, antiarrhythmic drugs may affect reentrant arrhythmias by prolonging conduction, converting unidirectional block into bidirectional block, or by improving conduction and abolishing unidirectional block.

In contrast to class IA and IC drugs, class IB agents do not substantially alter the effective refractory period or conduction velocity in normal ventricular myocardium. However, in the nondepressed myocardium, lidocaine might improve conduction of premature beats and eliminate unidirectional block. This effect is related to lidocaine's ability to shorten action potential duration. As a result, premature responses arising from incompletely repolarized fibers with less negative membrane potentials might arise from a more completely repolarized fiber in the presence of lidocaine. The $\dot{V}_{max}$ of this fiber starting from a more negative membrane potential would be increased. A more rapid rate of depolarization and the resulting increase in conduction velocity might prevent reentry. However, there is now a substantial body of evidence that lidocaine, by virtue of its differential effects on normal and abnormal partially depolarized myocardium, acts primarily by prolonging or blocking conduction in abnormal myocardium (Noneman and Jones, 1983). Additionally, lidocaine could minimize the dispersion of refractory periods between areas of diseased and normal myocardium. These and other potential effects of class I agents on the proposed electrophysiologic mechanisms of cardiac arrhythmias are summarized in Table 11-5.

Class IA and IC agents affect an increase in both the effective refractory periods and a reduction in the conduction velocity in ventricular myocardium. Whereas the magnitude of the increase in refractory periods is generally greater for class IA than IC agents, the slowing of conduction is far greater for class IC than IA agents. It is evident that these alterations in conduction and refractoriness

Table 11-5 Effects of Class I Antiarrhythmic Agents on Electrophysiologic Mechanisms of Cardiac Arrhythmias.

	Class		
Effect on Arrhythmia	IA	IB	IC
Suppression of enhanced automaticity	+	+	+
Suppression of abnormal automaticity	+	+	+
Suppression of triggered activity	−	−	−
Prevention of reentry by removing unidirectional block	−	+	−
Prevention of reentry by converting unidirectional block to bidirectional block	+	+	+

Key: + = effective; − = ineffective.

within the ventricular myocardium might promote bidirectional block and prohibit the propagation of impulses through a reentrant circuit. An increase in action potential duration and duration of refractoriness prevents reentrant excitation if the effective refractory period of some portion of the reentrant pathway prolongs, such that it exceeds, the transit time of an impulse within the circuit. The reported effect of procainamide on ventricular premature depolarizations supports this notion (Giardina, 1973). From these considerations regarding the antiarrhythmic mechanism of class IC agents, the potential for proarrhythmic effects can also be appreciated. The perpetuation of a reentrant arrhythmia requires that the effective refractory period of the tissues in the circuit be less than the product of the conduction velocity and the length of the circuit. Class IC agents such as flecainide, by decreasing conduction velocity more than the effective refractory period of various myocardial tissues, may, in theory, facilitate reentry. Although the precise mechanisms for proarrhythmic effects of class IC agents remain to be elucidated, the recent reports of worsening of arrhythmias associated with administration of these drugs emphasizes their potential toxicity (Lui et al., 1982; Hohnloser et al., 1983; Nathan et al., 1984).

To the extent that the calcium-dependent inward current mediates conduction through the normal A-V node, it is expected that agents which have no effect on this current would not affect conduction through or refractoriness in this tissue. As noted in Table 11-4, neither the conduction velocity nor the effective refractory period of the A-V node is affected significantly by class IA, IB, or IC agents. However, in patients with multiple functional pathways within the A-V node, both IA and IC agents have been noted to prolong selectively the effective refractory period of retrograde fast A-V nodal pathways with little effect on the effective refractory period of antegrade A-V nodal pathways (Gomes et al., 1979; Hellestrand et al., 1982). Flecainide in particular has been demonstrated to have a marked effect on the effective refractory period and conduction velocity of retrograde fast A-V nodal pathways. The theoretic implications regarding the potential efficacy of this agent for A-V nodal reentrant tachycardias are confirmed by preliminary trials of the drug in patients with this arrhythmia (Hellestrand et al., 1982). A-V nodal reentrant tachycardia was terminated acutely with intravenous flecainide in 8/9 patients in whom the arrhythmia could be reproduced during electrophysiologic studies. This termination was due to retrograde fast A-V nodal pathway block in seven patients and antegrade slow pathway block in one patient. The tachycardia cycle lengths were increased by an average of 33% by flecainide.

The effects of class I agents on antegrade and retrograde conduction and refractory periods of extranodal accessory pathways are summarized in Table 11-4. Although class IA agents prolong these parameters, and therefore, frequently are effective in terminating or preventing atrioventricular reciprocating tachycardias, the effects of class IC agents are more marked (Kasper et al., 1979; Mandel et al., 1973; Wellens and Durrer, 1973). In a recent report, in 18 patients with accessory A-V pathways, the antegrade and retrograde effective refractory period of the bypass tracts were increased significantly with complete antegrade block occurring in three patients and complete retrograde block in eight patients (Hellestrand et al., 1982). Orthodromic A-V reciprocating tachycardia was terminated successfully with flecainide in 12/14 patients. As would be expected, the tachycardia termination was due to retrograde accessory pathway block in the majority of cases (11 of 12 patients). Because of retrograde conduction delay in the accessory pathway, the tachycardia cycle length increased an average of 31% after flecainide administration. The drug also prevented reinitiation of the reciprocating tachycardia by programmed stimulation in 6/14 patients. Lorcainide has also been reported to be effective in the management of patients with preexcitation by similar effects on accessory pathways (Kasper et al., 1979).

By contrast, class IB drugs are less effective in prolonging conduction and refractoriness in anomalous A-V pathways (Rosen et al., 1972). Akhtar et al. (1981) reported that intravenous lidocaine had no effect or produced acceleration of the ventricular response during atrial fibrillation in a group of 10 patients with accessory pathways. The effective refractory period of the bypass tract could be determined by the extrastimulus technique after lidocaine in five patients. It showed no change in two patients, a decrease of 10–20 ms in two, and an increase of 50 ms in one. Reports exist of shortening of the antegrade effective refractory period of extranodal bypass tracts in patients receiving mexiletine; these observations need further investigation (McComish et al., 1977). It is evident from these electrophysiologic data that class IC agents are likely to prove more effective than class IA agents in the treatment of reentrant supraventricular tachycardia. Additionally, it is likely that type IB agents will be of little value in the therapy of this group of tachyarrhythmias.

The electrophysiologic effects of class I drugs on various clinical parameters of conduction and repolarization are presented in Table 11-6. These are largely predictable from the cellular electrophysiologic effects of these agents which have

Table 11-6 Clinical Electrophysiologic and Electrocardiographic Effects of Class I Drugs in Normal Cardiac Tissue.

	Intervals					
Class	A-H	H-V	P-R	QRS	Q-T	J-T
IA	↑↓	↑	0	↑	↑↑	↑↑
IB	0	0	0	0	0	0
IC	↑	↑↑	↑	↑↑	↑	0

Key: ↑ = increase; ↓ = decrease; ↑↓ = increase or decrease; 0 = no change; ↑↑ = marked increase.

been considered above. Class IB agents are generally free of significant clinical electrophysiologic effects in normal cardiac tissues. Class IA agents tend to have a more marked effect on repolarization than conduction. This is reflected in uniform increases in the Q-T interval on the surface electrocardiogram. Additionally, the J-T interval, an index of repolarization that controls for prolongation of the Q-T due to QRS widening (Q-T − QRS = J-T) is lengthened significantly by quinidine-like drugs. Class IC agents tend to have a far more marked effect on conduction and a lesser effect on repolarization. This is manifest as a prolongation of the A-H, H-V, P-R, and QRS intervals without a significant effect on the J-T interval (Duff et al., 1980).

Conclusion

Based on these electrophysiologic effects, conventional and investigational antiarrhythmics can be divided according to this modified classification system as shown in Table 11-7. These divisions are made on the basis of the predominant electrophysiologic effects of the agents. It should be emphasized that none of the various attempts to categorize antiarrhythmics satisfactorily accounts for all experimental and clinical observations. It is evident that for drugs whose electrophysiologic properties are characterized incompletely, such as ethmozin and aprindine, reevaluation may be necessary as more is learned about the agent (Kaverina et al., 1978). It is also apparent that difficulties with classification arise when agents have properties of more than one class. Aprindine, for example, has electrophysiologic effects of classes IA, IB, and IC. Thus, aprindine shortens the duration of the action potential and the effective refractory period of Purkinje fibers (Verdonck et al., 1974; Steinberg and Greenspan, 1976; Elharrar et al., 1977; Stoel and Hagemeijer, 1980). However, aprindine also slows the sinus rate and prolongs the refractory period and conduction through the A-V node, lengthens the A-H and H-V intervals and transmural left ventricular conduction time and increases the effective refractory periods of the ventricle (Elharrar et al., 1975). Sotalol, a class II β blocking agent, also has class III electrophysiologic effects in that it prolongs action duration. Despite these shortcomings, this classification emphasizes similarities among agents within one subgroup and electro-

Table 11-7 Modified Classification of Class I Drugs Based on Predominant Electrophysiologic Effects.

IA	IB	IC
Quinidine	Lidocaine	Flecainide
Procainamide	Mexiletine	Lorcainide
Disopyramide	Tocainide	Encainide
Pirmenol	Phenytoin	Propafenone
	Ethmozin	Indecainide

Table 11-8 Class I Drugs Efficacy for Various Clinical Arrhythmias.

Effect on Arrhythmia	Class		
	IA	IB	IC
Suppresses or terminates atrial fibrillation of flutter	++	−	+
Slows the rate of atrial flutter	++	−	+
Suppresses atrial premature beats	++	−	+
Suppresses automatic atrial tachycardias	+	−	+
Suppresses and terminates A-V nodal reentry	+	−	++
Suppresses and terminates A-V reciprocating tachycardia	+	±	++
Slows ventricular response with atrial fibrillation preexcitation	+	±	++
Suppresses ventricular premature beats	+	+	++
Suppresses and terminates ventricular tachycardia	+	+	+

Key: + = effective; − = ineffective; ± = partially effective; ++ = very effective.

physiologic differences between subgroups, thereby providing a more useful framework for the clinical use of antiarrhythmics. The proposed modifications of the original Vaughan Williams classification scheme have the merits of simplicity and clinical utility.

The observed efficacy of class I drugs for various proposed mechanisms of arrhythmias, as presented in Table 11-8, is largely predictable from the effects of these agents on conduction, refractoriness, automaticity, kinetics of onset of rate-dependent block, and other basic parameters previously discussed. From consideration of the unique electrophysiologic and clinical effects of class IA, IB, and IC drugs, it is generally possible to develop a strategy for the treatment of various categories of cardiac arrhythmias. As noted by Campbell (1983), consideration of the kinetics of interaction of class I drugs with the sodium channel in vitro may be of value in the practical management of arrhythmias. Recent work has supported the concept of "cross-tolerance" wherein drugs within a class show a similar spectrum of antiarrhythmic efficacy (Ferrick et al., 1982). If further observations support these concepts, then limiting drug trials to one agent from each group during serial drug testing could reduce considerably the number of trials undertaken in individual patients. Additionally, combined therapy with more than one agent from the same subgroup might be initiated only in refractory cases or to reduce noncardiac side effects when they occur with a single drug (Campbell, 1983).

It remains true that despite advances in our understanding of the mechanisms of cardiac arrhythmias, in some instances our limited knowledge of the precise electrophysiologic abnormalities accounting for an arrhythmia will frustrate a scientific approach to therapy. However, it is precisely for this reason that a thorough understanding of the electrophysiologic effects of these and other antiarrhythmic agents should be promoted by an appropriate classification system. Furthermore, investigations into the relationship of chemical structure to pharmacologic activity in the proposed classes of drugs may suggest characterization and synthesis of new, safer, and more potent compounds (Singh et al., 1983). With more relevant in vitro models, our understanding of arrhythmogenesis and antiarrhythmic effects will improve and should result in modifications of this classification. The recent resolution of the sodium currents at the level of the single ionic channel will permit direct analysis of many basic questions about the mechanisms of ion permeation (Grant et al., 1983). It is likely that, with the use of patch microelectrode techniques, the models of interaction of antiarrhythmic drugs with sodium channels will be placed on a firmer experimental basis. Based on our current knowledge of cellular cardiac electrophysiology, the mechanisms of various arrhythmias, and the effects of antiarrhythmic drugs, the division of class I drugs into three distinct subgroups is both scientifically reasonable and clinically useful.

Acknowledgments

This work was supported in part by grant 1R01-HL-25992 from the National Heart, Lung and Blood Institute and the National Institutes of Health, Bethesda, Maryland. Dr. Ruskin is the recipient of the American Heart Association Established Investigatorship 81-177, Dallas, Texas.

References

Abitol, H., Califano, J.E., Abate, C., Beilis, P., and Castellanos, H. 1983. Use of flecainide acetate in the treatment of premature ventricular contractions. Am Heart J 105:227–230.

Akhtar, M., Gilbert, C.J., and Shenasa, M. 1981. Effect of lidocaine on atrioventricular response via the accessory pathway in patients with Wolff-Parkinson-White syndrome. Circulation 63:435–441.

Anderson, J.L., Mason, J.W., Winkle, R.A., Meffin, P.J., Fowles, R.E., Peters, F. and Hamson, D.C. 1978. Clinical electrophysiological effects of tocainide. Circulation 57:685–691.

Anderson, J.L., Stewart, J.R., Perry, B.A., VanHamersfeld, D.D., Johnson, T.A., Conrad, G.J., Chang, S.F., Kvam, D.C., and Pitt, B. 1981. Oral flecainide acetate for the treatment of ventricular arrhythmias. N Engl J Med 305:473–477.

Arnsdorf, M.F., and Bigger, J.T. 1972. Effect of lidocaine hydrochloride on membrane conductance in mammalian cardiac Purkinje fibers. J Clin Invest 51:2252–2263.

Bassett, A.L., and Hoffman, B.F. 1971. Antiarrhythmic drugs: electrophysiological actions. Annu Rev Pharmacol 11:143–170.

Bigger, J.T. 1972. Antiarrhythmic drugs in ischemic heart disease. Hosp Pract 69–80.

Bigger, J.T. 1980. Management of arrhythmias. In: E. Braunwald, ed. Heart Disease: A Textbook of Cardiovascular Medicine. Vol. 1, pp. 691–743. Philadelphia: W.B. Saunders Company.

Bigger, J.T., and Mandel, W.J. 1970. Effect of lidocaine on the electrophysiological properties of ventricular muscle and Purkinje fibers. J Clin Invest 49:63–77.

Bigger, J.T., and Reiffel, J.A. 1979. Sick sinus syndrome. Annu Rev Med 30:91–118.

Campbell, T.J. 1983. Kinetics of onset of rate-dependent effects of Class I antiarrhythmic drugs are important in determining their effects on refractoriness in guinea-pig ventricle, and provide a theoretical basis for their subclassification. Cardiovasc Res 17:334–352.

Campbell, R.W.F., Henderson, A., Bryson, L.G., Reid, D.S., Sheridan, D.J., Rawlins, M.D., and Julian, D.G. 1981. Intravenous flecainide pharmacokinetics and efficacy. Circulation 64 (abstr) (suppl IV):265.

Chen, C.M., Gettes, L.S., and Katzung, B.G. 1975. Effect of lidocaine and quinidine on steady-state characteristics and recovery kinetics of (dV/dt) max in guinea pig ventricular myocardium. Circ Res 37:20–29.

Cheng, T.O., and Wadhwa, N. 1973. Sinus standstill following intravenous lidocaine administration. JAMA 223:790.

Cocco, G., and Strozzi, C. 1976. Initial clinical experience of lorcainide (RO 13-1042), a new antiarrhythmic agent. Eur J Pharmacol 14:105.

Davis, L.D., and Temte, J.V. 1969. Electrophysiological actions of lidocaine on canine ventricular muscle and Purkinje fibers. Circ Res 24:639–653.

Docouret, P. 1975. The effect of quinidine on membrane electrical activity in frog auricular fibers studied by current and voltage clamp. Br J Pharmacol 57:163–184.

Duff, H.J., Roden, D.M., Maffucci, R.J., Vesper, B., Lonard, G., Higgins, S.B., Oates, J.A., Smith, R.F., and Woosley, R.L. 1981. Suppression of resistant ventricular arrhythmias by twice daily dosing of flecainide. Am J Cardiol 48:1133–1140.

Elharrar, V., Bailey, J.C., Lathrop, D.A., and Zipes, D.P. 1977. Effects of aprindine HCL on slow channel action potentials and transient depolarizations in canine Purkinje fibers. Fed Proc 36(abstr):416.

Elharrar, V., Foster, P.R., and Zipes, D.P. 1975. Effects of aprindine HCL on cardiac tissues. J Pharmacol Exp Ther 195:201–205.

Ferrick, K.J., Bigger, J.T., Reiffel, J.A., Livelli, F.D., Gang, E.S., and Gliklich, J.I. 1982. Congruence in efficacy of procalinamide and quinidine for induced ventricular tachycardia (abstr). Circulation (suppl II) 66:142.

Gettes, L.S. 1979. On the classification of antiarrhythmic drugs. Mod Concepts Cardiovasc Dis 48:13–18.

Gettes, L.S. 1981. Physiology and pharmacology of antiarrhythmic drugs. Hosp Pract 89–101.

Giardina, E.G.V., and Bigger, J.T. 1973. Procainamide against re-entrant ventricular arrhythmias. Circulation 48:959–966.

Gomes, J.A.C., Dhatt, M.S., Rubenson, D.S., and Damato, A.N. 1979. Electrophysiological evidence for selective retrograde utilization of a specialized conducting system in A-V nodal reentrant tachycardia. Am J Cardiol 43: 687–698.

Granrud, G., Krejci, J., and Coyne, T. 1981. Sustained elimination of ventricular arrhythmias during chronic flecainide dosing. Circulation 64(abstr) (suppl IV):316.

Grant, A.D., Starmer, C.F., and Strauss, H.C. 1983. Unitary sodium channels in isolated cardiac myocytes of rabbit. Circ Res 53:823–829.

Harrison, D.C., Winkle, R.A., Sami, M., and Mason, J.W. 1980. Encainide: A new and potent antiarrhythmic agent. In: D.C. Harrison, ed. Cardiac Arrhythmias, A Decade of Progress. p. 327. Boston: G.K. Hall & Co.

Hauswirth, O., and Singh, B.N. 1979. Ionic mechanisms in heart muscle in relation to the genesis and the pharmacological control of cardiac arrhythmias. Pharmacol Rev 30:5–63.

Hellestrand, K.J., Bexton, R.S., Nathan, A.W., Beston, R.S., Spurrell, R.A.J., and Camm, A.M. 1982. Acute electrophysiological effects of flecainide acetate on cardiac conduction and refractoriness in man. Br Heart J 48:140–148.

Hodess, A.B., Follansbee, W.P., Spear, J.F., and Moore, E.N. 1979. Electrophysiological effects of a new antiarrhythmic agent, flecainide, on the intact canine heart. J Cardiovasc Pharmacol 1:427–439.

Hodges, M., Haughland, J.M., Granrud, G., Conard, G.J., Asinger, R.W., Mikell, F.L., and Krejci, J. 1982. Suppression of ventricular ectopic depolarizations by flecainide acetate, a new antiarrhythmic agent. Circulation 65: 879–885.

Hoffman, B.F. 1981. Relationships between effects on cardiac electrophysiology and antiarrhythmic efficacy. In: J. Morganroth, E.N. Moore, L.S. Dreifus, and E.L. Michelson, eds. The Evaluation of New Antiarrhythmic Drugs. The Hague: Martinus Nijhoff.

Hoffman, B.F., and Bigger, J.T. 1971. Antiarrhythmic drugs. In: J.R. DiPalma, ed. Drill's Pharmacology in Medicine. 4th ed. pp. 824–852. New York: McGraw-Hill.

Hoffman, B.F., Rosen, M.R., and Wit, A.L. 1975. Electrophysiology and pharmacology of cardiac arrhythmias. VII. Cardiac effects of quinidine and procainamide. Am Heart J 89:804–808.

Hohnloser, S., Zeiher, A., Hust, M.H., Wollschlager, H., and Just, H. 1983. Flecainide-induced aggravation of ventricular tachycardia. Clin Cardiol 6:103–135.

Horowitz, L.N., Josephson, M.E., and Farshidi, A. 1978. Human electropharmacology of tocainide, a lidocaine congener. Am J Cardiol 42:276–280.

Josephson, M.E., Caracta, A.R., and Lav, S.H. 1972. Effects of lidocaine on refractory periods in man. Am Heart J 84:778–756.

Kasper, W., Meinertz, T., Kersting, F., Lallgen, H., Lang, K., and Just, H. 1979. Electrophysiological actions of lorcainide in patients with cardiac disease. J Cardiovasc Pharmacol 1:343–352.

Kaverina, N.V., and Senova, Z.P. 1978. Ethmozin—a new preparation for treating cardiac rhythm disorders. In: Proceedings of the First US-USSR Symposium on Sudden Death. Yalta, Oct. 3–5, 1977. U.S. Department of HEW, PHS, NIH, DHEW Publication Number (NIH) 78:1470.

Keefe, D.L., Peters, F., and Winkle, R.A. 1982. Randomized double-blind placebo controlled crossover trial documenting oral lorcainide efficacy in suppression of symptomatic ventricular tachyarrhythmias. Am Heart J 103:511–518.

Kesteloot, H., and Stoobandt, R. 1977. Clinical experience with lorcainide (R 15 889), a new antiarrhythmic drug. Arch Int Pharmacodyn Ther 230:225–234.

Kupersmith, J., Antman, E.M., and Hoffman, B.F. 1975. In vivo electrophysiologic effects of lidocaine in canine acute myocardial infarction. Circ Res 36:84–91.

Lippestad, C.T., and Forfang, K. 1971. Production of sinus arrest by lignocaine. Br Med J 1:537.

Luckstead, E.F., and Tarr, M. 1972. Comparison of quinidine and bretylium tosylate effects on cardiac ionic currents. Fed Proc 31:818.

Lui, H.K., Lee, G., Dietrich, P., Low, R.I., and Mason, D.T. 1982. Flecainide-induced QT prolongation and ventricular tachycardia. Am Heart J 103:569–589.

Mandel, W.J., and Bigger, J.T. 1971. Electrophysiologic effects of lidocaine on isolated canine and rabbit atrial tissue. J Pharmacol Exp Ther 178:81–102.

Mandel, W., Laks, M., Obayaski, K., and Clifton, J. 1973. Electrophysiological features of the W.P.W. syndrome: Modification by procainamide. Circulation 48(suppl IV):195.

Mason, J.W., Winkle, R.A., Rider, A.K., Stinson, E.B., and Harrison, D.C. 1977. The electrophysiologic effects of quinidine in the transplanted human heart. J Clin Invest 59:481–489.

McComish, M., Robinson, C., Kitson, D., and Jewitt, D. 1977. Clinical electrophysiological effect of mexiletine. Postgrad Med J 53 (suppl 1): 85–91.

Moe, G.K. 1975. Evidence for reentry as a mechanism of cardiac arrhythmias. Rev Physiol Biochem Pharmacol 72:55–81.

Nathan, A.W., Hellestrand, K.J., Bexton, R.S., Banim, B.M., Spurell, A.J. and Camm, A.J., 1984. Proarrhythmic effects of the new antiarrhythmic agent flecainide. Am Heart J 107: 222–228.

Noneman, J.W., and Jones, M.R. 1983. Lidocaine. In: L. Gould, ed. Drug Treatment of Cardiac Arrhythmias. Vol 1, pp. 193–223. New York: Futura Publishing Company, Inc.

Olsson, S.B., and Evardsson, N. 1981. Clinical electrophysiologic study of antiarrhythmic properties of flecainide: Acute intraventricular delayed conduction and prolonged repolarization in regular spaced and premature beats using intracardiac monophasic action potential with programmed stimulation. Am Heart J 102:864–871.

Roos, J.C., Paalman, A.C.A., and Dunning, A.J. 1976. Electrophysiological effects of mexiletine in man. Br Heart J 38:61–72.

Rosen, J.R., Merker, C., and Pippenger, C.E. 1976. The effects of lidocaine on canine ECG and electrophysiologic properties of Purkinje fibers. Am Heart J 91:191–202.

Rosen, K.M., Barwolf, C., Ehsani, A., and Rahimtoola, S.H. 1972. Effects of lidocaine and propranolol on the normal and anomalous pathways in patients with pre-excitation. Am J Cardiol 30:801–809.

Rosen, M.R., Wit, A.L., and Hoffman, B.F. 1975. Electrophysiology and pharmacology of cardiac arrhythmias. Am Heart J 89:526–536; 665–674; 804–808.

Sami, M., Mason, J.W., Oh, G., and Harrison, D.C. 1979a. Canine electrophysiology of encainide, a new antiarrhythmic drug. Am J Cardiol 43:1149–1154.

Sami, M., Mason, J.W., Peters, F., and Harrison, D.C. 1979b. Clinical electrophysiologic effects of encainide, a newly developed antiarrhythmic agent. Am J Cardiol 44:526–532.

Schmid, P.G., Nelson, L.D., Mark, A.L., Heistad, D.D., and Abboud, F.M. 1974. Inhibition of adrenergic vasoconstriction by quinidine. J Pharmacol Exp Ther 188:124.

Seipel, L., and Breithardt, G. 1976. Sinus recovery time after disopyramide phosphate. Am J Cardiol 37(letter):1118.

Sekiya, A., and Vaughan Williams, E.M. 1963. A comparison of the antifibrillatory actions and effects on intracellular cardiac potentials of pronethalol, disopyramide and quinidine. Br J Pharmacol 26:473–481.

Singh, B.N., Collett, J.T., and Chew, C.Y.C. 1980. New perspectives in the pharmacologic therapy of cardiac arrhythmias. Progr Cardiovasc Dis 22:243–301.

Singh, B.N., and Hauswirth, O. 1974. Comparative mechanisms of action of antiarrhythmic drugs. Am Heart J 87:367–382.

Singh, B.N., and Vaughan Williams, E.M. 1971. Effect of altering potassium concentration on the action of lidocaine and diphenylhydantoin on rabbit atrial and ventricular muscle. Circ Res 29:286–297.

Somani, R. 1980. Antiarrhythmic effects of flecainide. Clin Pharmacol Ther 27:464–470.

Spear, J.F., and Moore, E.N. 1982. The contribution of cellular electrophysiology in the development of antiarrhythmic agents. Electropharmacology 5:238–250.

Steinberg, M.I., and Greenspan, K. 1976. Intracellular electrophysiological alterations in canine cardiac conducting tissue induced by aprindine and lidocaine. Cardiovasc Res 10:236–244.

Stoel, I., and Hagemeijer, F. 1980. Aprinidine: A review. Eur Heart J 1:147–156.

Swedberg, K., Pehrson, J., and Ryden, L. 1978. Electrocardiographic and hemodynamic effects of tocainide (W-36095) in man. Eur J Clin Pharmacol 14:15–19.

Vaughan Williams, E.M. 1970. Classification of antiarrhythmic drugs. In: E. Sandoe, E. Flenstead-Jensen, and K.H. Olsen, eds. Symposium on Cardiac Arrhythmias. pp. 449–472. Sodertalje, Sweden: AB Astra.

Vaughan Williams, E.M. 1975. Classification of antiarrhythmic drugs. J Pharmacol Ther 1:115–138.

Verdonck, F., Vereecke, J., and Vleugels, A. 1974. Electrophysiological effects of aprindine on isolated heart preparations. Eur J Pharmacol 26:338–347.

Vik-mo, H., Ohm, O.J., and Lund-Johansen, P. 1982. Electrophysiologic effects of flecainide acetate in patients with sinus nodal dysfunction. Am J Cardiol 50:1090–1094.

Weld, F.M., Coromilas, J., Rottman, J.N., and Bigger, J.T. 1982. Mechanisms of quinidine-induced depression of maximum upstroke velocity in ovine cardiac Purkinje fibers. Circ Res 50:369–376.

Wellens, H.J.J., and Durrer, D. 1973. Effect of procainamide and quinidine gluconate in Wolff-Parkinson-White Syndrome. Circulation 48(suppl IV):17.

Winkle, R.A., Meffin, P.J., Fitzgerald, J.W., and Harrison, D.C. 1976. Clinical efficacy and pharmacokinetics of a new orally effective antiarrhythmic, tocainide. Circulation 54:884-889.

Wittig, J., Harrison, L.A., and Wallace, A.G. 1973. Electrophysiological effects of lidocaine on distal Purkinje fibers of canine heart. Am Heart J 86:89.

EDITOR'S NOTES

Antiarrhythmic Effects of Conduction-Slowing Agents (Class I)

The hallmark of the discussions of class I antiarrhythmic drug is *diversity*, which was addressed by three different authors. In this regard, the concept that antiarrhythmic drugs can be categorized or identified by a major common mechanism of action has prevailed at least for a decade, as reviewed by Dr. Vaughan Williams. Indeed, the basic classification system remains largely intact although certain components of Dr. Vaughan Williams' drug classification system have been modified, reemphasized, or added to. For example, although class I agents represent the largest component of antiarrhythmic drugs utilized in clinical practice today, various agents have been added to this class since the original conception of the drug classification. Thus a subdivision of class I drugs has evolved that also has proven to be clinically useful. Similarly, the concept of a class III drug classification has only been fully appreciated during the last few years, largely due to the dramatic success of amiodarone in preventing life-threatening arrhythmias. Newer data concerning the fourth class of drug classifications, the so-called calcium antagonists, has also placed the limitations of this classification in proper perspective. Currently, from a perspective of antiarrhythmic efficacy, calcium antagonists are largely limited to supraventricular arrhythmia treatment, having failed to have a significant impact on the treatment of ventricular arrhythmias. Alternatively, their ultimate clinical application may be very broad, as suggested by the unexpected effect on cell coupling. Although it is apparent that most of the antiarrhythmic drugs possess one or more of the four classes of action, a newer class may be emerging that, by its relative degree of specificity, may constitute a separate class of action (class V). These drugs are the bradycardic agents and alinidine is an example. The clinical significance of this type of agent in the treatment of arrhythmias is, however, yet to be determined.

Dr. Vaughan Williams also suggests in his thought-provoking chapter that one must be cognizant of acute versus chronic effects of antiarrhythmic drugs. In this regard, the chronic effects of beta-blockers, for example, may primarily account for the putative efficacy of such agents in the treatment of postinfarction patients. Based on the acute effects of beta-blockers, one would not predict the observed changes in action potential duration in the chronic setting that implicate a class III action of these drugs. Furthermore, when considering other effects of prolonged beta-blockade such as increasing the capillarity of the ventricular myocardium, one is again reminded of the impact that complex drug effects have on the overall efficacy of a particular agent via nonelectrophysiologic effects. Thus, in addition to the primary electrophysiologic effects, such agents affect the autonomic nervous system, central nervous system, and hemodynamic function of the heart. Furthermore, their metabolism and rates of excretion vary widely.

Basic electrophysiologic measurements have defined three subgroups of drugs with relatively unique characteristics. The class IA agents, which include the classic antiarrhythmic drugs, quinidine and procainamide, appear to occupy an intermediate position in the spectrum of class I antiarrhythmic drugs. In contrast, IB drugs, exemplified by lidocaine and mexilitine, and class IC drugs, exemplified by encainide and flecainide, occupy the opposite points of the spectrum when effects on conduction and action potential duration are considered. Many of the electrophysiologic differences between agents in these groups can be explained by their relative *use* dependence, denoting the rapidity with which drugs become attached to and released from sodium channels versus the potency with which they depress conduction. For example, class IC drugs are relatively nonspecific but very potent conduction-depressing-type agents. Flecainide, an example of this drug classification, has shown such effects both in the animal and clinical setting. Class IC drugs generally tend to be very potent PVC suppressors. Based on previous discussions of the mechanism of conduction-related arrhythmias, one can envision a potential mechanism of action for conduction-slowing drugs that induces bidirectional conduction block. Unfortunately, many agents that slow conduction also tend to have closely coupled hemodynamic or myocardial depressing effects that, at times, limit the clinical application due to a narrow therapeutic to toxic ratio. Although all class I drugs share this property of conduction slowing, the degree of conduction slowing varies and, furthermore, may be accompanied by a change in refractoriness, indicated by the increased action potential duration demonstration by quinidine and procainamide. Thus quinidine exemplifies antiarrhythmic effects related to conduction slowing and refractoriness while flecainide demonstrates, as its primary effect, conduction-slowing effects.

The differing electrophysiologic effects of the three subgroups of class I drugs are also emphasized in the excellent discussion of this concept by Dr. Estes and his colleagues, particularly as related to the clinical electrophysiologic setting. These authors conclude that it is both scientifically sound and clinically useful to subdivide class I drugs into three distinct groups based upon their effect on action potential duration. Of important clinical consideration is the concept of employing agents from one subgroup versus combined therapy with more than one agent from the same or different subgroups. For example, one might readily predict that agents from the same subgroup may have more or less comparable efficacy. While there are certain quantitative differences, overall, this concept does seem to prevail. For example, if a particular patient does not respond to a class IA agent, this patient is unlikely to respond to another agent from class IA. In contrast, combining two agents that alter conduction or slow conduction dramatically may be unwise (e.g., combining a class IA and class IC agent), while combining a class IA with a class IB, the latter classification showing use dependence and less potent conduction slowing, may be more advisable. Indeed, preliminary evidence suggests that combinations of class IA and class IB may have a synergistic effect. Although such reasoning may prove correct in various situations, one must recognize that such approaches form only a guideline, and individual variations, regarding drug therapy responsiveness must be fully expected. In addition, when agents have properties of more than one class, further complications may materialize.

The diversity of effects among class I agents is also magnified when the effects are measured or considered in tissue of differing electrophysiology. Thus effects of these agents on normal tissue may be substantially different when compared to abnormal (usually ischemic) tissue. The alterations of membrane characteristics and basic electrophysiologic properties by diseased states may substantially alter the manifestations of antiarrhythmic drugs within a particular tissue. As an example, lidocaine has little demonstrable electrophysiologic effect in normal tissue; however, in ischemic tissue profound effects are seen, both in isolated tissue and whole animal preparations.

Based upon the observation that an antiarrhythmic drug usually possesses more than one effect common to all four drug classifications, it is important to maintain an appropriate perspective of the classification system, both from a conceptual and practical standpoint. On one hand, one should not overinterpret the practical application of the classification system, but utilize it as a general guide in differentiating among various drugs. For example, if a drug fails in therapy, one should consider utilizing a drug from a different class or subclass, rather than another drug from the original class that failed. Similarily, drug combinations can be more rationally chosen if one appreciates the additive electrophysiologic effects of the major classes of drugs. On the other hand, it is known that effects of different classes can be shown in a single drug. In this regard, one focuses on the *dominant* electrophysiologic effects of drugs in the different classes. For example, secondary or additional effects often are not apparent until higher doses of the drug are attained (e.g., the local anesthetic effect of propranolol). In the case of propanolol, the local anesthetic effect is not considered to be of clinical significance since such doses are not attained clinically. The mere existence of several classes of drug effects exemplifies the relative nonspecificity of existing drugs, emphasized by their "retrospective" classification. Thus, when the above qualifications are kept in mind, the Vaughan Williams classification system can be useful in guiding some of the considerations that are important in choosing an appropriate drug therapy. Until drugs can be developed with more specific effects on the myocardium or with truly singular electrophysiologic actions, the drug classification system should continue to be employed as a general guide and as a reference point in the overall process of delineating effective antiarrhythmic drug therapy.

B. Antiarrhythmic Effects of Adrenergic Blocking Agents (Class II)

Chapter 12

β-Adrenergic Blockade in the Treatment of Arrhythmias

William H. Frishman and Lawrence I. Laifer

Introduction

The introduction of β-adrenoceptor blocking drugs to clinical medicine 25 years ago ushered in a new era of pharmacologic intervention and revolutionized the management of cardiovascular disease. In addition to becoming a therapeutic mainstay for the treatment of hypertension, angina, and various arrhythmias, β-blockers have now been shown to reduce the risk of mortality post-myocardial infarction, and have numerous applications well beyond the cardiovascular sphere. The use of β-blockers in the treatment of arrhythmias will be discussed in this chapter. It is important first to review some basic pharmacologic concepts regarding β-adrenergic blocking drugs.

Pharmacologic Characteristics of β-Blockers

Based on the observation that the relative potency of a series of sympathomimetic amines varied with the effector organs or systems, Ahlquist, in 1948, postulated that there were two distinct types of adrenergic receptors which he classified as α- and β-receptors. β-Receptors were later divided in two groups: β_1-receptors in the heart, and β_2-receptors in the bronchi and blood vessels (Lands et al., 1967; Dunlop and Shank, 1968; Lefkowitz, 1974). Table 12-1 lists the distribution of these receptors in human tissues.

Table 12-1 Distribution of Adrenoreceptors.

Organ	Receptor	Effect of Stimulation
Heart	β_1	Increase in heart rate
	β_1	Increase in cardiac contractility
	β_1	Acceleration in conduction
Bronchi	β_2	Dilatation
Blood vessels	β_2	Dilatation
	α	Constriction
Eye	α	Dilatation
Gastrointestinal tract	α, β	Reduction in motility

Ahlquist's theory was viewed with much skepticism until 1958 when Powell and Slater discovered dichloroisoprenaline (DCI), the first β-blocking agent. The discovery that DCI selectively blocked those responses mediated by β-receptors gave credance to Ahlquist's views and was a pivotal development in human pharmacology. Although DCI was unsuitable for clinical use as a β-blocker because of its excessive β-stimulant (agonist) activity, the concept that β-blockade of the cardiac receptor might be useful in the therapy of angina led Black and Stephenson (1962) and others to develop β-blocking agents that would become effective antianginal drugs. It soon became evident that their therapeutic efficacy extended well beyond the control of angina to include treatment of arrhythmias, hypertension, and management of noncardiovascular disease.

Pharmacodynamic Properties

β-Blocking Potency β-Blocking drugs competitively inhibit the effects of catecholamines at β-adrenoreceptor sites, thereby diminishing the effect of any concentration of agonist on a sensitive tissue (Frishman, 1979). The dose-response curve is thus shifted to the right, and in the presence of a β-blocking drug, a higher concentration of agonist is required to evoke a given tissue response. One can assess the relative potency of a β-blocking agent by its inhibition of isoproterenol-induced tachycardia or by the amount of isoproterenol required to reverse the heart rate slowing effect of a given β-blocker (Waal-Manning, 1976). As seen in Table 12-2, on a milligram per mg basis, pindolol and timolol are the most potent, and acebutolol, labetalol, and sotalol are the least potent of the β-blocking drugs.

Structure-Activity Relationship The molecular structures of β-adrenergic blocking agents (Fig. 12-1) have features in common with isoproterenol, the β-adrenergic agonist. The affinity for the β-receptor appears to be determined by the size of the alkyl-substituted secondary or tertiary amine to the 2-C side chain. The larger the alkyl group, the greater the affinity for the β-receptor. The particular structure attaches to the receptor site, and the nature of the substituents on the aromatic ring determines whether the effects will be predominantly activation or blockade (Connolly et al., 1976). The configuration of the asymmetric β-carbon of the side chain is crucial for pharmacologic activity. β-Blocking drugs exist as pairs of optical isomers. However, almost all the β-blocking activity resides in the levorotatory isomer (Frishman, 1979; Barrett and Cullum, 1968). For example, the (−) levorotatory isomers of propranolol and alprenolol are up to 100 times more active than the (+) dextrorotatory isomers. Only the racemic mixture of each drug, consisting of equal parts of the two isomers, is available for clinical use. The different stereoisomers of β-adrenergic blocking drugs are useful for dif-

Table 12-2 Pharmacodynamic Properties and Cardiac Effects of β-Adrenoreceptor Blocking Drugs.

Drug	β_1-Blockade Potency Ratio (Propranolol = 1.0)	Relative β_1-Selectivity	Intrinsic Sympathomimetic Activity	Membrane-Stabilizing Activity	Resting Heart Rate	Exercise Heart Rate	Myocardial Contractility	Resting Blood Pressure	Resting Atrioventricular Conduction	Antiarrhythmic Effect
Acebutolol	0.3	+	+	+	↓	↓	↓	↓	↓	+
Atenolol	1.0	+	0	0	↓	↓	↓	↓	↓	+
Esmolol*		+ +	0	0	↓	NA	↓	↓	↓	+
Labetalol†	0.3	0	0	0	↓↔	↓	↓	↓	↓↔	+
Metoprolol	1.0	+	0	0	↓	↓	↓	↓	↓	+
Nadolol	1.0	0	0	0	↓	↓	↓	↓	↓	+
Oxprenolol	0.5–1.0	0	+ +	+	↓↔	↓	↓↔	↓	↓↔	+
Penbutolol	1.0	0	+ +	0	↓↔	↓	↓↔	↓	↓↔	+
Pindolol	6.0	0	+ + +	+	↓↔	↓	↓↔	↓	↓↔	+
Propranolol		0	0	+ +	↓	↓	↓	↓	↓	+
LA Propranolol	0.6–1.0	0	0	+ +	↓	↓	↓	↓	↓	+
Sotalol	0.3	0	0	0	↓	↓	↓	↓	↓	+
Timolol	6.0	0	0	0	↓	↓	↓	↓	↓	+
Isomer D-propranolol††		0	0	+ +	↔	↔	↓↔	↔	↓↔	+ −

*Esmolol is a new ultra-short acting β-blocker which is only available in intravenous form.
†Labetalol has additional α-adrenergic blocking properties and direct vasodilatory activity.
††Effects of D-propranolol occur with doses in human beings well above the therapeutic level. The isomer also lacks β-blocking activity
NA, not available; LA, long-acting.

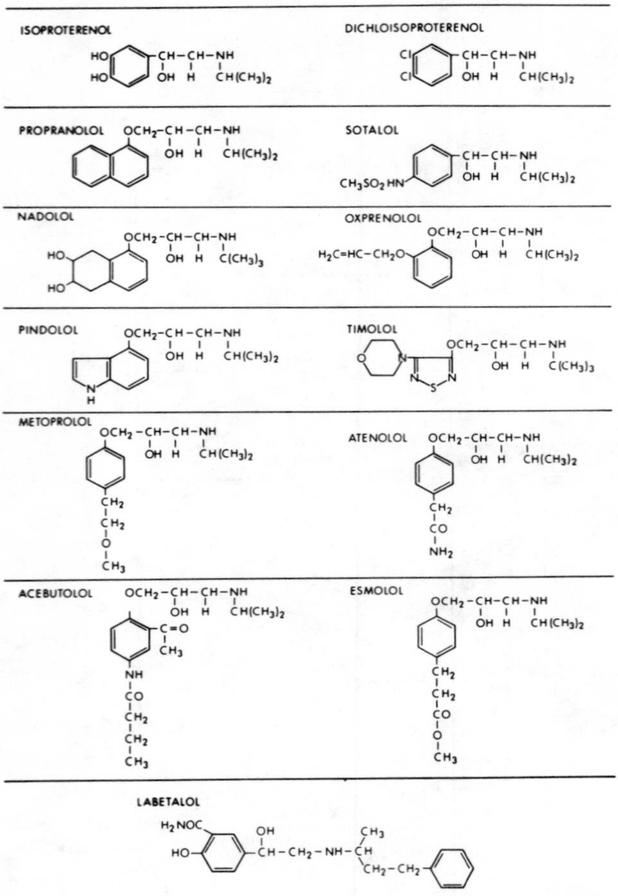

12-1 Molecular structures of isoproterenol and some β-adrenergic blocking drugs.

ferentiating between the effects of β-receptor blockade and other properties of the drug, but clinically, the (+) dextrorotatory isomers are of no therapeutic value (Connolly et al., 1976; Frishman, 1979).

Membrane-Stabilizing Activity Membrane-stabilizing activity, also known as "quinidine-like effect" or "local anesthetic" action, is unrelated to competitive inhibition of catecholamine action. It occurs equally in both optical isomers of the drug (Connolly et al., 1976). Membrane-stabilizing activity was demonstrated electrophysiologically in propranolol (Barrett and Cullum, 1968), oxprenolol (Brunner et al., 1970), and alprenolol (Basil et al., 1973) by a reduction in the rate of rise of the intracardiac potential without a change in the overall duration of the action or resting potential. The concentration of propranolol at which this effect has been demonstrated on human ventricular muscle in vitro is approximately 50–100 times the blood level associated with inhibition of exercise-induced tachycardia (Singh, 1973). The difference is even greater with other β-blockers. The antiarrhythmic effect of β-blockers is primarily due to β-blockade and not membrane-stabilizing activity (Singh and Jewitt, 1974); atenolol, metoprolol, nadolol, pindolol, sotalol, and timolol are all devoid of membrane-stabilizing activity, yet they all demonstrate an antiarrhythmic effect.

Intrinsic Sympathomimetic Activity (ISA) Certain β-adrenoreceptor blocking drugs have intrinsic sympathomimetic activity (also known as partial agonist activity). β-Blockers with ISA slightly activate the β-receptor, while preventing the access of natural or synthetic catecholamines to the receptor site. Dichloroisoprenaline, the first β-adrenoreceptor blocking drug, exhibited such marked partial agonist activity that it was unsuitable for clinical use (Connolly et al., 1976). However, compounds with less ISA are effective β-blocking drugs. Acebutolol, oxprenolol, penbutolol, and pindolol cause a very small agonist response, indicating that they partially stimulate as well as block the receptor. Atenolol, metoprolol, nadolol, propranolol, sotalol, and timolol, in contrast, do not produce any agonist response when they interact with β-receptors in the absence of primary agonists such as isoproterenol or epinephrine.

Whether the presence of partial agonist activity in a β-blocker confers any advantage in cardiac therapy is still a matter of some debate (Powell and Slater, 1974; Opie, 1980; Koch-Weser, 1979). β-Blockers with ISA cause less slowing of the heart rate at rest than propranolol or metoprolol, although the exercise-induced increase in heart rate is similarly blunted (Frishman et al., 1979b). They may also depress atrioventricular conduction less than β-blockers without ISA (Frishman and Silverman, 1979a). In general, β-blockers with ISA are as effective as β-blockers without ISA in the treatment of hypertension (Atterhog et al., 1976), effort angina (Frishman et al., 1979b), or arrhythmias (Aronow and Uyeyama, 1972). The partial agonist activity in a β-blocker may protect against peripheral vascular complications, bronchial asthma, and myocardial depression (Ablad et al., 1967; Frishman and Silverman, 1979b), but the evidence for this is preliminary and will require more definitive clinical trials.

Selectivity Lands et al., (1967) suggested that β-adrenoreceptors could be classified into two distinct types: β_1 (lipolysis and cardiac stimulation) and β_2 (bronchodilation and vasodilation). This subclassification has led to the development of agonist or antagonist drugs that are relatively selective at either β_1- or β_2-receptor sites (Dunlop and Shanks, 1968).

β_1-selective blocking agents (e.g., metoprolol) in low doses inhibit cardiac β_1-receptors but have less effect on vascular and bronchial β-adrenoreceptors. In higher doses, however, this selectivity is overcome and β_2-receptors are blocked as well (Koch-Weser, 1979). Because β_1-selective blockers have little inhibitory effect on the peripheral β_2-receptors, they possess two theoretical advantages. First, β_1-selective agents may be safer than nonselective β-blockers in patients with asthma or chronic obstructive pulmonary disease because adrenergic bronchodilation can still be mediated by the unblocked β_2-receptors. Clinical studies in patients with asthma showed a lower incidence of respiratory side effects with low dose β_1-selective agents than with equivalent doses or propranolol (Koch-Weser, 1979; Frishman, 1979; Sinclair, 1979). A second advantage of β_1-selective blockers is that they may not block the β_2-receptors that mediate arteriolar dilatation (Sannerstedt and Wasir, 1977), and thus, may prove advantageous in the treatment of hypertension. However, β_1-selectivity is a dose-dependent phenomenon that eventually disappears when larger doses, such as those usually required for the treatment of hypertension, are used (Letora et al., 1975; Fitzgerald, 1972). In contrast, β-blockers with intrinsic sympathomimetic activity maintain this effect without diminution even at higher doses (Imhof, 1974).

α-Blocking Activity Labetalol is a β-blocker with antagonistic properties at both α- and β-adrenoreceptors (Frishman and Halprin, 1979). Before labetalol, only antagonists acting at α- or β-adrenoreceptors, but not both, were available. Labetalol has been shown to be 6–10 times less potent than phentolamine at α-adrenoreceptors, 1.5–4 times less potent than propranolol at β-adrenoreceptors, and is itself 4–16 times less potent at α- than at β-adrenoreceptors (Frishman and Halprin, 1979).

Labetalol, like other β-blockers, has been shown to be a useful agent in the treatment of arrhythmias, hypertension, and angina pectoris (Frishman et al., 1981). However, unlike most β-blocking drugs, the additional α-adrenergic blocking actions of labetalol lead to a reduction in peripheral vascular resistance which may maintain cardiac output in patients (Frishman and Halprin, 1979).

Pharmacokinetic Properties

Absorption and Metabolism All the β-blocking drugs are well absorbed over a wide portion of the small intestine except for atenolol and nadolol (Table 12-3). Absorption is fairly rapid, with peak blood concentrations being achieved 1–3 h after administration (Frishman, 1979).

The β-adrenergic blocking drugs can be divided by their pharmacokinetic properties into two broad categories: those eliminated by hepatic metabolism, which

Table 12-3 Pharmacokinetic Properties of β-Adrenoreceptor Blocking Drugs.

Drug	Extent of Absorption	Extent of Bioavailability	Dose-dependent Bioavailability (Major first-pass hepatic metabolism)	Interpatient Variations in Plasma Levels	β-Blocking Plasma Concentrations	Protein Binding	Lipid Solubility*
	% of dose			–fold		%	
Acebutolol	≃70	≃50	No	7	0.2–2.0 μg/ml	30–40	Weak
Atenolol	≃50	≃40	No	4	0.2–5.0 μg/ml	<5	Weak
Esmolol†	DA	DA	DA		0.3–1.0 μg/ml		
Labetalol	>90	≃25	Yes	10	0.7–3.0 μg/ml	≃50	Weak
Metroprolol	>90	≃50	No	7	50–100 ng/ml	12	Moderate
Nadolol	≃30	≃30	No	7	50–100 ng/ml	≃30	Weak
Oxprenolol	≃90	≃40	No	5	80–100 ng/ml	80	Moderate
Pindolol	>90	≃90	No	4	5–15 ng/ml	57	Moderate
Practolol	>90	≃100	No	4–7	1.5–5.0 μg/ml	≃40	Weak
Propranolol	>90	≃30	Yes	20	50–100 ng/ml	93	High
LA Propranolol	>90	≃20	Yes	10–20	20–100 ng/ml	93	High
Sotalol	≃70	≃60	No	4	0.5–4.0 μg/ml	0	Weak
Timolol	>90	≃75	No	7	5–10 ng/ml	≃10	Weak

*Determined by the distribution ratio between octanol and water.
†Ultra-short acting β-blocker, only available in intravenous form.
DA, doesn't apply; LA, long-acting.

Table 12-4 Elimination Characteristics of Orally Active β-Adrenoreceptor Blocking Drugs.

Drug	Elimination Half-life	Total Body Clearance	Urinary Recovery of Unchanged Drug	Total Urinary Recovery	Predominant Route of Elimination*	Active Metabolites	Drug Accumulation in Renal Disease
	h	ml/min	% of dose				
Acebutolol	3–4	6–15	≃40	>90	RE	Yes	No
Atenolol	6–9	130	≃40	>95	RE	No	Yes
Esmolol†	≃10 min	285		>70	HM††	No	No
Labetalol	3–6	2,700	<1	>90	HM	No	No
Metoprolol	3–4	1,100	≃3	>95	HM	No	No
Nadolol	14–24	200	70	70	RE	No	Yes
Oxprenolol	2–3	380	2–5	70–95	HM	No	No
Pindolol	3–4	400	≃40	>90	RE (≃40% unchanged) & HM	No	No
Practolol	6–8	140	>90	>90	RE	No	Yes
Propranolol	3–4	1,000	<1	>90	HM	Yes	No
LA Propranolol	10	1,000	<1	>90	HM	Yes	No
Sotalol	8–10	150	≃60	>90	RE	No	Yes
Timolol	4–5	660	≃20	65	RE (≃20% unchanged) & HM	No	No

*RE, renal excretion; HM, hepatic metabolism.
†Ultra-short acting β-blocker, only available in intravenous form.
††Metabolized by blood, tissue, and hepatic esterases.
LA, long-acting.

tend to have relatively short plasma half-lives, and those eliminated by the kidney, which tend to have longer half-lives (Table 12-4). Propranolol and metoprolol are both lipid-soluble, are almost completely absorbed from the small intestine, and are largely metabolized by the liver. They tend to have highly variable bioavailability and relatively short plasma half-lives (Frishman, 1979; Johnson and Regardh, 1976), but because of lack of correlation between plasma half-life and pharmacologic effect, these drugs may be able to be administered twice or even once daily.

In contrast, drugs like atenolol and nadolol are more water-soluble, are absorbed incompletely through the gut, and are eliminated unchanged by the kidney (Frishman, 1979; Frishman, 1981b; Heel et al., 1979; Heel et al., 1980). They tend to have less variable bioavailability in patients with normal renal function, in addition to longer half-lives allowing one dose a day. This latter property may be helpful in patients who are noncompliant with β-blocker treatment.

Specific pharmacokinetic properties of individual β-adrenergic blockers (first-pass metabolism, active metabolites, lipid solubility, and protein binding) may be important to the clinician. When drugs with first-pass metabolism are taken orally, they undergo a great deal of hepatic biotransformation and relatively little drug may reach the systemic circulation. Depending on the extent of the first-pass effect, an oral dose of a β-blocker must be proportionately larger than an intravenous dose to produce the same clinical effects (Frishman, 1979). Some β-adrenergic blockers are transformed into pharmacologically active compounds, and the total pharmacologic effect therefore depends on both the amount of drug administered and its active metabolites (Frishman, 1979). Lipid solubility in a β-blocker has been associated with the ability of the drug to concentrate in the brain (Frishman, 1979; Opie, 1980; Cruickshank, 1980), and many side effects of these drugs (lethargy, mental depression, hallucinations, etc.) may be secondary to actions on the central nervous system (Frishman, 1981a). It is still unclear, however, whether drugs that are less lipid-soluble cause fewer of these adverse reactions. Some β-adrenergic blockers are extensively protein-bound in the plasma and alterations in protein level or binding may influence the pharmacologic effects of these drugs (Frishman, 1979; Koch-Weser and Sellers, 1976).

Electrophysiologic Effects

β-Adrenoreceptor blocking drugs have two main effects on the electrophysiologic properties of specialized cardiac tissue. The first effect of β-blockers results from the specific blockade of adrenergic stimulation of cardiac pacemaker potentials. This is undoubtedly important in the control of arrhythmias caused by enhanced automaticity. In concentrations causing significant inhibition of adrenergic receptors, the β-blockers produce little change in the transmembrane potentials of cardiac muscle. However, by competitively inhibiting adrenergic stimulation, β-blockers decrease the slope of phase 4 depolarization and the spontaneous firing rate of sinus or ectopic pacemakers, and thus decrease automaticity. Arrhythmias occurring in the setting of enhanced automaticity as seen in myocardial infarction, digitalis toxicity, hyperthyroidism, and pheochromocytoma, would therefore be expected to respond well to β-blockade.

The second electrophysiologic effect of β-blockers is one of membrane-stabilizing action, also known as the "quinidine-like" or "local anesthetic" action. This property is unrelated to inhibition of catecholamine action and is possessed equally by both the d- and l-isomers of the drugs (d-isomers have almost no β-blocking activity) (Levy and Richards, 1966). Characteristic of this effect is a reduction in the rate of rise of the intracardiac action potential without affecting the spike duration or the resting potential (Vaughan Williams and Papp, 1970). Associated features include an elevated electrical threshold of excitability, delay in conduction velocity, and a significant increase in the effective refractory period. This effect and its attendant changes have been explained by an inhibition of the depolarizing inward sodium current.

Sotalol is unique among the β-blockers in that it alone possesses class III antiarrhythmic properties, causing prolongation of the action potential period and thereby delaying repolarization (Edwardsson et al., 1980). Clinical studies have verified the efficacy of sotalol in the control of arrhythmias (Latour et al., 1977; Fogelman et al., 1972; Prakash et al., 1970; Simon and Berman, 1979; Burckhardt et al., 1983), but additional investigation will be required to determine whether its class III antiarrhythmic properties contribute significantly to its efficacy as an antiarrhythmic agent.

The most important mechanism underlying the antiarrhythmic effect of β-blockers (with the possible exclusion of sotalol) is felt to be β-blockade with resultant inhibition of pacemaker potentials. The contribution of membrane-stabilizing action does not appear to be clinically significant. This is born out by at least two separate lines of evidence. The plasma concentration of propranolol necessary for arrhythmia control is far less than the level required for membrane stabilization to occur. In vitro experiments with human ventricular muscle have shown that the concentration of propranolol required for membrane stabilization is 50–100 times the concentration usually associated with inhibition of exercise-induced tachycardia and at which only β-blocking effects occur (Coltart et al., 1970). Moreover, d-propranolol which possesses membrane-stabilizing properties but no β-blocking action, is a weak antiarrhythmic event in high doses, while β-blockers devoid of membrane-stabilizing action (atenolol, metoprolol, nadolol, pindolol, etc.) have been shown to be effective antiarrhythmic drugs.

Table 12-5 Antiarrhythmic Mechanisms for β-Blockers

1. β-Blockade
   - Electrophysiology: depress excitability; depress conduction
   - Prevention of ischemia: decrease automaticity; inhibit reentrant mechanisms
2. Membrane-stabilizing effects
   - Local anesthetic, "quinidine-like" properties: depress excitability; prolong refractory period; delay conduction
   - Clinically, probably not significant
3. Special pharmacologic properties (β-cardioselectivity, intrinsic sympathomimetic activity) do not appear to contribute to antiarrhythmic effectiveness

If, indeed, β-blockade is the major mechanism for the antiarrhythmic effect, with the contribution of membrane-stabilizing properties being negligible, then one would expect all β-blockers to be similarly effective at a comparable level of β-blockade. In fact, this appears to be the case. No superiority of one β-blocking agent over another in the therapy of arrhythmias has yet been demonstrated convincingly. Differences in overall clinical usefulness are related to their other associated pharmacologic properties (Table 12-5) (Gibson, 1974).

β-Blockers slow the rate of discharge of the sinus and ectopic pacemakers and increase the effective refractory period of the atrioventricular node by their β-adrenergic blocking actions. They also slow both antegrade and retrograde conduction in anomalous pathways (Frishman and Silverman, 1979a). Since all β-blockers studied thus far cause an increase in atrioventricular conduction time, advanced A-V block is a potential complication when β-blockers are used. Agents with partial agonist activity (intrinsic sympathomimetic activity) such as oxprenolol and pindolol, may provide some protection from the A-V conduction impairment induced by blockade (Giudicelli et al., 1975).

In high doses, β-blockers can induce sinus node dysfunction and lead to sinoatrial block or sinus arrest. These drugs are therefore best avoided in patients with "sick sinus syndrome," a condition which can be exacerbated by β-adrenergic blockade (Frishman and Silverman, 1979a).

Therapeutic Uses in Cardiac Arrhythmias

β-Adrenergic blocking drugs have become an important treatment modality for various cardiac arrhythmias (Table 12-6). While it has been acknowledged for a long time that β-blockers are more effective for supraventricular than ventricular arrhythmias, it has been appreciated only recently that these agents can be quite useful in the treatment of ventricular tachyarrhythmias in the setting of myocardial ischemia.

Table 12-6 Drug Interactions that May Occur with β-Adrenoreceptor Blocking Drugs.

Drug	Possible Effects	Precautions
Aluminum hydroxide gel	Decreases β-blocker absorption and therapeutic effect	Avoid β-blocker-aluminum hydroxide combination
Aminophylline	Mutual inhibition	Observe patient's response
Antidiabetic agents	Enhanced hypoglycemia: hypertension	Monitor for altered diabetic response
Calcium channel inhibitors (e.g., verapamil, diltiazem)	Potentiation of bradycardia, myocardial depression, and hypotension	Avoid use, although few patients show ill effects
Cimetidine	Prolongs half-life of propranolol	Combination should be used with caution
Clonidine	Hypertension during clonidine withdrawal	Monitor for hypertensive response; withdraw β-blocker before withdrawing clonidine
Digitalis glycosides	Potentiation of bradycardia	Observe patient's response; interactions may benefit angina patients with abnormal ventricular function
Epinephrine	Hypertension; bradycardia	Administer epinephrine cautiously; cardioselective β-blocker may be safer
Ergot alkaloids	Excessive vasoconstriction	Observe patient's response; few patients show ill effects
Glucagon	Inhibition of hyperglycemic effect	Monitor for reduced response
Halofenate	Reduced β-blocking activity; production of propranolol withdrawal rebound syndrome	Observe for impaired response to β-blockade
Indomethacin	Inhibition of antihypertensive response to β-blockade	Observe patient's response
Isoproterenol	Mutual inhibition	Avoid concurrent use or choose cardiac selective β-blocker
Levodopa	Antagonism of levodopa's hypotensive and positive inotropic effects	Monitor for altered response; interaction may have favorable results
Lidocaine	Propranolol pretreatment increases lidocaine blood levels and potential toxicity	Combination should be used with caution; use lower doses of lidocaine
Methyldopa	Hypertension during stress	Monitor for hypertensive episodes
Monoamine oxidase inhibitors	Uncertain, theoretical	Manufacturer of propranolol considers concurrent use contraindicated

Table 12-6 continued.

Drug	Possible Effects	Precautions
Phenothiazines	Additive hypotensive effects	Monitor for altered response especially with high doses of phenothiazine
Phenylpropranol-amine	Severe hypertensive reaction	Avoid use, especially in hypertension controlled by both methyldopa and β-blockers
Phenytoin	Additive cardiac depressant effects	Administer IV phenytoin with great caution
Quinidine	Additive cardiac depressant effects	Observe patient's response; few patients show ill effects
Reserpine	Excessive sympathetic blockade	Observe patient's response
Tricyclic Anti-depressants	Inhibits negative inotropic and chronotropic effects of β-blockers	Observe patient's response
Tubocurarine	Enhanced neuromuscular blockade	Observe response in surgical patients, especially after high doses of propranolol

Supraventricular Arrhythmias

These arrhythmias have a variable response to β-blockade. β-Blockers are not only therapeutically useful, but diagnostically important; by slowing a very rapid heart rate, the drug may permit an accurate ECG diagnosis of an otherwise puzzling arrhythmia.

Sinus Tachycardia This arrhythmia usually has an obvious cause (e.g., fever, hyperthyroidism, congestive heart failure) and therapy should be addressed to correction of the underlying condition. However, if the rapid heart rate itself is compromising the patient, for example, causing recurrent angina in a patient with coronary artery disease, then direct intervention with a β-blocker is effective and indicated therapy. Patients with heart failure, however, should not be treated with β-blockers unless they have been placed on diuretic therapy and digitalized, and then only with extreme caution.

Supraventricular Ectopic Beats As with sinus tachycardia, specific treatment of these extrasystoles is seldom required and therapy should be directed to the underlying cause. Although supraventricular ectopic beats are often the precursors of atrial fibrillation (especially in acute myocardial infarction, thyrotoxicosis, and mitral stenosis), there is no evidence that prophylactic administration of β-

blockers can prevent the development of atrial fibrillation. Supraventricular ectopic beats due to digitalis toxicity generally respond well to β-blockade. β-Blockers can be useful for those patients in whom supraventricular ectopic activity causes discomforting palpitations.

Paroxysmal Supraventricular Tachycardia (SVT) These may be divided into two groups: 1, Those related to abnormal conduction (e.g., reciprocating A-V nodal tachycardia, the reentrant tachycardias, as in the Wolff-Parkinson-White syndrome, in which there is abnormal conduction through an A-V nodal bypass tract), and 2, Those caused by ectopic atrial activity, as in digitalis toxicity. Since β-blockade delays A-V conduction (e.g., increased A-H interval in His bundle electrocardiograms) and prolongs the refractory period of the reentrant pathways, it is not surprising that many cases of paroxysmal supraventricular tachycardia respond to β-blockers. In acute episodes, vagal maneuvers after β-blockade may effectively terminate an arrhythmia when they may have been previously unsuccessful without β-blockade. Even when β-blockers do not convert an arrhythmia to sinus rhythm, by increasing atrioventricular nodal refractoriness, they will often slow the ventricular rate. Additionally, the use of β-blocking drugs still allows the option of direct current countershock cardioversion (which would be more hazardous if digitalis in high doses was used initially).

Atrial Flutter β-Blockade can be used to slow the ventricular rate (by increasing A-V block) and may restore sinus rhythm in a large percentage of patients. This is a situation in which β-blockade may be of diagnostic value: given intravenously, β-blockers slow the ventricular response and permit the differentiation of flutter waves, ectopic P waves, or sinus mechanism.

Atrial Fibrillation The major action of β-blockers in rapid atrial fibrillation is the reduction in the ventricular response by increasing the refractory period of the A-V node. While all β-blocking drugs have been effective in slowing ventricular rates in patients with atrial fibrillation, they are less effective than quinidine or DC cardioversion in the reversion of atrial fibrillation to sinus rhythm (although this can occur, especially when the atrial fibrillation is of recent onset).

β-Blockers must be used cautiously when atrial fibrillation occurs in the setting of a severely diseased heart which is dependent on high levels of adrenergic tone to avoid myocardial failure. These drugs may be particularly useful in controlling the ventricular rate in situations where this is difficult to achieve with maximally tolerated doses of digitalis (e.g., thyrotoxicosis, hypertrophic cardiomyopathy, mitral stenosis, etc.).

Many patients with paroxysmal atrial fibrillation or flutter may have "sick sinus" or "tachy-brady" syndrome, and administration of β-blockers may precipitate severe bradycardic episodes. These patients often require both antiarrhythmic therapy and a pacemaker.

Ventricular Arrhythmias

β-Adrenoreceptor blocking drugs can decrease the frequency or abolish ventricular ectopic beats in various conditions. They are particularly useful if these arrhythmias are related to excessive catecholamines (e.g., exercise, halothane anesthesia, pheochromocytoma, exogenous catecholamines), myocardial ischemia, or digitalis.

Premature Ventricular Contractions The response of these arrhythmias to β-blockade is variable. The best response can be expected to occur in ischemic heart disease, particularly when the arrhythmia is secondary to an ischemic event. Since β-blockers are effective in preventing ischemic episodes, arrhythmias generated by these episodes may be prevented.

β-Blockers are also quite effective in controlling the frequency of premature ventricular contractions (PVCs) in hypertrophic cardiomyopathy and in mitral valve prolapse. In these situations, a β-blocker is generally the antiarrhythmic drug of first choice.

Ventricular Tachycardia β-Blocking drugs should not be considered agents of choice in the treatment of acute ventricular tachycardia. Cardioversion or other antiarrhythmic drugs (lidocaine, quinidine, procainamide, etc.) should be the initial mode of therapy. β-Blockers have, however, been shown to be of benefit for prophylaxis against recurrent ventricular tachycardia, particularly if sympathetic stimulation appears to be a precipitating cause. There have been several reported studies showing the prevention of exercise-induced ventricular tachycardia by β-blockers; in many previous cases, there had been a poor response to digitalis or quinidine (Taylor and Halliday, 1965; Sloman and Stannard, 1967; Gettes and Surawicz, 1967).

Myocardial Infarction and Sudden Death

There is now conclusive evidence demonstrating a reduction in mortality following an acute myocardial infarction in those patients treated with β-blockers. The most convincing long term data have emerged from the Norwegian timolol trial (1981) and the Beta-Blocker Heart Attack Trial (BHAT) which employed propranolol hydrochloride (1982). The Norwegian trial involving 1,884 patients, demonstrated that timolol maleate, given orally 10 mg twice daily for an average of 17 and up to 33 months, reduced total mortality proportionately by 36%. The BHAT involving 3,837 patients, showed that propranolol, given orally 60–80 mg three times daily for an average of 25 and up to 39 months, reduced total mortality by 26%. As in the timolol study, the protective effect was primarily seen in the first 12–18 months of intervention.

When cause-specific mortality is analyzed in the β-blocker trials, it indicates that the reductions in total mortality were due to a reduction in cardiovascular deaths (Wilhelmsson et al., 1974; Vedin et al., 1975; Ahlmark et al., 1974; Ahlmark et al., 1976; Andersen et al., 1979; Barber et al., 1975; Multicentre International Study, 1975; Multicentre International Study, 1977; The Norwegian Multicenter Study Group, 1981; The Beta-Blocker Heart Attack Trial Research Group, 1982; Hansteen et al., 1982; Julian et al., 1982; Taylor et al., 1982b; Australian and Swedish Pindolol Study Group, 1983). Although different definitions of sudden death were employed in the trials, the benefit from β-blocker treatment appears to stem particularly from the prevention of these deaths. Pooled data from the seven trials reporting on sudden death (Wilhelmsson et al., 1974; Ahlmark et al., 1976; Multicentre International Study, 1975; Multicentre International Study, 1977; The Norwegian Multicenter Study Group, 1981; The Beta-Blocker Heart Attack Research Group, 1982; Hansteen et al., 1982; Julian et al., 1982) showed a 28% reduction in mortality compared to placebo, a 33% reduction in sudden cardiac death, and a reduction in nonsudden cardiac death of 20%. The reduction in sudden cardiac death would suggest a primary antiarrhythmic effect in explaining the beneficial action of β-blockers. By effecting β-blockade, these agents can attenuate cardiac stimulation by the sympathetic nervous system, and perhaps the potential for reentrant ventricular arrhythmias and sudden death (Pratt and Lichstein, 1982; Anderson et al., 1983). Experimental studies have shown that β-blockers raise the ventricular fibrillation threshold in the ischemic myocardium (Anderson et al., 1983). Placebo-controlled clinical trials have shown that β-blockers reduce the number of episodes of ventricular fibrillation and cardiac arrest during the acute phase of myocardial infarction (Rydén et al., 1983; Yusuf et al., 1983). The long term β-blocker post-myocardial infarction trials and other clinical studies have demonstrated that there is a significant reduction of complex ventricular arrhythmias (Julian et al., 1982; Hjalmarson et al., 1981; Lichstein et al., 1983; Koppes et al., 1980; von der Lippe and Lund-Johansen, 1981).

Although an antiarrhythmic effect of β-blockers is suggested by the reduction in sudden cardiac deaths, this along cannot explain the observed decrease in nonsudden cardiac death and the reduction in nonfatal reinfarctions. The latter two findings may well be a result of the anti-ischemic properties of β-blockers, which may also contribute to the beneficial effect of β-blocker therapy in survivors of myocardial infarction (Frishman et al., 1983).

Clinical Studies

Acebutolol

β_1-Selective with Partial Agonist and Membrane-Stabilizing Activity. Acebutolol (Sectral) is not approved for clinical use in arrhythmia.

In a double-blind study, Williams et al. (1979) demonstrated the efficacy of treating supraventricular tachyarrhythmias with intravenous acebutolol in 15 patients. In the 10 patients with atrial fibrillation, two with atrial flutter, two with multifocal atrial tachycardia, and one with premature atrial complexes, there was a significant reduction in heart rate 5 min after the drug was administered, with a peak reduction at 10–30 min. Two of ten patients with atrial fibrillation converted to normal sinus rhythm with β-blocker treatment.

Aronow et al. (1979b) demonstrated the efficacy of acebutolol in 20 patients with supraventricular tachyarrhythmias, five of whom had chronic obstructive pulmonary disease. All 10 patients with atrial fibrillation and six with atrial flutter slowed their ventricular rates by more than 15 beats/min. Atrial premature contractions were eliminated or reduced by greater than 75% in each of the two patients with this arrhythmia, and the one patient with multifocal atrial tachycardia converted to sinus rhythm. In this study, acebutolol was well tolerated by all five patients with chronic obstructive pulmonary disease.

Ahumada et al. (1979) assessed the effects of intravenous acebutolol on ventricular arrhythmias in 22 patients with acute myocardial infarction. The group of treated patients was matched with 22 control subjects for frequency of ventricular extrasystoles that was measured prior to any treatment with acebutolol. The acebutolol-treated patients showed a significant decrease in the frequency of ventricular extrasystoles and repetitive arrhythmias, while the matched controls failed to exhibit a similar decrement during the same time period.

In a double-blind cross-over clinical trial, Burckhardt and Raeder (1980) studied the effect of acebutolol on both the grade of ventricular arrhythmias and on the incidence of stress-induced arrhythmias in patients with chronic coronary artery disease. Overall, the acebutolol group showed an improvement in the average grade (using a modified Lown classification) from 3.2 ± 0.35 (placebo) to 1.4 ± 0.38 (acebutolol). During and after exercise, the incidence of ventricular arrhythmias in the placebo group decreased from 18.15 ± 7.7 ventricular premature beats (VPB) to 3.46 ± 1.7 VPB in the acebutolol group. Grading of exercise-induced arrhythmias fell from 1.92 ± 3.3 (placebo) to 0.69 ± 0.24 (acebutolol). There was, therefore, both an improvement in the grade of arrhythmias, as well as a significant decrease in VPBs during and after exercise on acebutolol.

To evaluate the long term suppression of ventricular arrhythmias by oral acebutolol, de Soyza et al. (1980) studied 20 patients with documented coronary artery disease. In a 4-week short term trial using an average total daily dose of 1,100 mg, 11 of 20 patients had greater than 70% reduction of PVCs from base-line. Nine of these eleven patients were continued in a long term acebutolol trial for 12 months; and in two-thirds, a greater than 80% reduction in PVC frequency was maintained at the end of 12 months.

In a double-blind randomized study in 20 patients, Aronow et al. (1979a) evaluated the effect of intravenous acebutolol versus saline solution on the frequency of PVCs. Intravenous acebutolol effected a 75% or greater reduction in PVCs in

18 of the 20 patients, while a similar reduction was not seen in any of the 12 patients given intravenous saline. The therapeutic effect of acebutolol lasted for at least 3.5 h in 70% of the patients. Aronow et al. (1980) also compared intravenous acebutolol to propranolol in a double-blind randomized study in 24 patients. In 10 of the 12 patients on propranolol or acebutolol, premature ventricular contractions were abolished or reduced by 75% or more. Singh et al. (1982) confirmed the comparative efficacies of propranolol and acebutolol for decreasing PVCs both at rest and with exercise.

de Soyza et al. (1982) examined 60 patients by 24-h ambulatory ECG monitoring to determine the efficacy of acebutolol in treating ventricular arrhythmias. In a randomized, double-blind, placebo-controlled study using acebutolol 200 and 400 mg three times daily, these investigators showed a greater than 70% reduction in premature ventricular contractions per h in greater than 50% of patients. The 400-mg dose appeared slightly more effective than the 200-mg dose in reducing ventricular ectopy.

In a randomized double-blind placebo-controlled study, Lui et al. (1983) assessed the efficacy of acebutolol in reducing ventricular ectopic beats. Of 25 patients studied, 11 had 70% or greater reduction in ventricular premature beats with acebutolol and 9 of the 11 responders had 90% or greater suppression. The mean reduction of paired ventricular premature beats was 71% on acebutolol (200 or 400 mg) and only 49% on placebo. In five patients, there was total abolition of paroxysmal ventricular tachycardia while on acebutolol.

Shapiro et al. (1982) compared the antiarrhythmic effects of acebutolol to slow-release quinidine sulfate for reducing premature ventricular contractions, in a double-blind randomized cross-over trial of 20 patients. There was no significant difference between the two treatment groups, with 9 of 20 in the acebutolol group and 8 of 20 in the quinidine group demonstrating a 75% reduction in premature ventricular contractions.

The antiarrhythmic significance of dosing intervals with acebutolol was assessed by Frick and Kala (1981) in a double-blind cross-over study of six hypertensive patients with daily ventricular arrhythmias. These investigators examined whether a once daily regimen of acebutolol (400 mg) was as effective as a twice daily regimen (200 mg) in controlling hypertension and arrhythmias. Both regimens were equally effective in reducing blood pressure and heart rate at rest and with exertion, and both significantly shortened the Q-Tc interval. However, only the twice daily dosage significantly decreased the incidence of ventricular ectopy (a sustained reduction of 50% throughout the 24 h), while the once daily regimen did not (a sustained reduction of only 7% over 24 h). The measured serum concentration of acebutolol was found to be twice as high on the twice daily regimen. In view of the same degree of β-blockade on both regimens (as measured by similar decreases in heart rate at both rest and exertion with both dosing intervals), it was concluded that the antiarrhythmic effect of acebutolol was better correlated with its plasma concentration rather than with the degree of clinically determined β-blockade.

Atenolol

β_1-Selective without Membrane-Stabilizing or Partial Agonist Activity. Atenolol (Tenormin) is not approved for clinical use in arrhythmia.

Winchester et al. (1978) treated 29 patients with supraventricular arrhythmias with two different intravenous β-blockers. Seventeen received intravenous atenolol 0.15 mg/kg for 20 min, and 12 received intravenous acebutolol 1.0 mg/kg for 15 min. Eleven of twelve patients with atrial flutter or fibrillation had their ventricular rate reduced to less than 100 beats/min, including one conversion to sinus rhythm. Of the 16 patients with paroxysmal supraventricular tachycardia, four had their heart rate slowed to less than 100 beats/min, five had no change in heart rate, and seven reverted to sinus rhythm. All six treatment failures occurred in patients with acute arrhythmias, whereas all patients with chronic arrhythmias responded. No differences in the antiarrhythmic efficacies of the two drugs were observed.

Rossi et al. (1983) assessed the efficacy of intravenous atenolol in the treatment of ventricular arrhythmias in 182 patients suspected of an acute myocardial infarction. Ninety-five patients were randomized to receive intravenous atenolol followed by oral treatment, and 87 patients received placebo. The treated patients had significantly fewer ventricular extrasystoles. Repetitive ventricular arrhythmias were detected in 64 control patients (74%) and in 55 placebo-treated patients (58%). R on T wave arrhythmias occurred in 58 control patients (67%), compared with only 25 treated patients. These investigators confirmed that early intravenous atenolol prevents ventricular arrhythmias in patients with suspected acute myocardial infarction.

Roland et al. (1978) used 24-h ECG tape recordings to determine the incidence of arrhythmias in 388 patients with suspected myocardial infarction who were receiving either propranolol, atenolol, or placebo. Seventy-six per cent of patients with a diagnosed myocardial infarction had ventricular arrhythmias compared to 24% of patients in whom a myocardial infarction was not substantiated. After monitoring patients for 6 weeks, the incidence of arrhythmias was similar with propranolol, atenolol, and placebo. There was no difference in the incidence or type of arrhythmias recorded between patients who died and those who were still alive at 6 weeks. These investigators hypothesized that since the β-blockers used in this study showed little evidence of antiarrhythmic activity, increasing the dosage would not be prudent because of the risk of hypotension.

In contrast to the findings of Roland et al. (1978), Yusuf et al. (1983) studied 477 patients suspected of having an acute myocardial infarction, and randomly assigned them treatment with intravenous and oral atenolol or placebo. Atenolol treatment significantly prevented the development of infarction compared to placebo, in patients who presented with no electrocardiographic changes. One hundred eighty of these patients were analyzed for ventricular arrhythmias by 24-h ECG monitoring. There was a significant reduction in the incidence of R on T ectopic beats in the atenolol-treated group (26%) compared to the 67% incidence in the placebo group. In the atenolol-treated patients, there was a significant reduction in repetitive ventricular arrhythmias, and a marginally significant reduction in supraventricular arrhythmias, most significantly in the incidence of atrial fibrillation. These investigators noted fewer cardiac arrests in the atenolol-treated group, but could not definitely implicate an antiarrhythmic effect for their observations.

Esmolol

β_1-Selective without Partial Agonist or Membrane-Stabilizing Activity. Esmolol (ASL-8052) is a new ultrashort-acting (half-life possibly 10 min) β-adrenergic blocker which is only available in intravenous form. It is still in the early stages of clinical testing and is not yet approved for clinical use in the United States.

Preliminary studies have shown the drug to be both effective and safe when used either as a pulse dose or drip infusion to treat various supraventricular and ventricular arrhythmias (Byrd et al., 1983; Byrd et al., in press).

Labetalol

Nonselective, β-Blocker with α_1-Adrenergic Blocking Activity, No Membrane or Partial Agonist Activity. Labetalol (Trandate, Normodyne) is not approved for clinical use in arrhythmia.

Preliminary studies have shown labetalol to be both safe and effective for treating hypertensive patients with varied supraventricular and ventricular arrhythmias. Mazzola et al. (1981) studied the acute antihypertensive and antiarrhythmic effect of labetalol in 26 patients, 11 of whom had arrhythmias which were comprised of: paroxysmal atrial fibrillation (three patients), sinus tachycardia (two patients), paroxysmal supraventricular tachycardia (three patients), slow atrial fibrillation (one patient), and ventricular tachycardia (two patients). Labetalol was given intravenously at a rate of 1 mg/min and restored sinus rhythm in all but two patients: there was no effect in the patient with slow atrial fibrillation, and one patient with paroxysmal atrial fibrillation died of complete heart block and low cardiac output. Romano et al. (1981) conducted a preliminary clinical trial on the hypotensive and antiarrhythmic effect of labetalol in 10 patients with essential hypertension and frequent PVCs. At a dose of 800 mg daily, labetalol significantly lowered blood pressure and produced a significant reduction in PVCs after 2 weeks. By the end of 4 weeks, the PVCs were almost completely suppressed.

Metoprolol

β_1-Selective without Partial Agonist or Membrane-Stabilizing Activity. Metoprolol (Lopressor, Betacore) is not approved for clinical use in arrhythmia.

Moller and Rehnquist (1979) treated 21 patients with paroxysmal supraventricular tachyarrhythmias, atrial flutter, and atrial fibrillation. Using 2–20 mg of intravenous metoprolol, approximately 50% of the patients with paroxysmal supraventricular tachycardia and atrial flutter converted to normal sinus rhythm, compared to one of eight patients with atrial fibrillation. Of those patients who did not convert to normal sinus rhythm, there was still a significant lowering of the ventricular rate.

These findings were confirmed by Rehnquist (1981) who performed a multicenter study involving 142 patients; 28 had paroxysmal atrial tachycardia, 35 had atrial flutter, and 79 atrial fibrillation. Using 5–15 mg of metoprolol intravenously, 57% of the patients with paroxysmal atrial tachycardia, 23% with atrial flutter, and 13% with atrial fibrillation converted to normal sinus rhythm. A ventricular rate reduction of more than 25%, or less than 100 beats/min was obtained in 68% of the patients, with an additional 18% showing a reduction of 10% in ventricular rate.

In a double-blind, placebo-controlled trial, Whitehead (1980) followed 60 dental patients who underwent general anesthesia. After induction, he noted a lower mean heart rate in the metoprolol group (86 beats/min) compared to placebo (98 beats/min). Runs of ventricular premature contractions occurred in 12 patients on placebo and in only four on metoprolol.

Pratt et al. (1983) evaluated the efficacy of metoprolol in suppressing complex ventricular arrhythmias in a single-blind, placebo-controlled 10-day protocol with continuous Holter monitoring of 20 patients. At a dose of 200 mg daily, metoprolol suppressed 60% of total PVCs and 84% of ventricular couplets. Of 10 patients who demonstrated ventricular tachycardia during placebo, metoprolol had total suppression in six patients and overall, effected a 94% reduction. During exercise testing, metoprolol demonstrated a 70% reduction in total PVCs, complete suppression of couplets in five of seven patients, and elimination of all exercise-induced ventricular tachycardia.

Metoprolol and its antiarrhythmic effects in post-myocardial infarction patients was studied by Olsson et al. (1981). In a double-blind trial using placebo or oral metoprolol, 100 mg twice daily, the investigators followed patients for 6 months after their myocardial infarcts. There was a significant decrease in malignant premature ventricular contractions at 1 month with metoprolol, which was not observed at 6 months.

Rydén et al. (1983) analyzed the effects of intravenous and oral metoprolol on ventricular arrhythmias in 1,395 patients suspected of having a myocardial infarction. In their double-blind, placebo-controlled, randomized study, patients received either placebo or 15 mg of metoprolol intravenously at the time of admission, and then 200 mg daily for 3 months. Metoprolol did not influence the occurrence of premature ventricular contractions or reduce the incidence of ventricular tachycardia episodes, but only 6 of the 23 patients with ventricular fibrillation were from the metoprolol group. It was suggested from these findings that metoprolol has a prophylactic effect against ventricular fibrillation in patients with acute myocardial infarction. In a further analysis of the above study in regard to the effects on mortality and morbidity, Hjalmarson et al. (1983) found that there was a decrease in the 3-month total mortality by 36% in the metoprolol-treated group (62 deaths in the placebo group versus 40 in the metoprolol group). This reduction in 3-month total mortality in the metoprolol group was independent of age, history of prior myocardial infarction, or history of prior chronic β-blocker therapy (before entry into the study). These investigators also noted a 35% reduction in late myocardial infarction in those patients in the metoprolol group. After 90 days of double-blind treatment, all patients were given open treatment with metoprolol. In a 1-year follow-up, it was found that there was still a difference in mortality between the original two groups after 90 days and 1 year. These findings suggest that in order to exert a beneficial effect, metoprolol therapy should be initiated during the early phase of a myocardial infarction.

Nadolol

Nonselective, without Partial Agonist Effects or Membrane-Stabilizing Activity. Nadolol (Corgard) is not approved for clinical use in arrhythmia.

As with other β-adrenoreceptor blocking drugs, nadolol has antiarrhythmic properties that stem from its ability to antagonize the effects of catecholamines on cardiac automaticity and conductivity (Frishman, 1981b; Evans et al., 1976). Although the electrophysiologic properties of nadolol are known, there are sparse clinical data on its effects on arrhythmia.

Vukovich et al. (1976) treated 29 patients with ventricular and supraventricular arrhythmias with sequential oral doses of placebo and nadolol. A reduction or remission of arrhythmias was observed in approximately two-thirds of the patients. Arrhythmias that responded favorably to nadolol therapy included ventricular bigeminy and trigeminy, paroxysmal supraventricular tachycardia, and sinus tachycardia. The patients with atrial flutter or fibrillation did not convert to normal sinus rhythm with nadolol therapy, but did demonstrate a reduced ventricular response.

In a single-blind, cross-over study (Myburgh et al., 1983), the efficacy of nadolol versus sotalol was compared in the suppression of PVCs in 22 patients with chronic ventricular arrhythmias. Both drugs significantly suppressed ventricular ectopy and there was no statistically significant prolongation of the Q-Tc interval.

Nadolol might prove extremely useful in long term management of cardiac arrhythmias because of its long plasma half-life that requires once daily administration; however, more clinical data will be required to establish the efficacy of a single daily dose of nadolol or any other long-acting β-blocker in patients with arrhythmias.

Oxprenolol

Nonselective, with Partial Agonist Activity and Membrane-Stabilizing Activity. Oxprenolol (Trasicor, Iset) is not approved for clinical use in arrhythmia.

Sandler et al. (1971) studied the efficacy of intravenous and oral oxprenolol for the treatment of various cardiac arrhythmias in 43 patients with acute myocardial ischemia or infarctions. Thirteen of twenty-seven episodes of paroxysmal supraventricular tachycardia were controlled. Only two of six episodes of supraventricular ectopics were abolished by oxprenolol. None of the seven episodes of atrial fibrillation reverted to sinus rhythm, and in only three of the seven patients did the ventricular rate fall below 100 beats/min. Oxprenolol abolished premature ventricular contractions in 13 of 18 episodes, and two of three patients with idioventricular rhythm converted to normal sinus rhythm. Both patients with ventricular tachycardia failed to respond to oxprenolol treatment, and developed a hypotensive reaction.

Fuccella and Imhoff (1969) examined the efficacy of oral oxprenolol treatment in 98 patients with cardiac arrhythmias. Fifteen of twenty-two patients with sinus tachycardia converted to sinus rhythm and six of the remaining seven had a decrease in heart rate. Of six patients with paroxysmal atrial fibrillation, the attacks completely disappeared in three, and decreased in frequency in another two. Of the 28 patients with chronic atrial fibrillation, only in four did the fibrillation disappear, but in 19, a decrease in heart rate was observed. Since only six patients with atrial flutter were treated, no conclusion could be drawn regarding the efficacy of oxprenolol for this arrhythmia. Six of eight patients with supraventricular extrasystoles experienced a complete disappearance of this arrhythmia, with the two remaining patients experiencing a decrease in frequency. Of the 16 patients with ventricular extrasystoles, five had a complete disappearance of the arrhythmia, with six of the remaining patients experiencing a decreased incidence.

The effects of oxprenolol were examined in a large placebo-controlled trial in 1,103 survivors of an acute myocardial infarction (Taylor et al., 1982b). An antiarrhythmic effect with oxprenolol could explain the reduction in mortality observed when drug treatment was started within 4 months of the infarction.

Pindolol

Nonselective with Partial Agonist Activity and No Membrane-Stabilizing Activity. Pindolol (Visken) is not approved for the treatment of arrhythmia.

Multiple clinical trials have shown pindolol, with partial agonist activity, to be as efficacious as propranolol for the treatment of supraventricular arrhythmias (Frishman, 1983; Levi and Proto, 1972).

Frishman et al. (1979a) evaluated intravenous and oral pindolol in 18 patients with supraventricular tachyarrhythmias (paroxysmal atrial tachycardia, atrial fibrillation and flutter) who had been responsive to propranolol treatment, but where long term maintenance with propranolol was not possible because of drug-induced bronchospasm. All 18 patients failed to respond to an initial intravenous placebo, after which they received intravenous pindolol (0.4–1.4 mg). Six of seven patients with paroxysmal supraventricular tachycardia converted to normal sinus rhythm. In the six patients with atrial fibrillation, three converted to normal sinus rhythm, and three demonstrated only ventricular rate slowing. Of the two patients with atrial flutter, one converted to normal sinus rhythm, and one had no response. Both patients with junctional tachycardia converted to normal sinus rhythm as did the one patient with multifocal atrial tachycardia. The 16 patients who responded to intravenous pindolol therapy received oral therapy (2.5–10 mg every 6 h), and on this regimen, a long term antiarrhythmic benefit was maintained in 12 of 16 patients.

Aronow and Vyeyama (1972) studied the efficacy of intravenous pindolol in 30 patients with various cardiac arrhythmias. All seven patients with atrial fibrillation reduced their ventricular rate, with two patients converting to normal sinus rhythm. A rapid ventricular rate was reduced in six of seven patients with atrial flutter. Three of these seven patients converted to atrial fibrillation, two of whom were converted to normal sinus rhythm. One patient with atrial tachycardia became hypotensive after the second dose of pindolol. Two patients with atrioventricular junctional tachycardia, three with sinus tachycardia, and three with atrial premature contractions, were converted to normal sinus rhythm. Paroxysmal repetitive ventricular tachycardia due to digitalis toxicity was abolished in one patient. Pindolol abolished or greatly reduced frequent premature ventricular beats in 10 out of 14 patients. Thus, pindolol was useful for the treatment of cardiac arrhythmias in 24 of these 30 patients.

Podrid and Lown (1982) studied 43 patients to determine the efficacy of pindolol in treating ventricular arrhythmias. Of these patients, 23 had coronary heart disease, five had valvular disease, and 15 had no demonstrable heart disease. The efficacy of pindolol during acute and maintenance therapy was assessed by ambulatory ECG monitoring and treadmill exercise testing. Pindolol was most effective in preventing ventricular arrhythmias provoked by exercise, suppressing premature ventricular beats in 53% of patients. Eighty per cent of patients without demonstrable heart disease had suppression of exercise-induced arrhythmias while they were receiving pindolol, whereas patients with coronary heart disease had a 50% suppression rate. These investigators concluded that pindolol was most effective when ventricular arrhythmias occur with exercise, especially in patients with no structural heart disease. However, pindolol has a limited role as a monotherapy for suppressing ventricular arrhythmias in patients with known coronary artery disease.

Pindolol's effective suppression of exercise-induced arrhythmias was corroborated by Samek and Roskamm (1982) who studied both the antianginal and antiarrhythmic effects of pindolol in 521 patients who had a myocardial infarction 5–6 months earlier. The patients were exercised on a bicycle ergometer with simultaneous ECG recording, both on the day prior to drug testing and 2 h after oral ingestion of 5 mg pindolol. Of the 66 patients in the pretreatment group who developed PVCs during exercise, 44 either reverted to normal rhythm or had a decrease in ectopy; a finding which was found to be statistically highly significant.

A recent electrophysiologic study demonstrated that pindolol's effect on the ventricular fibrillation threshold was not as pronounced as with other β-blockers. This study suggested that β-blockers with partial agonism may not be as effective in preventing sudden death (Anderson et al., 1983).

Propranolol

Nonselective with Membrane-Stabilizing Activity, No Partial Agonist Activity. Propranolol (Inderal) is approved in intravenous and oral form for the treatment of supraventricular tachyarrhythmias. There have been multiple studies confirming the effectiveness of oral and intravenous propranolol for these arrhythmias (Singh and Jewitt, 1974; Harrison et al., 1965; Schamroth, 1966; Irons et al., 1967). Recent studies have also demonstrated the efficacy of the drug for treating ventricular arrhythmias (Lichstein et al., 1983; Hansteen et al., 1982; Tewari et al., 1982; Woosley et al., 1979).

Frieden et al. (1968) treated 30 patients with sustained or recurrent atrial arrhythmias who were treated unsuccessfully with agents such as digoxin, quinidine, diphenylhydantoin, and procainamide. In all 10 patients with atrial fibrillation, the ventricular rate slowed to less than 100 beats/min; three were converted to normal sinus rhythm. Seven of twelve patients with paroxysmal supraventricular arrhythmias were maintained in sinus rhythm with infrequent attacks, and the other five had no attacks for 22 months. Three of four patients with persistent sinus tachycardia were treated successfully with propranolol. Four patients in the study were unable to tolerate the drug because of gastrointestinal side effects and excessive bradycardia.

For the elective therapy of cardiac arrhythmias during an acute myocardial infarction, Lemberg et al. (1970) reported favorably on the use of propranolol. The arrhythmias included atrial fibrillation, atrial flutter, paroxysmal tachycardia, and ventricular tachycardia. A majority of the patients responded to a total intravenous dose of less than 5 mg of propranolol.

Propranolol has also been shown to be an effective agent to prevent supraventricular tachyarrhythmias that frequently occur after coronary artery bypass surgery (Salazar et al., 1979; Oka et al., 1980; Mohr et al., 1981; Silverman et al., 1982). Many of these arrhythmias are caused by the abrupt withdrawal of propranolol just prior to surgery.

In assessing the correct propranolol dose for arrhythmia treatment, Woosley et al. (1979) have suggested that higher oral doses of propranolol be used than those needed to treat hypertension. In a study of 32 patients with chronic high frequency ventricular arrhythmias, dosages were increased sequentially until arrhythmia suppression was achieved, side effects appeared, or a maximum dosage of 960 mg/day was reached. At dosages of less than 160 mg/day, only 33% responded with a 70% or greater decrease in ventricular ectopic beats. At daily dosages of 200–640 mg, an additional 40% responded. Since the response rate for this clinical trial was higher than that observed in other studies, the investigators stressed the need for a more individualized approach to patient therapy.

These same investigators (Woosley et al., 1979) also showed that the plasma concentration needed for ventricular arrhythmia treatment was higher than that needed for β-blockade. This raises the possibility that a mechanism such as membrane stabilization activity may be clinically important. It was also noted that suppression of renin release also occurs at the high dosage level and, therefore, might play a role in arrhythmia suppression.

Gibson and Sowton (1969) reviewed 125 controlled cases of resting ventricular arrhythmia treated with propranolol 25 mg intravenously, or 30–120 mg orally/day. Ventricular arrhythmias were suppressed in 44% and decreased in an additional 13% of the patients.

Nixon et al. (1978) studied the efficacy of propranolol in decreasing the frequency of exercise-induced ventricular ectopic activity in 15 patients. Using individually titrated doses, 10 patients had an effective reduction in exercise-induced ventricular ectopy. Propranolol therapy abolished ventricular tachycardia in four patients, and ventricular couplets in 8 of 12 patients.

Tewari et al. (1982) studied the effects of propranolol versus verapamil on exercise-induced arrhythmias in 65 patients, 38 of whom had coronary artery disease. Total suppression of ventricular ectopy occurred in 31% of the patients while on propranolol as compared to only 17% while on verapamil. Propranolol was able to effect a reduction from grade II to either grade I or 0 in 68.6% of patients with grade II (or higher) ventricular ectopic arrhythmias in contrast to verapamil which was only effective in 35% of these patients. When the 65 patients were separated into groups of coronary artery disease and noncoronary artery disease, both drugs were more effective in the coronary artery disease group.

Koppes et al. (1980) evaluated the use of propranolol in treating premature ventricular beats in 32 patients within 2 months of an uncomplicated acute myocardial infarction. All patients at base-line had more than 30 premature ventricular beats/h with bigeminy, couplets, multifocal complexes, or ventricular tachycardia. With an average dose of 160 mg of propranolol daily, a significant decrease in the frequency and complexity of premature ventricular beats was noted compared to control. During treatment, 50% of patients had a 70% or greater suppression of premature ventricular beats, and in 41% of patients, a 90% or greater suppression of premature ventricular beats was observed. Koppes suggested that a decrease in ventricular arrhythmias induced by propranolol may have a favorable effect in reducing the risk of sudden cardiac death.

In the β-Blocker Heart Attack Trial, the largest controlled study of its kind to date, Lichstein et al. (1983) evaluated the effects of propranolol and placebo on ventricular arrhythmias in survivors of an acute myocardial infarction. Ventricular arrhythmia was defined as a premature ventricular complex frequency of more than 10/h/day with ambulatory ECG monitoring. The ambulatory ECG was recorded at base-line before treatment, and again 6 weeks later. At base-line, 8.0% of patients randomized to propranolol and 9.1% of patients randomized to placebo had ventricular arrhythmias. The frequency of ventricular arrhythmias at 6 weeks in the propranolol-treated group was 14.9% compared to 27.3% in the placebo-treated group. In those patients with arrhythmias at base-line, only 56% (14/25) of the propranolol-treated patients compared to 69% (20/29) of the placebo-treated patients continued to have ventricular arrhythmias. It was also observed that at 6 weeks, 12% of the propranolol-treated patients compared to 23.5% of the placebo-treated patients developed arrhythmias that were not observed during the base-line study.

Hansteen (1983) studied 560 high risk survivors of acute myocardial infarction at 12 Norwegian hospitals. The main purpose of this randomized, double-blind study was to determine the efficacy and safety of propranolol 160 mg/day on the incidence of sudden cardiac death over a 12-month treatment period. A 52% reduction in the rate of sudden cardiac death was noted with propranolol treatment compared to placebo (11 deaths in the propranolol group compared to 23 in the placebo group). The incidence of ventricular arrhythmias was also noted to be more frequent in the placebo-treated patients when compared to patients receiving propranolol.

Sotalol

Nonselective, without Membrane Activity or Partial Agonist Activity. Sotalol (Sotacor) differs electrophysiologically from other β-blockers, since in high concentrations, it prolongs the duration of the action potential in ventricular muscle and Purkinje fibers. Sotalol thus possesses the properties of a class III antiarrhythmic agent, in addition to the class II antiarrhythmic actions shared by all other β-adrenoreceptor blocking drugs. Sotalol at high doses prolongs the ECG Q-T interval, which can predispose to reentrant ventricular arrhythmias by enhancing temporal dispersion. The drug is not approved for clinical use in the United States.

Latour et al. (1977) studied the efficacy of intravenous sotalol using doses of 20–60 mg in 20 patients with various cardiac arrhythmias. Sotalol was beneficial in both patients with sinus tachycardia and in four of seven patients with other supraventricular tachyarrhythmias. The drug was particularly efficacious in lidocaine-resistant ventricular arrhythmias where it was effective in 9 of 11 patients.

Fogelman et al. (1972) treated 34 patients with cardiac arrhythmias of varying etiology with 20 mg of intravenous sotalol. Five of the six patients with paroxysmal supraventricular tachycardia and none of the five patients with atrial flutter reverted to normal sinus rhythm. In the four patients with an acute onset of atrial ectopia, complete abolition of ectopic beats occurred in three, and in the fourth, the incidence of ectopic beats was decreased from 50 to 4 ectopic beats/min. In four of six patients with the acute onset of premature ventricular contractions, the ectopic beats were abolished, and in the remaining two, they were reduced. Two of three patients with chronic ventricular arrhythmias demonstrated a reduced incidence of premature ventricular contractions, while the third patient had an increase in the ectopy from 9 to 20 beats/min. Three of the five patients with the acute onset of atrial fibrillation converted to normal sinus rhythm, with the cardiac rate slowing in the remaining two. None of the nine patients with chronic atrial fibrillation converted to normal sinus rhythm, but the cardiac rate was significantly reduced in seven of the nine patients. No patient with ventricular tachycardia reverted to sinus rhythm with sotalol treatment. These investigators concluded that sotalol was effective for the treatment of supraventricular tachycardias, the acute onset of atrial and ventricular ectopias, and the acute onset of atrial fibrillation.

Prakash et al. (1970) studied the antiarrhythmic efficacy of sotalol in 18 patients with supraventricular arrhythmias and in seven patients with ventricular arrhythmias. Four of six patients with paroxysmal supraventricular tachycardia converted to normal sinus rhythm. In an additional six patients with episodic supraventricular tachycardia, sotalol prevented further recurrences in two. Two of six patients with atrial flutter converted to normal sinus rhythm, but in the other four patients with atrial flutter and in another patient with atrial fibrillation, the ventricular response was slowed from an average of 150 to 60 beats/min. In one patient with paroxysmal atrial fibrillation and in another with paroxysmal ventricular tachycardia, sotalol prevented recurrences in both. In one of two patients, sotalol decreased the frequency of premature atrial contractions, and in five patients with premature ventricular contractions, it abolished the arrhythmias in one and reduced the frequency of the ectopia in the other four. These investigators concluded that sotalol is a moderately effective antiarrhythmic drug.

Simon and Berman (1979) studied 38 patients with various cardiac arrhythmias for an average period of 5.9 months. Of the 38 patients, 16 received intravenous sotalol, cardioversion, or both, to restore sinus rhythm; 13 patients responded to intravenous sotalol alone. Eleven of these thirteen (84.6%) converted to normal sinus rhythm. Nineteen of the twenty-two patients who received oral therapy were well controlled with restoration of sinus rhythm; similarly, sinus rhythm was established in nine of nine patients with paroxysmal supraventricular tachycardia, one of one with atrial flutter, three of four with atrial fibrillation, two of three with paroxysmal ventricular tachycardia, and four of five with premature ventricular contractions. Overall, 35 of 38 patients showed improvement of their arrhythmias on sotalol therapy. Of the three patients who did not improve, two had atrial fibrillation and one had premature ventricular contractions. After discontinuing oral sotalol therapy for 1–3 months, 14 of the original 38 patients were given a second course of sotalol treatment for an additional period of up to 9 months. Three of the six patients with paroxysmal supraventricular tachycardia abolished their arrhythmia, while the other three demonstrated a reduced frequency of the arrhythmia. Of the four patients with paroxysmal ventricular tachycardia, one experienced a decreased severity, and in three patients all arrhythmic episodes ceased. The three patients with atrial fibrillation, and the one with atrial flutter were converted to normal sinus rhythm.

In a placebo-controlled, double-blind, cross-over study, Burckhardt et al. (1983) studied the effects of sotalol on ventricular arrhythmias in patients with chronic ischemic heart disease. Using 24-h Holter monitoring, there was an improvement in maximum Lown class in 7 of 14 patients by 1.7 ± 0.3 classes. These seven responders initially had class IVA and IVB arrhythmias on placebo. There was also a significant decrease in the total number of hours of grade 3 and 4 arrhythmias in all 14 patients. Of the five patients who remained in the same Lown class, the number of hours in grade 3 and 4 arrhythmias were reduced and their PVC-to-PVC coupling intervals increased (417.5 ± 26.2 to 498.0 ± 38.0 ms). These findings are important in that they show that sotalol had a significant effect on high grade ventricular arrhythmias. This study also revealed a highly significant correlation between antiarrhythmic response and Q-T_c interval prolongation (five of the seven patients who improved their Lown class had a prolongation of their Q-T_c interval and two patients' Q-T_c interval remained unchanged), and therefore suggest that the beneficial effect of sotalol on high grade ventricular arrhythmias is a result of Q-T_c interval prolongation.

In a multicenter, double-blind, randomized study, Julian et al. (1982) studied the effect of sotalol 320 mg once daily, compared with placebo in 1,456 patients who survived an acute myocardial infarction. Treatment was started 5–14 days after infarction, and patients were followed for 12 months. The mortality rate was 7.3% in the sotalol group, compared to 8.9% in the placebo group. The mortality was 18% lower in the sotalol compared to the placebo group, but the difference was not statistically significant. This study suggested that the class III antiarrhythmic effects of sotalol are not clinically important, since β-blockers lacking this property appear to show comparable efficacy in postinfarction therapy.

Timolol

Nonselective, without Membrane-Stabilizing Activity or Partial Agonist Activity. Timolol (Blocadren) is not approved for clinical use in arrhythmia.

In a randomized, double-blind study of 88 patients, Tonkin et al. (1981) assessed the efficacy of timolol (10 mg twice daily) administered within 10.74 h ($\pm$ 5.07 h) of onset of acute myocardial infarction. After discharge from the hospital, the patients were reevaluated at 3 and 12 months. Timolol did not demonstrate any reduction in mortality rate, infarct size, or incidence of arrhythmias (except for sinus tachycardia).

The Norwegian Multicenter Study Group (1981) demonstrated a reduction in the incidence of total mortality, nonfatal reinfarction, and sudden death after 1 year of treatment with timolol in survivors of an acute myocardial infarction. In a subproject of the above study, von der Lippe and Lund-Johansen (1981) analyzed the effect of timolol on late ventricular arrhythmias. Eighty-one patients at high risk (groups I and II) who had survived a first infarction or reinfarction were randomized within 7 to 28 days after their myocardial infarction to either placebo (44 patients) or timolol (37 patients). Twenty-four-hour Holter monitoring was done 1 day before randomization, and 3 days, 1 month, and 6 months after initiation of therapy. During this period, the number of patients with complex ventricular arrhythmias (ventricular couplets, bigeminy, ventricular tachycardia, early cycle PVCs), as well as the average number of PVCs per h, significantly increased only in the placebo group. It appears that high risk patients, post-myocardial infarction have an increased severity and incidence of ventricular arrhythmias which, in this study, were effectively inhibited by timolol.

Adverse Effects: Contraindications

The adverse effects of β-blocking drugs can be divided into two categories: 1, those that result from known pharmacologic consequences of β-adrenoreceptor blockade, and 2, other reactions apparently unrelated to β-blockade.

Side effects of the first type are widespread because of the ubiquitous nature of the sympathetic nervous system in the control of metabolic and physiologic function. These include asthma, heart failure, hypoglycemia, heart block, intermittent claudication, and Raynaud's phenomenon. Side effects of the second category are rare and include an unusual oculomucocutaneous reaction and the possibility of carcinogenesis.

Adverse Cardiac Effects Related to β-Adrenoreceptor Blockade

Cardiac Failure β-Adrenoreceptor blockade may cause congestive heart failure 1, in an enlarged heart with impaired myocardial function where excessive sympathetic drive is essential to maintain it on a compensated Starling curve, or 2, if the stroke volume is restricted and tachycardia is needed to maintain cardiac output.

Any β-blocking drug may be associated with the development of heart failure, particularly in patients with underlying myocardial dysfunction. Furthermore, it is possible that an important component of heart failure may be accounted for by increases in peripheral resistance produced by nonselective agents. A recent study (Taylor et al., 1982a) has addressed the claim that β-blockers with intrinsic sympathomimetic activity are less likely to precipitate heart failure. Four intravenous β-blockers were given to 24 patients with coronary artery disease and their effects on left ventricular function were measured. Although all four drugs depressed left ventricular (LV) function, practolol and oxprenolol, which have intrinsic sympathomimetic activity, caused significantly less depression of LV function than propranolol or metoprolol, which lack this property. β_1-Selective blockers (practolol, metoprolol) had a measurable hemodynamic advantage.

β-Blockers should therefore be avoided in patients with significantly impaired myocardial function. If necessary, however, digitalis and diuretics may be used in conjunction with a β-blocker, preferably one having intrinsic sympathomimetic activity.

Atrioventricular Conduction Delay and Sinus Node Dysfunction Slowing of the resting heart rate is a normal response to treatment with a β-blocking drug. Healthy individuals can sustain a heart rate of 50 without impairment. Drugs with intrinsic sympathomimetic activity do not lower the resting heart rate to the same degree as propranolol. However, all β-blocking drugs are contraindicated in patients with "sick sinus syndrome," unless an artificial pacemaker is present.

If there is a partial or complete atrioventricular conduction defect, use of a β-blocking drug may lead to a serious bradyarrhythmia. Compounds which have intrinsic sympathomimetic activity appear to cause less impairment of atrioventricular conduction.

β-Blocker Withdrawal Exacerbation of angina, and in some cases acute myocardial infarction, have been reported following the abrupt cessation of propranolol therapy after chronic administration in patients with coronary artery disease (Adlerman et al., 1974). A "rebound" effect has not been as clearly defined with the other β-blocking agents. However, discontinuation of any β-blocker therapy should be done gradually and cautiously in patients with ischemic heart disease.

Adverse Noncardiac Side Effects Related to β-Adrenoreceptor Blockade

Effect on Ventilatory Function The bronchodilator effects of catecholamines on the bronchial β-receptors are prevented by β-blockade with nonselective agents (Dunlop and Shanks, 1968). Compounds with intrinsic sympathomimetic activity and/or cardioselectivity are less likely to increase airway resistance in asthmatics than propranolol (Beumer and Hardonk, 1972–73; Singh et al., 1976; Skinner et al., 1976). β-Selectivity is not absolute, however, and may diminish with higher doses. Therefore, in general, all β-blockers should be avoided in patients with active bronchospastic disease.

Peripheral Vascular Effects Cold extremities and absent pulses have been described as occurring more frequently in patients receiving β-blockers for hypertension, compared with methyldopa (Waal-Manning, 1976). In some instances, vascular compromise has been severe enough to cause cyanosis and impending gangrene (Frolich et al., 1969). This effect is due to the reduction in cardiac output and blockade of β-adrenergic mediated skeletal muscle vasodilation, resulting in unopposed α-adrenoreceptor vasoconstriction (Lundvall and Jarholt, 1976). β-Blocking drugs with β_1-selectivity or intrinsic sympathomimetic activity will not affect peripheral vessels to the same degree as propranolol. Raynaud's phenomenon is one of the more common side effects of propranolol treatment (Simpson, 1974; Zacharias et al., 1972), and it too, is probably related to nonselective β-blockade.

Patients with peripheral vascular disease who suffer from intermittent claudication often report worsening of symptoms when treated with β-blocking drugs (Rodgers et al., 1976). It is yet to be determined whether drugs with cardioselectivity or intrinsic sympathomimetic activity can protect against this side effect.

Glucose Metabolism In man, mobilization of muscle glycogen is a β-receptor mediated function, while mobilization of liver glycogen depends on α-receptor stimulation (Porter, 1969; Antonis et al., 1967). As a result, β-receptor blocking drugs (especially nonselective blockers) may retard recovery from insulin-induced hypoglycemia. In humans, it has been shown that propranolol can delay the return of blood glucose values to normal after insulin-induced hypoglycemia (Abramson et al., 1966). Likewise, if liver glycogen is reduced by fasting or illness, the concomitant administration of β-blocking drugs may prolong recovery from hypoglycemia since alternative stores cannot be readily mobilized (Dollery et al., 1969). Severe hypoglycemia reactions have been described during therapy with β-blocking drugs, in both insulin-dependent diabetic as well as nondiabetic patients (Abramson et al., 1966; Reveno and Rosenbaum, 1968). Propranolol has been shown to produce blunting of the hyperglycemic response to exercise in normal volunteers (Allison et al., 1969). These hypoglycemic effects may be less marked with β_1-selective agents and agents with intrinsic sympathomimetic activity (which may partially stimulate β_2-receptors) (Deacon and Barnett, 1975).

Additionally, β-blockers cause a marked diminution in the manifestations of sympathetic discharge associated with hypoglycemia, and this interference with compensatory responses to hypoglycemia can mask some "warning signs" of this condition (Lloyd-Mostyn and Oram, 1975).

Central Nervous System Effects Dreams, hallucinations, insomnia, and depression can occur during therapy with β-blockers (Simpson, 1974). These symptoms are evidence of drug entry into the central nervous system (CNS) and are especially common with the highly lipid-soluble β-blockers (propranolol, alprenolol) which presumably penetrate the CNS better.

Other Effects Diarrhea, nausea, gastric pain, constipation, and flatulence have been seen occasionally with all β-blockers. Hematologic reactions are rare: rare cases of purpura (Stephens, 1966) and agranulocytosis (Nawabi and Ritz, 1973) have been described with propranolol.

Adverse Effects Unrelated to β-Adrenoreceptor Blockade

Oculomucocutaneous Syndrome; Sclerosing Peritonitis A characteristic immune reaction, the oculomucocutaneous syndrome, affecting singly or in combination eyes, mucous and serous membranes, and the skin, often in association with a positive antinuclear factor, has been reported in patients treated with practolol, and has led to the curtailment of its use (Wright, 1975; Waal-Manning, 1975). Close attention has been focused on this syndrome because of fears that other β-adrenoceptor blocking drugs may be associated with this syndrome. Sclerosing peritonitis is another apparent immunologic complication that has been reported following protracted oral practolol therapy.

Carcinogenicity Pronethanol, the first β-adrenoreceptor blocking drug to achieve wide use, was withdrawn by its manufacturers because, in doses 10 times the maximum therapeutic concentration, it caused thymic tumors and lymphosarcomata in mice, although not in rats or dogs (Paget, 1963). More recently, tolamolol and pamatolol, two cardioselective β-adrenoreceptor blocking drugs, were withdrawn from clinical trials because they caused mammary tumors in mice and rats at high doses (Status Report on β-Blockers, 1978). The relevance of these findings to causation of tumors in man is difficult to evaluate, since the doses were high and the relationship between malignant tumors in animals and man has not been defined.

Drug Interactions

β-Blockers may often be administered as part of combined antiarrhythmic therapy, or may be one of several agents in a patient's overall therapeutic regimen. They may be used together with digitalis to control the ventricular rate in atrial fibrillation or flutter or to convert the rhythm to sinus rhythm. Combinations of β-blocking drugs and quinidine have been tried in attempts to convert atrial fibrillation to sinus rhythm and to maintain sinus rhythm after successful conversion. Since β-blockade appears to be the major factor in the antiarrhythmic effects of β-blockers and the "quinidine-like" (membrane-depressant) actions appear negligible, it would seem logical that such combined therapy would have a beneficial additive effect. Several studies have demonstrated a high rate of conversion of atrial fibrillation to sinus rhythm with combined quinidine-β-blocker therapy, including arrhythmias that were resistant to quinidine therapy alone (Sterns and Borman, 1969; Reynolds and Vander Ark, 1967; Fors et al., 1971). Such combined therapy has also helped maintain sinus rhythm after cardioversion (Levi and Proto, 1970).

β-Blockers along with quinidine or procainamide may also be given for resistant ventricular arrhythmias, especially in patients with coronary artery disease. Caution must be used for the possible exacerbation of congestive heart failure because of additional cardiac depressant effects.

Increasing numbers of patients may be on combined therapy with β-blockers and the new calcium channel blocking agents, for the treatment of ischemic heart disease and tachyarrhythmias. These patients may be particularly susceptible to severe bradycardia, congestive heart failure or hypotension; combined therapy must be administered with caution.

Table 12-6 summarizes drug interactions that may occur with β-blocking drugs.

Toxicity and Treatment of Toxicity

The β-adrenoreceptor blocking drugs have many associated adverse effects when used in the therapeutic dose range. With the growing application of these drugs in clinical practice, cases of attempted suicide and accidental overdosage resulting in bradycardia, hypotension, low cardiac output, cardiac failure, and cardiogenic shock have been reported (Editorial, 1978). Bronchospasm may also occur, and respiratory depression can develop, perhaps as a result of severe circulatory impairment or from a central drug effect. In severe intoxications, the myocardium may become relatively refractory to pharmacologic and electrical stimulation, and death occurs in asystole (Editorial, 1978). Changes in mental status, convulsions, and coma have been seen in patients with β-blocker overdosage.

Sotalol intoxication differs from that seen with other β-blockers. In addition to hypotension and bradycardia, patients have significantly prolonged corrected Q-T intervals with severe ventricular tachyarrhythmias. Neuvonen et al. (1981) reported on six patients with sotalol intoxication (of 2.4–8 g) with the above findings. In five of the six, serious ventricular arrhythmias were seen, including multifocal ventricular extrasystoles and bigeminy (five patients), several episodes of ventricular tachycardia (four patients), and short periods of ventricular fibrillation (two patients). Of all the β-blockers, sotalol alone has class III antiarrhythmic activity (in addition to class II), and the finding of malignant ventricular arrhythmias with sotalol intoxication therefore should not be too surprising, since it is known that a prolonged Q-T interval predisposes to reentrant arrhythmias.

The major goals of treatment of β-blocker poisoning are: 1, to remove quickly any ingested tablets; 2, to counteract life-threatening cardiovascular and pulmonary effects; and 3, to treat central nervous system disturbances. These patients should be managed with intensive supportive care in facilities equipped for continuous cardiac monitoring and ventilatory support. The clinical manifestations of intoxication are usually seen within 1–2 h after ingestion, and because of the prolonged effects of β-blockers in the body, may persist for several days. Sudden rapid deterioration with cardiovascular collapse is common.

If ingestion is recent, emesis should be initiated to remove unabsorbed tablets. If the patient is comatose or convulsing, endotracheal intubation should be performed, followed by gastric lavage with a large bore tube. Activated charcoal can be given orally or by lavage, and sodium or magnesium sulfate can be given orally as a cathartic. Hemodialysis is unlikely to rid the body of propranolol, since the drug is greater than 95% protein-bound.

Patients should be monitored carefully for bradycardia and atrioventricular conduction defects. Should these occur, atropine in a dose of 0.5–3.0 mg intravenously should be given to reduce unopposed vagal activity. If this is unsuccessful, isoproterenol infusion at a dosage rate of 4 mg/min may be useful, although occasionally higher infusion rates have been required. Glucagon, which increases heart rate and improves atrioventricular conduction by nonadrenergic mechanisms, may be useful in patients unresponsive to isoproterenol (Glick et al., 1968). Glucagon is administered as an initial intravenous bolus of 50 mg/kg infused over 1 min, followed by an intravenous infusion of 1–5 mg/h. A temporary transvenous pacemaker should be inserted if heart block or severe bradycardia cannot be readily controlled by pharmacologic means.

Glucagon, in addition to its electrophysiologic effects, activates adenyl cyclase and enhances myocardial contractility by mechanisms different from catecholamines; its inotropic effect is not blocked by β-blockers (Glick et al., 1968; Parmley, 1971; Kosinski and Malindazak, 1973). It is felt to be the initial drug of choice for myocardial depression and hypotension in β-blocker self-poisoning, although epinephrine and norepinephrine have both been proven efficacious (Glick et al., 1968; Parmley, 1971; Kosinski and Malindazak, 1973).

The physician should rapidly establish effective respiratory function in patients, creating an artificial airway if necessary. Adequate tidal volume should be maintained. Although rare in self-poisoning, severe bronchoconstriction may require isoproterenol inhalation in larger than usual doses. Aminophylline can be given as an initial 5–6 mg/kg intravenous bolus over 15–20 min, followed by a continuous infusion of 0.9 mg/kg/h, maintaining serum aminophylline levels at 10–20 mg/ml. A β_2-adrenoreceptor stimulating drug (e.g., terbutaline) can also be administered.

Hypoglycemia, a rare complication of β-adrenoreceptor blocker self-poisoning, can be treated with glucose and/or glucagon. Seizure activity can be seen in β-adrenoreceptor blocker overdosage. Hypotension, hypoxia, or hypoglycemia should be corrected, and intravenous diazepam has proven to be effective in controlling seizure activity in several patients.

Acknowledgments

Reprinted in part from Frishman, W.H. 1984. Clinical Pharmacology of the β-Adrenoceptor Blocking Drugs. 2nd Ed. Norwalk: Appleton-Century-Crofts. In Press, with permission.

References

Ablad, B., Brugard, M., and Elk, L. 1967. Pharmacologic properties of H56/28, a β-adrenergic receptor antagonist. Acta Pharmacol Toxicol (suppl 2) 25:9–40.

Abramson, E.A., Arky, R.A., and Woeber, L.A. 1966. Effects of propranolol on the hormonal and metabolic responses to insulin induced hypoglycemia. Lancet 2:1386–1388.

Adlerman, E.L., Coltart, D.J., Wettach, G.E., and Harrison, D.C. 1974. Coronary artery syndromes after sudden propranolol withdrawal. Ann Intern Med 81:925–927.

Ahlmark, G., and Saetre, H. 1976. Long-term treatment with beta-blockers after myocardial infarction. Eur J Clin Pharmacol 10:77–83.

Ahlmark, G., Saetre, H., and Korsgren, M. 1974. Reduction of sudden death after myocardial infarction. Lancet 2:1563.

Ahlquist, R.P. 1948. A study of the adrenotropic receptors. Am J Physiol 153:586–599.

Ahumada, G.G., Karlsberg, R.P., Jaffe, A.S., Ambos, H.D., Sobel, B.E., and Roberts, R. 1979. Reduction of early ventricular arrhythmia by acebutolol in patients with acute myocardial infarction. 41(6):654–659.

Allison, S.P., Chamberlain, M.I., and Miller, J.E. 1969. Effects of propranolol on blood sugar, insulin and free fatty acids. Diabetologia 5:339–342.

Andersen, M.P., Frederiksen, J., Jurgensen, H.J., Pedersen, F., Bechsgaard, P., Hansen, D.A., Nielsen, B., Pedersen-Bjergaard, O., and Rasmussen, S.L. 1979. Effect of alprenolol on mortality among patients with definite or suspected acute myocardial infarction. Lancet 2:865–868.

Anderson, J.L., Rodier, H.E., and Green, L.S. 1983. Comparative effects of beta-adrenergic blocking drugs on experimental ventricular fibrillation threshold. Am J Cardiol 51:1196–1202.

Antonis, A., Clark, M.L., Hodge, R.L., Molony, M., and Pickington, T.R.E. 1967. Receptor mechanisms in the hyperglycaemic response to adrenaline in man. Lancet 1:1135–1137.

Aronow, W.S., Turbow, M., Lurie, M., Whittaker, K., and Van Camps, S. 1979a. Treatment of premature ventricular complexes with acebutolol. Am J Cardiol 43(1):106–108.

Aronow, W.S., and Uyeyama, R.R. 1972. Treatment of arrhythmias with pindolol. Clin Pharmacol Ther 13:15–22.

Aronow, W.S., Van Camp, S., Turbow, M., Whittaker, K., and Lurie, M. 1979b. Acebutolol in supraventricular arrhythmias. Clin Pharmacol Ther 25:149–153.

Aronow, W.S., Wong, R., Plasencia, G., Landa, D., and Turbow, M. 1980. Effect of acebutolol and propranolol on premature ventricular complexes. Clin Pharmacol Ther 28(1):28–31.

Atterhög, J.H., Duner, H., and Pernow, B. 1976. Experience with pindolol, a β-receptor blocker in the treatment of hypertension. Am J Med 60:872–876.

Australian and Swedish Pindolol Study Group. The effect of pindolol on the two years mortality after complicated myocardial infarction. Eur Heart J 4:367–375.

Barber, J.M., Boyle, D. McC., Chaturvedi, N.C., Singh, N., and Walsh, M.J. 1976. Practolol in acute myocardial infarction. Acta Med Scand (suppl) 587:213–219.

Barrett, A.M., and Cullum, V.A. 1968. The biological properties of the optical isomers of propranolol and their effect on cardiac arrhythmias. Br J Pharmacol 34:43–55.

Basil, B., Jordan, R., Loveless, A.H., and Maxwell, D.R. 1973. β-Adrenoceptor blocking properties and cardioselectivity of M and B 17,803A. Br J Pharmacol 48:198–211.

The β-Blocker Heart Attack Trial Research Group. 1982. A randomized trial of propranolol in patients with acute myocardial infarction. JAMA 247:1707–1714.

Beumer, H.M., and Hardonk, H.J. 1972–73. Effects of β-adrenergic blocking drugs on ventilatory failure in asthmatics. Eur J Clin Pharmacol 5:77–80.

Black, J.W., and Stephenson, J.S. 1962. Pharmacology of a new adrenergic β-receptor blocking compound (nethalide). Lancet 2:311–314.

Brunner, H., Hedwall, P.R., and Maier, R., 1970. Pharmacologic pro aspects of oxprenolol. Postgrad Med J (Nov Suppl) 5–14.

Burckhardt, D., Pfisterer, M., Hoffman, A., Burkart, F., Emmenegger, H., Jost, M., Boili, P., and Buehler, F.R. 1983. Effects of the beta-adrenoceptor blocking agent sotalol on ventricular arrhythmias in patients with chronic ischemic heart disease. A placebo-controlled, double-blind crossover study. Cardiology 70(suppl 1):114–121.

Burckhardt, D., and Raeder, E.A. 1980. The effect of acebutolol on cardiac arrhythmias in patients with chronic coronary artery disease. Am Heart J 99(4):443–445.

Byrd, R.C., Sung, R.J., Mark, J., Newlands, J., and Parmley, W.C. 1983. Efficacy of ASL-8052 (a short-training beta-adrenergic blocking agent) for control of ventricular rate in atrial flutter or atrial fibrillation. Clin Res 31:172A.

Byrd, R.C., Sung, R.J., Marks, J., and Parmley, W.W. 1984. Safety and efficacy of esmolol (ASL-8052: an ultrashort-acting beta-blocking agent) for control of ventricular rate in supraventricular tachycardias. J Am Coll Cardiol 3(2 pt. 1):392–399.

Coltart, D.J., Gibson, D.G., and Shand, D.G. 1970. Plasma propranolol levels associated with suppression of ventricular ectopic beats. Br Med J 3:731–734.

Connolly, M.E., Keusting, F., and Dollery, C.T. 1976. The clinical pharmacology of β-adrenoreceptor blocking drugs. Progr Cardiovasc Dis 19:203–234.

Cruickshank, J.M. 1980. The clinical importance of cardioselectivity and lipophilicity in beta-blockers. Am Heart J 100:160–178.

Deacon, S.P., and Barnett, D. 1976. Comparison of atenolol and propranolol during insulin-induced hypoglycemia. Br Med J 2:7–9.

de Soyza, N., Kane, J.J., Murphy, M.L., Laddu, A.R., Doherty, J.E., and Bissett, K. 1980. The long-term suppression of ventricular arrhythmia by oral acebutolol in patients with coronary artery disease. Am Heart J 100(5):631–635.

de Soyza, N., Shapiro, W., Chandraratna, P.A., Aronow, W.S., Laddu, A.R., and Thopson, C.H. 1982. Acebutolol therapy for ventricular arrhythmia: randomized placebo-controlled, double-blind multicenter study. Circulation 65:1129–1135.

Dollery, C.T., Paterson, J.W., and Connolly, M.E. 1969. Clinical pharmacology of β-blocking drugs. Clin Pharmacol Ther 10:765–799.

Dunlop, D., and Shanks, R.G. 1968. Selective blockade of adrenoceptive beta-receptors in the heart. Br J Pharmacol Chemother 32: 201–218.

Editorial. 1978. Self-poisoning with β-blockers. Br Med J 1:1010–1011.

Edwardsson, N., Hirsch, I., Emanuelsson, H., Ponten, J., and Olsson, S.B. 1980. Sotalol-induced delayed ventricular repolarization in man. Eur Heart J 1(5):335–343.

Evans, D.B., Peschka, M.T., Lee, R.J., and Laffan, R.J. 1976. Anti-arrhythmic action of nadolol, a β-adrenergic receptor blocking agent. Eur J Pharmacol 35:17–27.

Fitzgerald, J.D. 1972. Cardioselective β-adrenergic blockade. Proc R Soc Med 65:761–764.

Fogelman, F., Lightman, S.L., Sillett, R.W., and NcNicol, M.W. 1972. The treatment of cardiac arrhythmias with sotalol. Eur J Clin Pharmacol 5:72–76.

Fors, W.J., Vander Ark, C.R., and Reynolds, E.W. 1971. Evaluation of propranolol and quinidine in the treatment of quinidine resistant arrhythmias. Am J Cardiol 27:190.

Frick, M.H., and Kala, R. 1981. Antiarrhythmic significance of dosing intervals in beta-receptor blocking therapy of hypertension with acebutolol. Am J Cardiol 48(5):911–916.

Frieden, J., Rosenblum, R., Enselberg, C.D., and Rosenberg, A. 1968. Propranolol treatment of chronic intractable supraventricular arrhythmias. Am J Cardiol 22:711–717.

Frishman, W.H. 1979. Clinical pharmacology of the new β-adrenergic blocking drugs. Part 1. Pharmacodynamic and pharmacokinetic properties. Am Heart J 97:663–670.

Frishman, W.H. 1981a. β-Adrenoceptor antagonists. New drugs and new indications. N Engl J Med 305: 500–506.

Frishman, W.H. 1981b. Nadolol—a new β-adrenoceptor antagonist. N Engl J Med 305: 678–682.

Frishman, W.H., Davis, R., Strom, J., Elkayam, U., Stampfer, M., Ribner, H., Weinstein, J., and Sonnenblick, E. 1979a. Clinical pharmacology of the new beta-adrenergic blocking drugs. Part 5. Pindolol (LB-46) therapy for supraventricular arrhythmia: a viable alternative to propranolol in patients with bronchospasm. Am Heart J 98:393–398.

Frishman, W.H., Furberg, C.D., and Friedewald, W.T. 1983. β-Adrenergic blockade for survivors of acute myocardial infarction. N Engl J Med 310:830–837.

Frishman, W.H. 1983. Pindolol: a new β-adrenoceptor antagonist with partial agonist activity. N Engl J Med 308:940–944.

Frishman, W.H., and Halprin, S. 1979. Clinical pharmacology of the new beta-adrenergic blocking drugs. Part 7. New horizons in beta-adrenoceptor blockade therapy: labetalol. Am Heart J 98:660–665.

Frishman, W.H., Kostis, J., Strom, J., Hossler, M., Elkayam, U., Goldner, S., Silverman, R., Davis, R., Weinstein, J., and Sonnenblick, E. 1979b. Clinical pharmacology of the new β-adrenergic blocking drugs. Part 6. A comparison of pindolol and propranolol in treatment of patients with angina pectoris. The role of intrinsic sympathomimetic activity. Am Heart J 98:526–535.

Frishman, W.H., and Silverman, R. 1979a. Clinical pharmacology of the new β-adrenergic blocking drugs. Part 2. Physiologic and metabolic effects. Am Heart J 97:797–807.

Frishman, W.H., and Silverman, R. 1979b. Clinical pharmacology of the new β-adrenergic blocking drugs. Part 3. Comparative clinical experience and new therapeutic applications. Am Heart J 98:119–131.

Frishman, W.H., Strom, J., Kirschner, M., Poland, M., Klein, N., Halprin, S., LeJemtel, T.H., Kram, H., and Sonnenblick, E.H. 1981. Labetalol therapy in patients with system hypertension and angina pectoris: effects of combined alpha and beta-adrenoreceptor blockade. Am J Cardiol 48:917–928.

Frohlich, E.D., Tarazi, R.C., and Dustan, H.P. 1969. Peripheral arterial insufficiency: a complication of beta-adrenergic blocking therapy. JAMA 208:2471–2472.

Fuccella, L.M., and Imhoff, P. 1969. Experience with a new beta-receptor blocking agent (Trasicor) in the management of cardiac arrhythmias. Pharmacol Clin 1:123.

Gettes, L.S., and Surawicz, B. 1967. Long-term prevention of paroxysmal arrhythmias with propranolol therapy. Am J Med Sci 254:256–265.

Gibson, D., and Sowton, E. 1969. The use of beta-adrenergic receptor blocking drugs in dysrhythmias. Progr Cardiovasc Dis 12:16–39.

Gibson, D.G. 1974. Pharmacodynamic properties of β-adrenergic receptor blocking drugs in man. Drugs 7:8–38.

Giudicelli, J.F., Lhoste, F., and Bossier, J.R. 1975. β-Adrenergic blockade and atrioventricular conduction impairment. Eur J Pharmacol 31:216–225.

Glick, G., Parmley, W., Wechsler, A.S., and Sonnenblick, E.H. 1968. Glucagon. Circ Res 22:789.

Hansteen, V. 1983. Beta-blockade after myocardial infarction: The Norwegian propranolol study in high-risk patients. Circulation 67(suppl 1):57–60.

Hansteen, V., Moinichen, E., Lorensten, E., Anderson, A., Strom, O., Soiland, K., Dyrbekk, D., Refsum, A.M., Tromsdal, A., Knudsen, K., Elka, C., Barken, A., Jur, J., Smith, P., and Hoff, P.I. 1982. One year's treatment with propranolol after myocardial infarction: preliminary report of Norwegian Multicentre Trial. Br Med J 284:155–160.

Harrison, D.C., Griffin, J.R., and Fiene, T.J. 1965. Effects of beta-adrenergic blockade with propranolol in patients with atrial arrhythmias. N Engl J Med 273:410–415.

Heel, R.C., Brogden, R.N., Pakes, G.E., Speight, T.M., and Avery, G.S. 1980. Nadolol: a review of its pharmacological properties and therapeutic efficacy in hypertension and angina pectoris. Drugs 20:1–23.

Heel, R.C., Brogden, R.N., Speight, T.M., and Avery, G.S. 1979. Atenolol: a review of its pharmacological properties and therapeutic efficacy in angina pectoris and hypertension. Drugs 17:425–460.

Hjalmarson, Å., Elmfeldt, D., Herlitz, J., Holmberg, S., Malek, I., Nyberg, G., Rydén, L., Swedberg, K., Vedin, A., Waagstein, F., Waldenstrom, A., Waldenstrom, J., Wedel, H., Wilhelmsen, L., and Silhelmsson, C. 1981. Effect on mortality of metoprolol in acute myocardial infarction. A double-blind randomized trial. Lancet 2:823–827.

Hjalmarson, Å., Herlitz, J., Holmberg, S., Rydén, L., Swedberg, K., Vedin, A., Waagstein, F., Waldenstrom, A., Waldenstrom, J., Wedel, H., Wilhelmsen, L., and Wilhelmsson, C. 1983. The Goteborg metoprolol trial. Effects on mortality and morbidity in acute myocardial infarction. Circulation 67(suppl 1):26–32.

Imhof, P.R. 1974. Characterization of β-blockers as antihypertensive agents in the light of human pharmacology studies. In: W. Schweizer, ed. β-Blockers: Present Status and Future Prospects. pp 40–50. Bern: Huber.

Irons, G.V., Ginn, W.N., and Orgain, E.S. 1967. Use of a beta-adrenergic receptor blocking agent (propranolol) in the treatment of cardiac arrhythmias. Am J Med 43:161–170.

Johnson, G., and Regardh, C.G. 1976. Clinical pharmacokinetics of β-adrenoreceptor blocking drugs. Clin Pharmacokin 1:233–263.

Julian, D.G., Presscott, R.J., Jackson, F.S., and Szekely, P. 1982. Controlled trial of sotalol for one year after myocardial infarction. Lancet 1:1142–1147.

Koch-Weser, J. 1979. Metoprolol. N Engl J Med 301:698–703.

Koch-Weser, J., and Sellers, E.M. 1976. Binding of drugs to serum albumin. N Engl J Med 294:311–316, 526–531.

Koppes, G.M., Beckmann, C.H., and Jones, F.G. 1980. Propranolol therapy for ventricular arrhythmias two months after acute myocardial infarction. Am J Cardiol 46:322–328.

Kosinski, E.J., and Malindazak, G.S., Jr. 1973. Glucagon and isoproterenol, in reversing propranolol toxicity. Arch Intern Med 132: 840–843.

Lands, A.M., Arnold, A., McAulliff, J.P., Luduena, F.P., and Brown, T.G. 1967. Differentiation of receptor systems activated by sympathomimetic amines. Nature 214: 597–598.

Latour, Y., Dumont, G., Brosseau, A., and Lelorie, J. 1977. Effects of sotalol in twenty patients with cardiac arrhythmias. Int J Clin Pharmacol 15:275–278.

Lefkowitz, R.J. 1974. Selectivity in β-adrenergic response. Circulation 49:783–785.

Lemberg, L., Castellanos, A., and Arcebal, A.G. 1970. The use of propranolol in arrhythmias complicating acute myocardial infarction. Am Heart J 80:479–487.

Letora, J.J.L., Mark, A.L., Johannsen, U.J., Wilson, W.R., and Abboud, F.M. 1975. Selective β_1 receptor blockade with oral practolol in man. J Clin Invest 56:719–724.

Levi, G.F., and Proto, C. 1970. Combined treatment of atrial fibrillation with propranolol and quinidine. Cardiology 55:249–254.

Levi, G.F., and Proto, C. 1972. Combined treatment of atrial fibrillation with quinidine and beta-blockers. Br Heart J 34:911–914.

Levy, J.V., and Richards, V. 1966. Inotropic and chronotropic effects of a series of β-adrenergic blocking drugs: some structure activity relationships. Proc Soc Exp Biol Med 122:373–379.

Lichstein, E., Morganroth, J., Harrist, R., and Hubble, E. 1983. Effect of propranolol on ventricular arrhythmias. The Beta-Blocker Heart Attack Trial. Circulation 67(suppl 1): 5–10.

Lloyd-Mostyn, R.H., and Orams, S. 1975. Modification by propranolol of cardiovascular effects of induced hypoglycemia. Lancet 2:1213–1215.

Lui, H.K., Lee, G., Dhurandhar, R., Hungate, E.J., Laddu, A., Dietrich, P., and Mason, D.T. 1983. Reduction of ventricular ectopic beats with oral acebutolol: a double-blind, randomized crossover study. Am Heart J 105(5):722–726.

Lundvall, J., and Jarholt, J. 1976. Beta-adrenergic dilator component of the sympathetic vascular response in skeletal muscle. Acta Physiol Scand 96:180–192.

Mazzola, C., Ferrario, N., Calzavara, M.P., Guffanti, E., and Vaccarella, A. 1981. Acute antihypertensive and antiarrhythmic effects of labetalol. Curr Ther Res 29:613–633.

Miller, R.R., Olson, H.G., Amsterdam, E.A., and Mason, D.T. 1975. Propranolol withdrawal rebound phenomenon: exacerbation of coronary events after abrupt cessation of antianginal therapy. N Engl J Med 293:416–418.

Mohr, R., Smolinsky, A., and Goor, D. 1981. Prevention of supraventricular tachyarrhythmia with low dose propranolol after coronary bypass. J Thorac Cardiovasc Surg 81:840–845.

Moller, B., and Rehnquist, N. 1979. Metoprolol in the treatment of supraventricular tachyarrhythmias. Ann Clin Res 11:34–41.

Multicentre International Study 1975. Improvement in prognosis of myocardial infarction by long-term beta-adrenoreceptor blockade using practolol. Br Med J 3:735–740.

Multicentre International Study 1977. Reduction in mortality after myocardial infarction with long-term beta-adrenoreceptor blockade. Suppl Rep Br Med J 2:419–421.

Myburgh, D.P., Smith, R., Diamond, T.H., Faitelson, H.L., and Sommers, D.K. 1983. A comparison of the efficacy of sotalol and nadolol in the suppression of ventricular ectopic beats. S Afr Med J 63(8):263–265.

Nawabi, I.U., and Ritz, N.D. 1973. Agranulocytosis due to propranolol. JAMA 223:1376–1377.

Neuvonen, P.J., Elonen, E., Vuorenmaa, T., and Laakso, M. 1981. Prolonged Q-T interval and severe tachyarrhythmias, common features of sotalol intoxication. Eur J Clin Pharmacol 20:85–89.

Nixon, J.V., Pennington, W., Ritter, W., and Shapiro, W. 1978. Efficacy of propranolol in the control of exercise induced or augmented ventricular ectopic activity. Circulation 57:115.

Norwegian Multicenter Study Group 1981. Timolol induced reduction in mortality and reinfarction in patients surviving acute myocardial infarction. N Engl J Med 304:801–807.

Oka, Y., Frishman, W.H., Becker, R., Kadish, A., Strom, J., Matsumoto, M., Orkin, L., and Frater, R. 1980. Clinical pharmacology of the new beta-adrenergic blockers. Part 10. Beta-adrenergic blockade and coronary artery surgery. Am Heart J 99:255–269.

Olsson, G., Rehnquist, N., Ludman, L., and Melcher, A. 1981. Metoprolol after acute myocardial infarction: effects on ventricular arrhythmias and exercise tests during six months. Acta Med Scand 210(1–2):59–65.

Opie, L.H. 1980. Drugs and the heart. β-Blocking agents. Lancet 1:693–698.

Paget, G.E. 1963. Carcinogenic actions of pronethalol. Br Med J 2:1266–1277.

Parmley, W.W. 1971. The role of glucagon in cardiac therapy. N Engl J Med 285:801–802.

Podrid, P.J., and Lown, B. 1982. Pindolol for ventricular arrhythmias. Am Heart J 104: 491–496.

Porter, D. 1969. Sympathetic regulation of insulin secretion. Its relation to diabetes mellitus. Arch Intern Med 123:252.

Powell, C.E., and Slater, I.H. 1974. Blocking of inhibitory adrenergic response. Circulation 49:783–785.

Prakash, R., Allen, H.N., Condo, F., Matloff, J.M., Swan, H.J.C., and Parmley, W.W. 1970. Clinical evaluation of the antiarrhythmic effects of sotalol. Am J Cardiol 26:654.

Pratt, C., and Lichstein, E. 1982. Ventricular antiarrhythmic effects of beta-adrenergic blocking drugs: a review of mechanism and clinical studies. J Clin Pharmacol 22:335–347.

Pratt, C.M., Yepsen, S.C., Bloom, M.G., Taylor, A.A., Young, J.B., and Quinones, M.A. 1983. Evaluation of metoprolol in suppressing complex ventricular arrhythmias. Am J Cardiol 52(1):73–78.

Rehnquist, N. 1981. Clinical experience with I.V. metroprolol in supraventricular tachyarrhythmias—a multicenter study. Ann Clin Res 13(suppl 30):68–72.

Reveno, W.S., and Rosenblum, H. 1968. Propranolol hypoglycemia. Lancet 1:920.

Reynolds, E.W., and Vander Ark, C.R. 1967. Treatment of quinidine resistant arrhythmias with combined use of quinidine and propranolol. Circulation (suppl II) 36:221–226.

Rodgers, J.C., Sheldon, C.D. Lerskin, R.A., and Livingston, W.R. 1976. Intermittent claudication complicating beta-blockade. Br Med J 1:1125.

Roland, J.M., Wilcox, R.G., Bank, D.C., Edwards, B., Fentem, P.H., and Hampton, J.R. 1978. Effect of beta-blockers on arrhythmias during six weeks after suspected myocardial infarction. Br Med J 11:518.

Romano, S., Orfei, S., and Pozzoni, L. 1981. Preliminary clinical trial on hypotensive and antiarrhythmic effect of labetalol. Drugs Exp Clin Res 7:65.

Rossi, P.R.F., Yusuf, S., Ramsdale, D., Furse, L.Y., and Sleight, P. 1983. Reduction of ventricular arrhythmias by early intravenous atenolol in suspected acute myocardial infarction. Br Med J 286:506–510.

Rydén, L., Ariniego, R., Arnman, K., Herlitz, J., Hjalmarson, A., Holmberg, S., Reyes, C., Smedgard, P., Svedberg, K., Vedin, A., Waagstein, F., Waldenstrom, A., Wilhelmsson, C., Wedel, H., and Yamamoto, M. 1983. A double-blind trial of metoprolol in acute myocardial infarction. Effects on ventricular tachyarrhythmias. N Engl J Med 308: 614–618.

Salazar, C., Frishman, W.H., Friedman, S., Patel, J., Lin, Y.T., Oka, Y., Frater, R., and Becker, R.M. 1979. β-Blockade for supraventricular tachycardia post-coronary artery surgery. A propranolol withdrawal syndrome. Angiology 30:816–819.

Samek, L., and Roskamm, H. 1982. Antianginal and antiarrhythmic effects of pindolol in postinfarct patients. Br J Clin Pharmacol 13(suppl 2):297s.

Sandler, G., and Pistevos, A.C. 1971. Use of oxprenolol in cardiac arrhythmias associated with acute myocardial infarction. Br Med J 1:254–257.

Sannerstedt, R., and Wasir, H. 1977. Acute hemodynamic effects of metoprolol in hypertensive patients. Br J Pharmacol 4:23–26.

Schamroth, L. 1966. Immediate effects of intravenous propranolol on various cardiac arrhythmias. Am J Cardiol 18:438–443.

Shapiro, W., Park, J., and Koch, G. 1982. Variability of spontaneous and exercise induced ventricular arrhythmias in the absence and presence of treatment with acebutolol or quinidine. Am J Cardiol 49:445–454.

Silverman, N., Wright, R., and Levitsky, S. 1982. Efficacy of low dose propranolol in preventing post operative supraventricular tachyarrhythmias. Ann Surg 196:194–197.

Simon, A., and Berman, E. 1979. Long term sotalol therapy in patients with arrhythmias. J Clin Pharmacol 19:547–556.

Simpson, F.O. 1974. β-Adrenergic receptor blocking drugs in hypertension. Drugs 7:85–105.

Sinclair, D.J.M. 1979. Comparison of effects of propranolol and metoprolol on airways obstruction in chronic bronchitis. Br Med J 1:168.

Singh, B.N. 1973. Clinical aspects of the antiarrhythmic action of β-receptor blocking drugs. Part 2. Clinical pharmacology. N Zeal Med J 78:529–535.

Singh, S.N., DiBianco, R., Davidov, M.E., Gottdiever, J.S., Johnson, W.L., Laddu, A.R., and Fletcher, R.D. 1982. Comparison of acebutolol and propranolol for the treatment of chronic ventricular arrhythmia. Circulation 65:1356–1364.

Singh, B.N., and Jewitt, D.E. 1974. β-Adrenergic receptor blocking drugs in cardiac arrhythmias. Drugs 7:426–461.

Singh, B.N., Whitlock, R.M.L., Combes, R.H., Williams, F.H., and Haris, E.A. 1976. Effects of cardioselective β-adrenoreceptor blockade on specific airways resistance in normal subjects and in patients with bronchial asthma. Clin Pharmacol Ther 19:493–501.

Skinner, C., Gaddu, J., and Palmer, K.N.V. 1976. Comparison of effects of metoprolol and propranolol on asthmatic airway obstruction. Br Med J 1:504.

Sloman, G., and Stannard, M. 1967. β-Adrenergic blockade and cardiac arrhythmias. Br Med J 4:508–512.

Status Report on β-Blockers. 1978. FDA Drug Bulletin. 8:13.

Stephens, S.A. 1966. Unwanted effects of propranolol. Am J Cardiol 18:463–472.

Sterns, S., and Borman, J.B. 1969. Early conversion of atrial fibrillation after open heart surgery by combined propranolol and quinidine treatment. Isr J Med Sci 5:102–107.

Taylor, R.R., and Halliday, E.J. 1965. β-Adrenergic blockade in the treatment of exercise-induced paroxysmal ventricular tachycardia. Circulation 32:778–782.

Taylor, S.H., Silke, B., Ebbutt, A., Sutton, G.C., Prout, B.J., and Burley, D.M. 1982b. A long-term prevention study with oxprenolol in coronary heart disease. N Engl J Med 307:1293–1301.

Taylor, S.H., Silke, B., and Lee, P.S. 1982a. Intravenous β-blockade in coronary heart disease: is cardioselectivity or intrinsic sympathomimetic activity hemodynamically useful? N Engl J Med 306:631–635.

Tewari, S.C., Das, B.K., Parashar, S.K., Prabhakaran, S.N., Grover, D.N., and Rastogi, D.S. 1982. Exercise induced ventricular arrhythmias and effects of suppressive therapy with propranolol and verapamil. Indian Heart J 34(3):162–165.

Tonkin, A.M., Joel, S.E., Reynolds, J.L., Aylwrd, P.E., Heddle, W.P., McRitchie, R.J., West, M.J., and Chalmers, J.P. 1981. Beta-blockade in acute myocardial infarction. Inability of relatively late administration to influence infarct size and arrhythmia. Med J Aust 2:145–146.

Vaughan Williams, E.M., and Papp, J. 1970. The effect of oxprenolol on cardiac intracellular potentials in relation to its antiarrhythmic local anesthetic and other properties. Postgrad Med J 46:22–32.

Vedin, A., Wilhelmsson, C., and Werko, L. 1975. Chronic alprenolol treatment of patients with acute myocardial infarction after discharge from hospital. Effects on mortality and morbidity. Acta Med Scand (suppl) 575:1–40.

von der Lippe, G., and Lund-Johansen, P. 1981. Effect of timolol on late ventricular arrhythmias after acute myocardial infarction. Acta Med Scand (suppl) 651:253–258.

Vukovich, R.A., Sasahara, A., Zombrano, P., Beldo, J., Godin, P., and Brannick, L. 1976. Antiarrhythmic effects of a new beta-adrenergic blocking agent, nadolol. Clin Pharmacol Ther 19:118.

Waal-Manning, H. 1975. Problems with practolol. Drugs 10:336–341.

Waal-Manning, H.J. 1976. Hypertension: which β-blocker? Drugs 12:412–441.

Whitehead, M.H., Whitmarsh, V.B., and Horton, J.N. 1980. Metoprolol in anaesthesia for oral surgery. The effect of pretreatment on the incidence of cardiac dysrhythmias. Anesthesia (8):779–782.

Wilhelmsson, C., Vedin, J.A., Wilhelmsen, L., Tibblin, G., and Werko, L. 1974. Reduction of sudden deaths after myocardial infarction by treatment with alprenolol. Preliminary results. Lancet 2:1157–1160.

Williams, D.O., Tatelbaum, R., and Most, A.S. 1979. Effective treatment of supraventricular arrhythmias with acebutolol. Am J Cardiol 44:521–525.

Winchester, M., Jackson, G., Meltzer, R.S., Bowden, R.E., Mace, J.G., Winkle, R.A., and Harrison, D.C. 1978. Intravenous atenolol and acebutolol in the treatment of supraventricular arrhythmias. Circulation 58(suppl 2):49.

Woosley, R.L., Kornhauser, D., Smith, R., Reele, S., Higgins, S.B., Nies, A.S., Shand, D.G., and Oates, J.A. 1979. Suppression of chronic ventricular arrhythmias with propranolol. Circulation 60:819–827.

Wright, P. 1975. Untoward effect associated with practolol administration. Oculomucocutaneous syndrome. Br Med J 1:595–598.

Yusuf, S., Sleight, P., and Rossi, P. 1983. Reduction in infarct size, arrhythmias, and chest pain by early intravenous beta-blockade in suspected acute myocardial infarction. Circulation 67(suppl 1):32–41.

Zacharias, F.J., Coven, K.J., Prestt, J., Vickers, J., and Wall, B.G. 1972. Propranolol in hypertension: a study of long term therapy, 1964–1970. Am Heart J 83:755–761.

Chapter 13

Clinical Antiarrhythmic Effects of Adrenergic Blocking Agents (Class II)

Joel Morganroth

Principles of Antiarrhythmic Study Design

It is now quite clear that patients who suffer electrical instability and concomitant left ventricular dysfunction are at the highest risk for sudden cardiac death (Morganroth, 1981). The majority of patients in this high risk group have chronic ventricular arrhythmias in which ventricular ectopy may be very frequent (hundreds to three thousand ventricular premature complexes/h/24 h) or complex (nonsustained ventricular tachycardia usually less than 15 s). The indication for treatment of chronic ventricular arrhythmias in this group of patients is to prevent sudden cardiac death since these arrhythmias produce no hemodynamic consequence or important symptoms. Ambulatory electrocardiographic monitoring and exercise testing are appropriate noninvasive tests to determine therapeutic efficacy and the ambulatory out-patient setting is a suitable study environment.

A smaller subgroup of patients will present with acute hemodynamically significant ventricular arrhythmias. The hemodynamic symptoms are usually on the basis of paroxysmal sustained ventricular tachycardia or occasionally nonsustained ventricular tachycardia in patients with more seriously disturbed left ventricular function. The indication for treatment in this group is the elimination of hemodynamic symptoms and also the hope of prevention of sudden cardiac death, an event that occurs with high frequency in this patient group. Electrophysiologic testing utilizing programmed stimulation with serial drug studies is an appropriate means to determine therapeutic efficacy. These patients should be treated in a sophisticated in-hospital monitored facility. Some patients will have such poor left ventricular function (e.g., left ventricular ejection fraction <0.20) and persistent complex sustained ventricular arrhythmias that little hope exists in altering their prognosis. It is hoped that patients with at least chronic ventricular arrhythmias and moderate left ventricular dysfunction (e.g., ejection fraction >0.20 <0.40) may respond to proper mechanical and electrical therapy with reduction in sudden cardiac death. The challenge of sudden cardiac death prevention may be considered the most important problem in modern day cardiology since this entity is the leading cause of death in the western world in which over 400,000 individuals annually suffer premature demise.

It is only in recent years that factors defining the efficacy of antiarrhythmic drugs have been clearly defined. In patients with chronic ventricular arrhythmias without hemodynamically significant symptoms, the most appropriate endpoint of drug efficacy should be the prevention of sudden cardiac death. The pharmacologic endpoint of significant statistical reduction in ventricular ectopic frequency has, of course, been the most widely applied efficacy definition to the study of new antiarrhythmic agents. Studies using antiarrhythmic agents to decrease ventricular ectopy with the hope of preventing sudden cardiac death have suffered from a high drop-out rate due to drug toxicity, subtherapeutic doses of antiarrhythmic agents employed in the trials, and methodologic and design flaws. With newly available class IC and class III agents which demonstrate much greater efficacy and safety profiles, and a better understanding of the proper conduct of multicenter clinical trials, studies emerging in the 1980's should answer the important question of whether treatment of chronic ventricular ectopy does improve survival.

Antiarrhythmic drug efficacy when assessed in individual patients must take into consideration the high degree of spontaneous variability that exists in chronic ventricular ectopic frequency (Morganroth et al., 1978). This high rate of spontaneous variability demands that proper statistical methodologies be used to evaluate drug-testing protocols and that proper attention be given to the design of such trials. Various statistical methodologies in clinical settings have shown that an appropriate definition for drug efficacy be used when comparing ambulatory ECG Holter monitoring data obtained on drug therapy to base-line placebo control data, a minimum of 75% reduction in mean hourly ectopic frequency is necessary to insure that the observed decrease was due to the therapy and not to the consequence of spontaneous variability. Data analysis in such drug-testing studies should be presented in terms of the per cent of individual patients responding with this level of reduction rather than the pooling of patient data on placebo and drug therapy. This latter practice will result in masking proper evaluation of efficacy and safety data such as the frequency of proarrhythmic effects.

Protocol designs using the above-cited methodology should be conducted primarily using the minimum entrance criteria of at least 30 premature ventricular complexes (PVCs)/h/24 h on at least two 24-h Holter monitoring sessions taken on placebo (Morganroth, 1981). Prior antiarrhythmic drugs should be discontinued for at least 7 days before placebo and at each dosage level, 24–48 h of Holter monitoring should be obtained. When a 75% reduction in frequency (and usually a 100% reduction in complex arrhythmia frequency) is obtained, the efficacious dose will be defined. During a final placebo period, one should expect to see at least a 50% return to the initial placebo base-line PVC frequency; although, in our experience, we frequently observe the lack of such a return in approximately

10–15% of patients. Such patients probably represent those with a high level of spontaneous variability of PVC frequency. The antiarrhythmic drug trials can be conducted using cross-over or parallel design models since the potential for carry-over effect is minimal when objective ambulatory monitoring data rather than symptomatic endpoints are used as efficacy criteria. Short term (over days to weeks) efficacy trials are preferrable to avoid underlying changes in cardiovascular status and/or frequency of ventricular arrhythmia, although long term efficacy and safety studies (months to years) are essential to define continuing beneficial effects. Comparative trials using a standard released antiarrhythmic agent are also needed. Reintroduction of placebo periods at approximately 6 months on long term therapy is recommended to insure continued presence for the need to continue antiarrhythmic agents.

Role of Adrenergic Blocking Agents in the Treatment of Ventricular Arrhythmias

Since their availability in clinical medicine, β-blocking agents have not been considered "first choice" agents for the treatment of ventricular ectopy. Electrophysiologic studies demonstrate that adrenergic blocking agents will block the catecholamine-induced increase in phase 4 depolarization in automatic cells, and thus β-blockers were a clinically useful antiarrhythmic class in patients whose ventricular ectopy occurred in settings such as the use of volatile anesthesia and in certain patients with ischemic induced ventricular ectopy usually noted on exercise. Other conditions, such as hypertrophic cardiomyopathy and mitral valve prolapse, in which β-blocking agents have a primary role in general therapy might also be used for treatment of ventricular arrhythmias. Clinical cardiologists have, however, often employed the class II β-adrenergic blocking agents as adjunctive therapy with the traditional class I antiarrhythmic drugs in ventricular arrhythmic therapy.

Table 13-1 details the clinical trials that in recent years have defined the efficacy of β-blocking agents in the suppression of patients with nonhemodynamically significant chronic ventricular arrhythmias in which proper statistical methodologies and trial designs have been employed (see above). These studies have used either homogeneous populations in which patients had predominantly coronary artery disease or mitral valve prolapse, or more commonly have employed populations with mixed cardiac conditions including idiopathic or no structural heart disease cases. Efficacy criteria have ranged from 70–75% reduction in PVCs and all these trials have used an adequate dose of the β-blocking agent at which β-adrenergic blockade should occur (Winkle et al., 1978; Winkle et al., 1977; Pratt et al., 1980; Woosley et al., 1979; de Soyza et al., 1980;

Table 13-1 Oral β-Blocking Agents in Chronic Ventricular Ectopy: Efficacy Determined by Holter Monitoring

Reference	Diagnosis	Drug	Efficacy		Comments	
Winkle et al., 1978	Mixed	Propranolol	2/16	(50%)	>70%*	240†
Winkle et al., 1977	Mitral valve prolapse	Propranolol	5/9	(56%)	>75%	40–320
Pratt et al., 1980	Coronary artery disease	Metoprolol	7/13	(54%)	>75%	100–200
Woosley et al., 1979	Mixed††	Propranolol	24/32	(75%)	>70%	up to 960
de Soyza et al., 1980	Mixed	Acebutalol	11/20	(55%)	>70%	300
Koppes et al., 1980	Acute myocardial infarction	Propranolol	18/32	(56%)	>70%	80–480
Schlemann et al., 1983	Mixed	Nadolol	7/13	(54%)	>75%	80–640
Morganroth, 1983	Mixed	Atenolol	7/12	(58%)	>70%	50–200
Podrid and Lown, 1982	Mixed	Pindolol	21/42 15/45	(50%)¶ (33%)£#	50–90%	20–80

*Percentage reduction required to define drug efficacy.
†Dose range studied in milligrams per day.
††Several cardiac diseases studied.
¶Acute.
£#Chronic Drug Testing.

Koppes et al., 1980; Schlemann et al., 1983; Morganroth et al., 1983; Podrid and Lown, 1982). As can be seen from Table 13-1, the average number of patients responding to β-adrenergic drug therapy in these trials is approximately 50–60%. Similar trials in which class I agents, such as quinidine, disopyramide and procainamide have been used to demonstrate a response rate of approximately 50–75% (Panidis and Morganroth, 1982). Thus, the class II β-adrenergic blocking agents should be considered only somewhat less effective than the traditional class I membrane-stabilizing antiarrhythmic drugs in reducing chronic PVC frequency. Side effect profiles of the β-adrenergic blocking agents are quite low and usually are less than 5% of patients studied. This is in marked contrast to the average of 20–30% side effects (which usually demand discontinuation of the drug) expected with the use of class I antiarrhythmic agents.

Table 13-2, correlates the pharmacologic properties of the β-blocking agents studied in Table 13-1, and relates them to their approximate efficacy in patients tested with chronic ventricular arrhythmias (Morganroth, 1983). Irrespective of the degree or nature of the presence of these pharmacologic properties, all β-adrenergic blocking agents demonstrated an approximate 50% efficacy rate in patients tested suggesting that none of these various properties alter the antiarrhythmic effect of this class. Thus, the antiarrhythmic effect on PVC frequency may be considered a class effect of the β-blockers.

Table 13-2 Comparisons among β-Blockers in Ventricular Ectopy (PVC) Suppression.

Drug	Cardioselectivity	Intrinsic Sympathomimetic Activity	Membrane Effect	PVC Response Rate
Propranolol	−	−	+	About 50%
Metoprolol	+	−	−	About 50%
Nadolol	−	−	−	About 50%
Atenolol	+	−	−	About 50%
Acebutalol	+	+	+	About 50%
Pindolol	−	+	−	About 50%

+ = present; − = absent

Use of β-Adrenergic Blocking Agents in Patients with Life-Threatening Arrhythmias

Patients with paroxysmal sustained ventricular tachycardia or ventricular fibrillation are appropriately studied in the electrophysiologic laboratory in an in-hospital monitored setting. These patients, in general, have severe underlying disturbance in cardiac function, and studies conducted in this group using solely β-adrenergic blocking agents have demonstrated poor responses. The adjunctive use of these agents with other classes of antiarrhythmic drugs, such as class IA antiarrhythmic agents anecdotally has improved efficacy. While some investigators have found better results with β-adrenergic blocking agents which approximate class I agent profiles, the adjunctive use of β-blockers with other antiarrhythmic drugs has been more successful. Sotalol, a class III agent with β-blocking properties and marked effects on repolarization, has been reported to be highly efficacious in patients with recurrent sustained ventricular tachyarrhythmias and may, therefore, prove to be a most useful drug in this setting (Senges et al., 1982).

β-Adrenergic Blocking Agents in the Prevention of Sudden Cardiac Death

Recently, three major cooperative clinical trials have been conducted demonstrating that β-adrenergic blocking agents used in patients immediately after acute myocardial infarction, have short term (90 day) and long term (mean 30 months) effectiveness on reducing sudden cardiac death (The Norwegian Multicenter Study Group, 1981; Hjalmarson et al., 1981; BHAT Research Group, 1982). Potential mechanisms of action for the decrease in mortality in these β-blocker trials post-myocardial infarction have not been elucidated. Possible mechanisms for this reduction include the primary antiarrhythmic effect of these agents or their ability to protect the myocardium during subsequent ischemia and/or infarction. Possible prevention of recurrent coronary occlusion or combinations of these mechanisms may also be operative. Unfortunately, little data are available evaluating specifically the antiarrhythmic effectiveness of the β-blockers (propranolol, timolol, and metoprolol) in these trials.

In the metoprolol trial (Rydén et al., 1983), patients were treated with 15 mg of metoprolol intravenously on admission to the coronary care unit with acute myocardial infarction and then dosed for 3 months at a 100-mg b.i.d. of metoprolol. This was a randomized, double-blind, parallel study in which half of the patients received metoprolol and the other half received matching doses of placebo. Six hundred and ninety-eight patients were treated with metoprolol and 697 were treated with doses of placebo. Base-line comparisons between the two groups demonstrated comparable clinical and objective findings. The antiarrhythmic data are quite revealing. This study documented that there were 17 out of 697 episodes of ventricular fibrillation in the placebo group compared to only 6 out of 698 in those patients on metoprolol. This was a highly statistically significant ($p < 0.01$) difference. In addition, the metoprolol group demonstrated a marked decrease in the requirement for lidocaine therapy for emergent ventricular ectopy in the coronary care unit (16 out of 698) compared to the placebo group (38 out of 697) ($p < 0.01$.)

Preliminary information has been also available on the effect of propranolol on arrhythmias in the β-blocker heart attack trial (Morganroth et al., 1982; Lichstein et al., 1983). This was a 31 center placebo controlled, double-blind randomized trial involving 3,837 post-myocardial infarction patients. Propranolol was prescribed to 1,916 and placebo to 1,921. These agents were administered after base-line evaluation which occurred from the 5th–21st day post-myocardial infarction. After randomization in this period, follow-up averaged 30 months. This trial demonstrated an approximate 25% decrease in mortality in those patients randomized to propranolol compared to placebo. Approximately 50% of the deaths in this trial (as is true in most trials of this nature) are due to sudden cardiac death, suggesting that an arrhythmia may potentially be the primary mechanism causing this reduction. In this trial, ambulatory Holter monitoring was performed in patients at base-line and in a randomized subset of approximately 25% of the population at 6 weeks. Sixteen hundred and forty-one out of 1,916 patients randomized to propranolol (85.6%) had successful 24-h Holter monitoring data at base-line compared to 1,630/1,921 patients randomized to placebo (84.9%), a nonsignificant difference. At 6 weeks, 407 patients on placebo and 419 patients on propranolol underwent a second 4-h monitoring period.

Irrespective of whether patients were on antiarrhythmic agents or not (approximately 15% of patients were on antiarrhythmic agents in this trial), the frequency of ventricular arrhythmia classes at base-line (Table 13-3) were comparable in patients who entered either the propranolol or placebo group. Table 13-4, demonstrates the frequency of ventricular arrhythmia classes in these two groups and shows no significant differences even when those patients on currently approved antiarrhythmic agents are excluded. When comparing 6-week to base-line Holter monitoring data in this study, there was an approximate 3-fold increase in the prevalence of ventricular arrhythmia in those patients on placebo. Table 13-5 demonstrates that in those patients on propranolol, a statistically significant blunting of the ventricular arrhythmia frequency occurs suggesting an antiarrhythmic effect.

Preliminary data have demonstrated that patients in this trial in whom successful reduction of ventricular arrhythmias occurred had a 0% prevalence of sudden cardiac death compared to approximately 7–8% in those in whom ventricular arrhythmias were not suppressed. Since this trial was not designed to determine the mechanism of sudden cardiac death prevention, these data are only to be considered preliminary (Morganroth et al., 1983).

Table 13-3 Results of Ambulatory ECG Monitoring in All Patients at Base-Line in the β-Blocker Heart Attack Trial.

Arrhythmia	Propranolol (N = 1,678)	Placebo (N = 1,863
PVC >10	13.6%	12.9%
PVC >30	6.9	6.9
PVC >10 + VC/VT	8.0	7.3
PVC >30 + VC/VT	5.1	4.7
VC/VT	20.9	20.4
PVC >0	82.9	84.5

PVC, premature ventricular complex; VC, ventricular couplets; VT, ventricular tachycardia.
N = number of patients.

Table 13-4 Ventricular Arrhythmias at Base-Line in β-Blocker Heart Attack Trial Patients.

Arrhythmia	All Patients (N = 3,837)	All Patients Excluding Those on Antiarrhythmic Agents
PVC >0	83.6	83.1
PVC >10	13.2	11.5
PVC >10 + VC/VT	7.7	6.7
PVC >30	6.9	5.7
PVC >30 + VC/VT	4.8	4.1
VC/VT	20.3	19.6

PVC, premature ventricular complex; VC, ventricular couplets; VT, ventricular tachycardia.

Table 13-5 Ambulatory ECG Monitoring at Base-Line and at 6 Weeks in Patients in the β-Blocker Heart Attack Trial.

	Base-Line	6 Weeks
Placebo	33/407 (8.1%)	104/407 (25.6%)
Propranolol	30/419 (7.2%)	61/419 (14.6%)
	Z = 0.05	Z = 3.95

β-Blocking agents have important effects on ventricular fibrillation threshold. In a canine coronary artery ligation model, using a wide dose range and stimulation technique to define the ventricular fibrillation threshold for several β-adrenergic blocking agents, Anderson et al. (1983) demonstrated that there was an approximate 6-fold increase in ventricular threshold in these animals, in both the nonischemic and ischemic setting. They postulated that the efficacy of β-adrenergic blocking agents in sudden cardiac death prevention was related to blockade of microreentry and prevention of ventricular fibrillation. In contrast, class I membrane-stabilizing antiarrhythmic agents may be more important in suppressing macroreentry which generates ventricular tachycardia.

Conclusions

It is quite evident from the data presented above, that the class II β-adrenergic blocking agents should be considered antiarrhythmic agents. In patients with chronic ventricular arrhythmias, the frequency of suppression of PVCs by β-blockers is comparable to that of other more standard antiarrhythmic agents (e.g., class I drugs), yet the tolerance level of the β-blocker class is much higher.

A marked reduction in sudden cardiac death has been demonstrated in patients subjected to long term cooperative clinical trials with β-blockers in the early post-myocardial infarction period. The mechanism by which β-blockers effect this important reduction is unknown, but an antiarrhythmic action can be demonstrated in these studies. Since sudden cardiac death is primarily due to ventricular tachyarrhythmias which degenerate into ventricular fibrillation, and since β-adrenergic blocking agents have an important effect on ventricular arrhythmia frequency and ventricular fibrillation threshold, one can hypothesize that the reduction in sudden cardiac death prevalence due to β-blocking agents (which are the only agents to date that have shown prevention of sudden cardiac death) results from their antiarrhythmic properties. Obviously, further research is required to clarify these issues.

References

Anderson, J.L., Rodier, H.E., and Green, L.S. 1983. Comparative effects of Beta-adrenergic blocking drugs on experimental ventricular fibrillation threshold. Am J Cardiol 7:1196–1202.

Beta-Blocker Heart Attack Trial Research Group. 1982. A randomized trial of propranolol in patients with acute myocardial infarction. I. Mortality results. JAMA 247:1707–1882.

de Soyza, N., Kane, J.J., Murphy, M.L., Laddu, A.R., Doherty, J.E., and Bissett, J.K. 1980. The long-term suppression of ventricular arrhythmias by oral-acebutolol in patients with coronary artery disease. Am Heart J 100:631.

Hjalmarson, A., Elmfeldt, D., Herlitz, J., Malek, I., Rydén, L., Vedin, A., Waldenström, A., Wedal, H., Elmfeldt, D., Holmberg, S., Nyberg, G., Swedberg, K., Waagstein,F.,

Waldenström, J., Wilhelmsen, L., and Wilhelmsson, C. 1981. Effect on mortality in acute myocardial infarction: a double-blind randomized trial. Lancet 2:823–827.

Koppes, G.M., Beckmann, C.H., and Jones, F.G. 1980. Propranolol therapy for ventricular arrhythmias two months post acute myocardial infarction. Am J Cardiol 46:322.

Lichstein, E., Morganroth, J., Harrist, R., and Hubble, E. for BHAT Study Group. 1983. Effect of propranolol on ventricular arrhythmia. The Beta-blocker Heart Attack Trial Experience. Circulation 67:II–I 5–1 II.

Morganroth, J., Michelson, E.L., Horowitz, L.N., Josephson, M.E., Pearlman, A.S., and Dunkman, W.B. 1978. Limitations of routine long-term electrocardiographic monitoring to assess ventricular ectopic frequency. Circulation 58:408.

Morganroth, J. 1981. How to evaluate a new antiarrhythmic drug: The challenge of sudden cardiac death. In: J. Morganroth, E.N. Moore, L.S. Dreifus, and E.L. Michelson, eds. The Evaluation of New Antiarrhythmic Drugs. The Hague: Martinus Nijhoff.

Morganroth, J., Lichstein, E., Hubble, R., and Harrist, R. 1982. Effect of propranolol on ventricular arrhythmias in the beta-blocker heart attack trial. Circulation 66:II–328.

Morganroth, J. 1983. Beta-blocking agents in the treatment of ventricular arrhythmias. In: J. Morganroth, and E.N. Moore, eds. The Evaluation of Beta-Blockers and Calcium Antagonist Drugs. The Hague: Martinus Nijhoff.

Morganroth, J., Lichstein, E., Hubble, E., and Harrist, R. 1983. Reduction of chronic ventricular arrhythmias and sudden cardiac death in patients post myocardial infarction. Clin Res 31:207A.

Morganroth, J. 1983. Short term evaluation of atenolol in hospitalized patients with chronic ventricular arrhythmias. Drugs 5:181–185.

Panidis, I., and Morganroth, J. 1982. Short- and long-term therapeutic efficacy of quinidine sulfate for the treatment of chronic ventricular arrhythmias. J Clin Pharmacol 22:379–384.

Podrid, P.J., and Lown, B. 1982. Pindolol for ventricular arrhythmias. Am Heart J 104:491–496.

Pratt, C.M., Matlack, J., Carney, S., Waggoner, A.D., Wichemeyer, W.W., Martin, F., and Miller, R.R. 1980. Effect of metoprolol in suppression of ventricular ectopic beats. Circulation 62:III.

Ryden, L., Ariniego, R., Arnman, K., Herlitz, J., Hjalmarson, A., Holmberg, S., Reyes, C., Smedgard, P., Svedberg, K., Vedin, A., Waagstein, F., Waldenstrom, A., Wilhelmsson, C., Wedel, H., and Yamamoto, M. 1983. A double-blind trial of metoprolol in acute myocardial infarction. N Engl J Med 308:614–618.

Schlemann, M., Morganroth, J., and Reid, P. 1983. Beta-blockade for suppression of high grade ventricular arrhythmias. J Am Coll Cardiol 1:613.

Senges, J., Lengfelder, W., Jauernig, R., Czygan, E., Brachmann, J., Rigos, I., and Kubler, W. 1982. Comparative effects of sotalol, metoprolol and quinidine on sustained ventricular tachycardia. Circulation 66: II–142.

The Norwegian Multicenter Study Group. 1981. Timolol-induced reduction in mortality and reinfarction in patients surviving acute myocardial infarction. N Engl J Med 304:801–807.

Winkle, R.A., Lopes, M.G., Goodman, D.J., Fitzgerald, J.W., Schroeder, J.S., and Harrison, D.C. 1977. Propranolol for patients with mitral valve prolapse. Am Heart J 93:422.

Winkle, R.A., Gradman, A.H., Fitzgerald, J.W., and Bell, P.A. 1978. Antiarrhythmic drug effect assessed from ventricular antiarrhythmic reduction in the ambulatory ECG and treadmill test. Comparison of propranolol, procainamide, and quinidine. Am J Cardiol 42:473.

Woosley, R.L., Kornhause, D., Smith, R., Reele, S., Higgins, S.B., Nies, A.S., Shand, D.G., and Oates, J.A. 1979. Suppression of chronic ventricular arrhythmias with propranolol. Circulation 60:819.

EDITOR'S NOTES

Antiarrhythmic Effects of Adrenergic Blocking Agents (Class II)

Widespread acceptance of beta-blocking drugs has had a significant impact on the treatment of arrhythmias and, in particular, the postmyocardial infarction patient. Although beta-blocking agents have been characterized by varying effects in addition to basic beta-blockade (e.g., membrane-stabilizing activity, intrinsic sympathomimetic activity, etc.), most studies agree that the major antiarrhythmic effect appears to reside with the beta-blocking activity. Therefore, the electrophysiologic effects of beta-blocking drugs in usual clinical doses appear to be manifest as antagonism of sympathetic neurotransmitters.

The most intriguing recent clinical application of these agents has been in the postinfarction patient. A number of beta-blocking agents have been found to reduce the incidence of reinfarction and sudden cardiac death following myocardial infarction. Since properties such as selectivity, intrinsic sympathomimetic activity, and membrane-stabilizing effects did not appear to influence the beta-blocking drugs' ability to affect the postinfarction complications, the concept that the antisympathetic activity of these drugs is of primary importance in the clinical outcome was further supported. However, several caveats do apply. Although it is outside the scope of this discussion to specifically review the various beta-blocking trials, their overall outcome did suggest that only about 25% of the post-myocardial infarction patients responded positively to beta-blocking drug therapy. Furthermore, the time of treatment onset postinfarction may have significant implications for the therapeutic impact of such agents. In addition, when considering the antiarrhythmic efficacy of beta-blockers per se, it would appear evident that these agents do not possess a high degree of efficacy in complex or life-threatening arrhythmias (e.g., ventricular tachycardias, etc.). Concerning antiarrhythmic therapy, these agents may serve more as an adjunct to primary antiarrhythmic drug therapy rather than a replacement, although in certain settings beta-blocking antiarrhythmic therapy may be indicated. One area in need of further clarification and research concerns the question as to what extent the sympathetic nervous system provides the "trigger" for the arrhythmogenic event, and in this regard, can beta-blocking drugs effectively block this "triggering event"?

Lastly, since beta-blocking therapy is more often chronic therapy rather than acute, one must be cognizant of the overall effects that these drugs may induce over long periods of time. While on one hand it may be that long-term or chronic therapy is essential for obtaining drug efficacy, on the other hand, known alteration in the lipid profile induced by beta-blockers or other side effects may predispose the already compromised patient to further complications.

C. Antiarrhythmic Effects of Agents Which Selectively Prolong Action Potential Duration (Class III)

Chapter 14

Cardiac Electrophysiologic Effects of Specific Class III Substances

Mitchell I. Steinberg and Eric L. Michelson

Introduction

Reentry appears to be the predominant electrophysiologic mechanism for the malignant ventricular arrhythmias occurring clinically (Josephson et al., 1978a; 1978b) or in experimental animals (Scherlag et al., 1970; El-Sherif et al., 1975), especially in the presence of chronic ischemia. Ventricular tachycardia may cause serious hemodynamic embarrassment or may degenerate into ventricular flutter or fibrillation. The initiation and maintenance of reentrant arrhythmias require a suitable electrophysiologic substrate, including areas of slow conduction (El-Sherif et al., 1975; 1982), unidirectional block, reduced refractoriness (Allessie et al., 1977), and the appropriate interplay among these factors (Moe, 1975). The pharmacologic therapy and prophylaxis of these arrhythmias remain a challenge. Of the numerous ways that drugs might prevent or interrupt a reentrant rhythm, one straightforward means would be increasing refractoriness within the reentrant loop without slowing conduction (Han, 1971; Wit et al., 1974). This has provided the electrophysiologic basis for designating as class III compounds those that selectively prolong action potential duration (APD) without significantly affecting the maximum rate of rise of the action potential ($\dot{V}_{max}$) and, hence, conduction velocity (Vaughan Williams, 1974; Hauswirth and Singh, 1979).

The theoretical framework for the potential usefulness of class III drugs was established early in this century by Mines (1914) and others (see Wit and Cranefield [1978] for review) who demonstrated that both slow conduction and shortened refractory period were requirements for continuous excitation of cardiac tissues leading to chaotic rhythm disorders both in isolated tissues and intact hearts. In the early 50's, it was demonstrated that low doses of veratrum alkaloids could selectively prolong APD and reduce the excitability of the dog heart (Brooks et al., 1955). Kaumann and Aramendiá (1968) demonstrated antifibrillatory effects of sotalol apparently distinct from of its β-blocking ability. Singh and Vaughan Williams (1970a) and Strauss et al. (1970) described the electrophysiologic properties of amiodarone and sotalol and suggested that class III activity might be involved in their mechanism of action. Independently, other investigators recognized that bretylium could, in contrast to other known antiarrhythmic drugs, selectively prolong the APD of cardiac tissues (Wit et al., 1970; Bigger and Jaffe, 1971). Since then, a wide variety of compounds have been described purporting to possess predominantly class III properties in cardiac tissues (Table 14-1).

Table 14-1 Agents Reported to Have Class III Electrophysiologic Properties.

Bretylium	ATX II
Clofilium	Amiloride
Sotalol	N-Acetylprocainamide
Nifenalol (INPEA)	Goniopora Toxin
Melperone	4-Aminopyridine
Amiodarone	TEA (and analogs)
Bunaphatine	Phenylephrine
Anthopleurin A	Veratrine
Meobentine	

Although it is true that these substances prolong APD and refractoriness, rarely is this activity unaccompanied by other electrophysiologic or pharmacologic activities. For example, bretylium is a potent adrenergic blocking agent (Boura and Green, 1959); amiodarone may slow conduction velocity (Waleffe et al., 1978; Hamer et al., 1983) and interfere with the rate of rise of the action potential (Rosenbaum et al., 1976; Mason et al., 1983); melperone is an α-antagonist that may produce reflex sympathetic stimulation (Platou et al., 1982a; 1982b); sotalol and nifenalol (INPEA) are β-receptor blocking agents (Singh and Vaughan Williams, 1970b; 1971). An excellent review of the varied pharmacologic and electrophysiologic properties of several clinically used class III agents has appeared recently (Bexton and Camm, 1982).

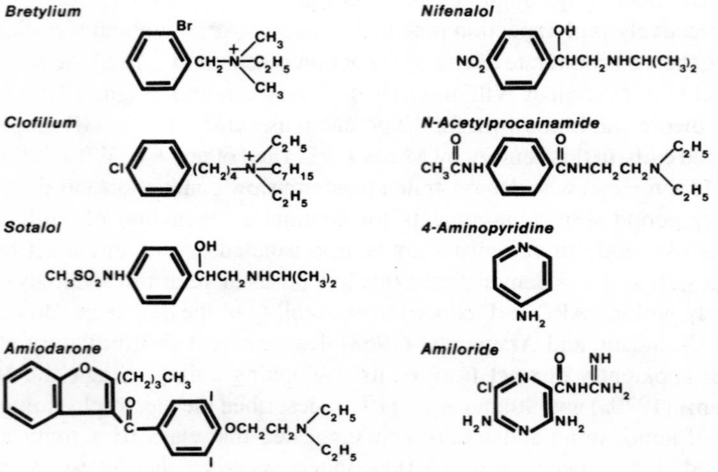

14-1 Molecular formulae of structures possessing class III activity.

The molecular structures of some of the more extensively studied class III drugs are shown in Figure 14-1. There seem to be few if any specific structural similarities among these agents, and at first glance, there appears little to guide the rational development of compounds within this class. This is probably not too surprising when one considers the variety of ways that drugs could interact potentially with ionic channels in the membrane to cause a selective increase in APD and refractory period (Table 14-2). However, small quaternary ammonium ions are well known to inhibit outwardly directed potassium currents in a variety of excitable tissues (Armstrong and Hille, 1972; Armstrong, 1975). In particular, tetraethylammonium ion (TEA) has been shown to prolong the APD of cardiac tissues (Haldimann, 1963; Ochi and Nishiye, 1974), although its potency is low, and in any case, TEA is hardly effective when applied extracellularly (Maruyama et al., 1980; Ito and Surawicz, 1981). Therefore, we examined a group of simple quaternary ammonium ions for their ability to prolong selectively APD duration of canine Purkinje fibers when superfused in vitro (Sullivan et al., 1978). In the present paper, we will demonstrate the strict structure-activity relationships, as determined in vitro, that govern specific class III activity within this group of drugs and show that such specificity in vitro can be extended to intact animal models as well.

Table 14-2 Possible Cellular Mechanisms for Class III Activity.

1. Delay in inactivation of rapid sodium current
   a. Marine toxins
   b. Veratrine alkaloids
2. Inhibition of background outward potassium currents
   a. Quaternary ammonium ions (TEA)
   b. 4-Aminopyridine
   c. Cesium, barium ions
3. Inhibition of delayed rectification (I_{x_1})
   a. Certain quaternary ions
4. Prolongation of the slow inward currents (Na^+ or Ca^{++})

Methodologies Employed

Studies in Vitro

Conventional microelectrode methodology was employed. The tissues were stimulated through bipolar Teflon-coated stainless steel electrodes at a basic cycle length of 1000 ms with square wave pulses of 0.5-ms duration at 1.5-times threshold voltage. Electronic differentiation was used to obtain the maximum rate of rise of the upstroke of the action potential ($\dot{V}_{max}$). APDs and refractory periods were measured by and on-line computer (DEC, PDP-11/45, coupled to an analog/digital converter; sampling frequency 50 μs for 10 ms; then 1 ms for the next 800 ms). Values of APD are reported at 95% of full repolarization (APD_{95}).

All drugs were dissolved in Tyrode's solution before being added to the superfusate. All the quaternary and tertiary amines described in this report were synthesized at Lilly Research Laboratories by Dr. B.B. Molloy and Mr. K. Hauser.

Studies in Vivo

Normal Dogs Ventricular effective refractory period (VERP) and contractility measurements were performed under halothane anesthesia. The right endocardial VERP was determined by applying square wave, constant current stimuli (l-ms duration) at a basic rate of 150 beats/min. The amplitude of the basic driving stimulus (S_1) was set at 1.5-times threshold, and the amplitude of the premature stimulus (S_2) was set at twice S_1. After 20 S_1 impulses, a premature S_2 impulse was inserted, and the next S_1 suppressed. S_2 was first initiated early in electrical systole during ventricular refractoriness and gradually delayed by 1-ms increments until a propagated ventricular response was obtained on the surface ECG. The VERP was defined as the longest S_1, S_2 interval that failed to elicit a propagated response. At least two VERP measurements were made 2 min apart and were averaged for each experimental determination.

Chronically Infarcted Dogs The method used to determine the excitability characteristics of normal and infarcted ventricle has been described (Michelson et al., 1980; 1981). Using unipolar cathodal stimulation (2-ms duration) at twice threshold intensity, intramyocardial plunge electrode sites were identified from which sustained tachyarrhythmias could be initiated reproducibly using one to three ventricular extrastimuli during ventricular pacing. Unipolar cathodal strength-interval curves were constructed from measurements of excitability and refractoriness at each pacing site (normal and infarct zones) before and after the initiation and termination of arrhythmias to confirm that the preparation was unchanged and suitable for evaluation of drug responses. Animals prepared in this manner have been demonstrated previously to have reproducible and sustained ventricular arrhythmias having characteristics similar to those induced in man in the clinical laboratory. Animals with ventricular tachycardia were returned to sinus rhythm by programmed pacing; animals with ventricular fibrillation were countershocked (20–40 watt s) to restore sinus rhythm. After determining baseline electrophysiologic parameters, either 200, 400, and 800 μg/kg of clofilium (Lily 150378) was infused iv over a 5-min period. Over the next 2–4 h, the effects of the drug on excitability, refractoriness, and conduction within normal and infarcted myocardium were monitored. In all studies in vivo, the ECG was monitored continuously, as well as blood pressure and heart rate.

Structure Activity Relationships in Vitro

The effect of changing the carbon length of the alkyl substituent of the phenylbutyl dimethylammonium nucleus is shown in Figure 14-2. Two peaks of activity were apparent; the ethyl and heptyl analogs showed the most activity. Further studies confirmed that a four-carbon link between the phenyl group and the ammonium ion head provided optimal activity, and that triethyl substitution of the quaternary nitrogen increased potency more than either trimethyl or tripropyl substitution (Fig. 14-3). Substitutions in the para position of the phenyl ring tended to increase potency somewhat, while ortho substitution, especially when both ortho positions were occupied, drastically reduced activity.

As shown on the bottom of Figure 14-3, the N-heptyldiethyl analog possessed an EC_{20} of 2.3×10^{-8} M (the concentration that increased APD by 20%) and was one of the more potent substances examined. Substituting a p-nitro or p-chloro (e.g., Lily 150378, known generically as clofilium) substituent on the phenyl ring, however, further increased potency (Fig. 14-4, left). The tertiary amine an-

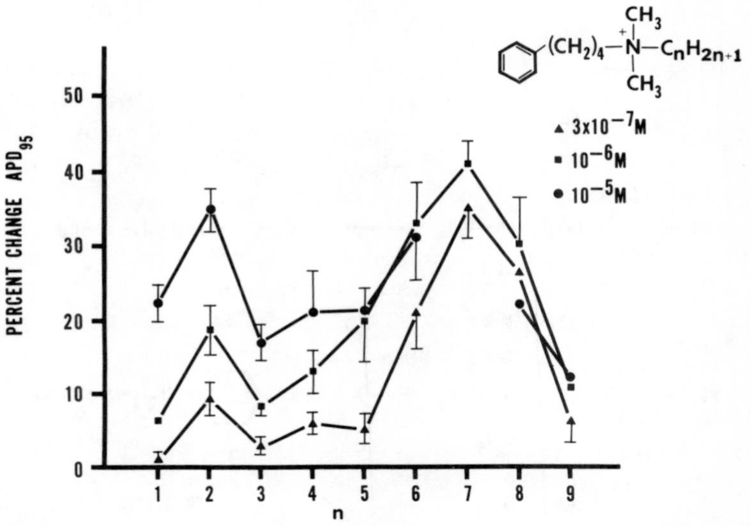

14-2 The effect of changing the N-alkyl substituent on action potential duration. Ordinate: Increase in Purkinje fiber action potential duration measured at 95% of full repolarization (APD_{95}). Abscissa: Number of carbon atoms in methylene chain (n). Drugs were superfused at the concentrations indicated. The values are mean ± SE of at least three experiments (two observations where standard error bars are absent).

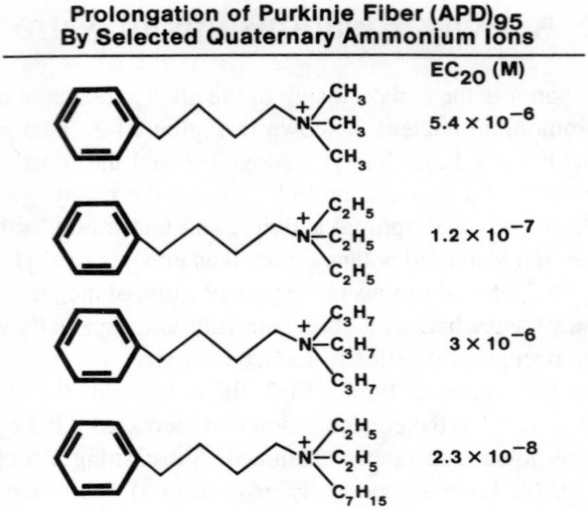

14-3 The effect of N-trialkyl substitution on Purkinje fiber action potential duration. The molar concentration producing a 20% increase in APD_{95} is shown on the right (EC_{20}).

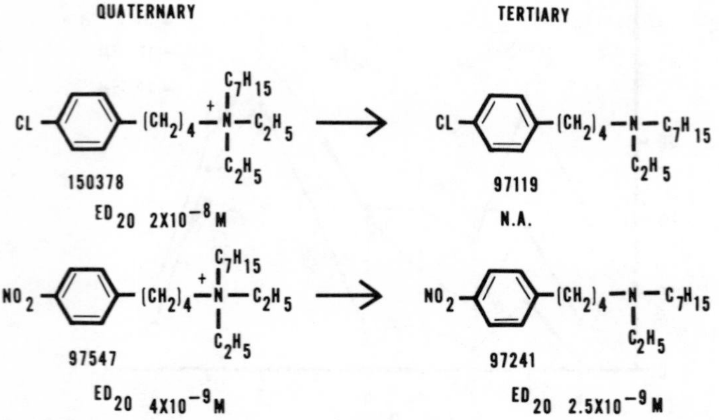

14-4 Relative potency of p-phenyl-substituted quaternary and tertiary amine analogs. ED_{20} refers to the concentration prolonging Purkinje fiber action potential duration by 20%. Conversion of the p-chlorophenyl-substituted quaternary analog to the tertiary amine abolishes activity (N.A.).

alogs were generally inactive, but it was surprising to find that in the p-phenyl nitro-substituted series, tertiary amines were at least as potent as the corresponding quaternary analogs. In fact, compound 97241 (Fig. 14-4, bottom right) is one of the most potent substances that directly effects the electrical activity of cardiac tissues (EC_{20}, 2.5×10^{-9} M). Full dose-response curves comparing the potency of 97241 and clofilium are shown in Figure 14-5. The changes in APD described for these analogs (either quaternary or tertiary amines) were unaccompanied by changes in the rate of rise of phase 0 or other cellular electrical parameters.

Electrophysiology in Vivo

The selective increase in APD and refractoriness obtained in vitro with these potent class III substances, is characterized in vivo by a significant increase in VERP and the QT_c interval (Steinberg et al., 1984). These effects on refractoriness are unaccompanied by changes in conduction indices (i.e., P-R, A-H, or H-V interval, or QRS duration). For both the quaternary and tertiary class III agents, we generally found a good correlation between the potency in prolonging the APD determined in vitro and increasing the VERP in normal dogs in vitro (compare Figs. 14-5 and 14-6).

Since it is well known that ischemia can influence the response to drugs (see Singer et al., 1981), the effects of clofilium on the chronically infarcted myocardium were compared with its effects on the normal zone in the chronic canine myocardial infarction model. As shown in Table 14-3, clofilium (0.2–0.8 mg/kg, iv) increased left ventricular VERP in both normal and infarct zones, the increase being greater in the latter. An example of the effect of clofilium on the strength-interval curve obtained from chronically infarcted and normal areas is shown in

Table 14-3 Ventricular Effective Refractory Period Increase after iv Clofilium.*

Dose mg/kg	Increase in Effective Refractory Period** Normal Sites	Infarct Sites
0.2	14 ± 2†	26 ± 2††
(3)	(8)	(14)
0.4	13 ± 1†	32 ± 2††
(6)	(13)	(32)
0.8	24 ± 4†	53 ± 5††
(3)	(6)	(15)

* Dogs with chronic infarcts (see "Materials and Methods") were paced at a cycle length of 300 ms and ventricular refractoriness was determined by the extrastimulus technique using plunge electrodes. Values were mean ± SE of the number of dogs or sites indicated in parentheses.

**P value infarct versus normal sites: $p < 0.01$ (Student's "t" test, unpaired data.)

†P value versus base-line: $p < 0.01$ (Student's "t" test, paired data).

††P value versus base-line: $p < 0.001$ (Student's "t" test, paired data).

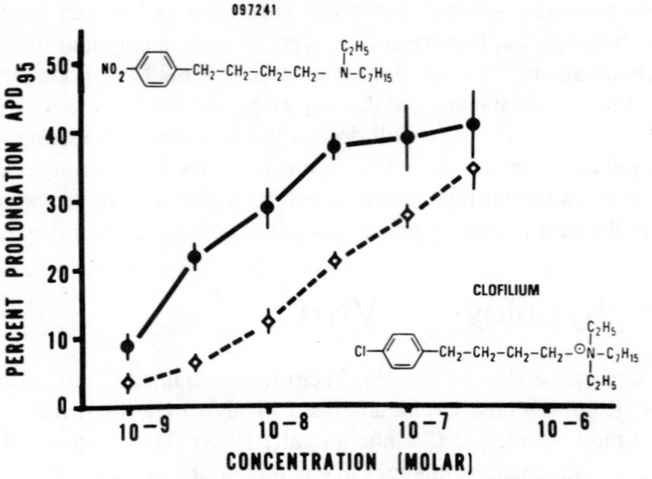

14-5 Relative potency of quaternary and tertiary amine class III substances in prolonging APD_{95}. Compounds were superfused at the concentration indicated on the abscissa. EC_{50} determined by probit analysis was 3.2×10^{-9} and 1.7×10^{-8} M for 97241 and clofilium, respectively. All values are mean ± SE from 4–51 experiments.

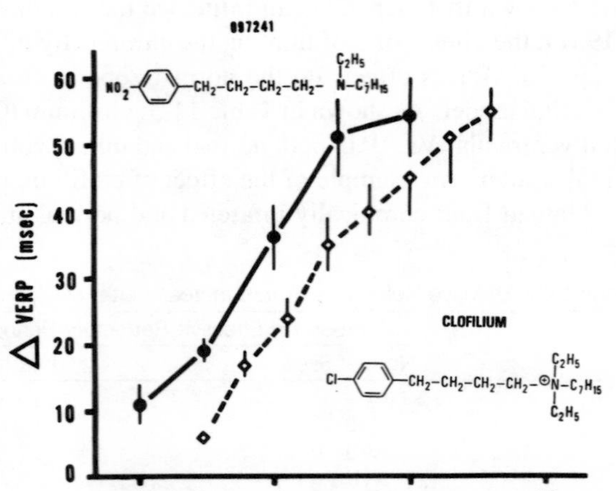

14-6 Relative potency of quaternary and tertiary amine class III drugs in prolonging ventricular effective refractory period (VERP) in halothane-anesthetized normal dogs. Ordinate: the increase in VERP from base-line values (174 ± 4 and 178 ± 3 ms for 97241 and clofilium, respectively). Abscissa: cumulative iv dose. Dogs were paced from the right ventricular apex at 150 beats/min, and VERP was determined with an intracavitary bipolar catheter using the extrastimulus technique. All values are mean ± SE of from 5–19 experiments. ED_{50} determined by probit analysis was 0.041 and 0.175 mg/kg for 97241 and clofilium, respectively.

Figure 14-7. The increase in relative and absolute refractoriness of the ventricle was unaccompanied by significant changes in threshold current at the longest coupling intervals in the normal zone, although small increases (0.15–0.25 mA) were seen in the ischemic zone. Furthermore, neither local conduction velocity in ischemic or normal zones nor global conduction (surface ECG parameters) was influenced by the drug. Following a 5–20 min latency period after the end of the infusion, clofilium (0.4–1.0 mg/kg) either prevented or made it more difficult to induce VT or fibrillation using triple extrastimuli inserted during the vulnerable period of the heart. Of 15 dogs that were inducible electrically before clofilium, nine were noninducible after the drug, five had VT/VF slowed, while only one animal showed no effect (unpublished data for six dogs given 1.0 mg/kg of clofilium were kindly supplied by G. Kopia).

We also studied another potent but structurally very different class III substance, anthopleurin A. Its effects on VERP and contractility (estimated as dP/dt_{max}) were compared with clofilium (Fig. 14-8). The polypeptide increased refractoriness to about the same extent as clofilium, but anthopleurin A, in contrast, caused much greater increases in contractility for a given increase in refractoriness. The increases in contractility and refractoriness were unaccompanied by significant changes in conduction intervals (except for prolonged QT_c) or blood pressure.

The potent and specific electrophysiologic properties of these class III substances, as demonstrated in animal studies, prompted the initial testing of one of them (clofilium) in patients undergoing programmed stimulation (Platia and Reid, 1984; Greene et al., 1983). As anticipated from the preclinical data, the agent increased both atrial and ventricular refractoriness and QT_c interval without changing conduction velocity indices (Steinberg et al., 1983). In about 40% of patients the drug either made it more difficult or prevented the induction of VT. However, in about 10% of patients undergoing programmed testing, an increase in the ease of arrhythmia induction or the development of spontaneous tachycardia occurred following iv dosing. On the other hand, in patients with spontaneous, but hemodynamically stable VT, some rather dramatic drug responses were seen. For example, Figure 14-9 shows the suppression of VT in a patient following a single iv dose of 0.3 mg/kg of clofilium. In this patient with incessant VT, the drug was effective in suppressing VT for almost two days. Similar results were obtained in two other spontaneous VT patients (information kindly supplied by Dr. H. Leon Greene).

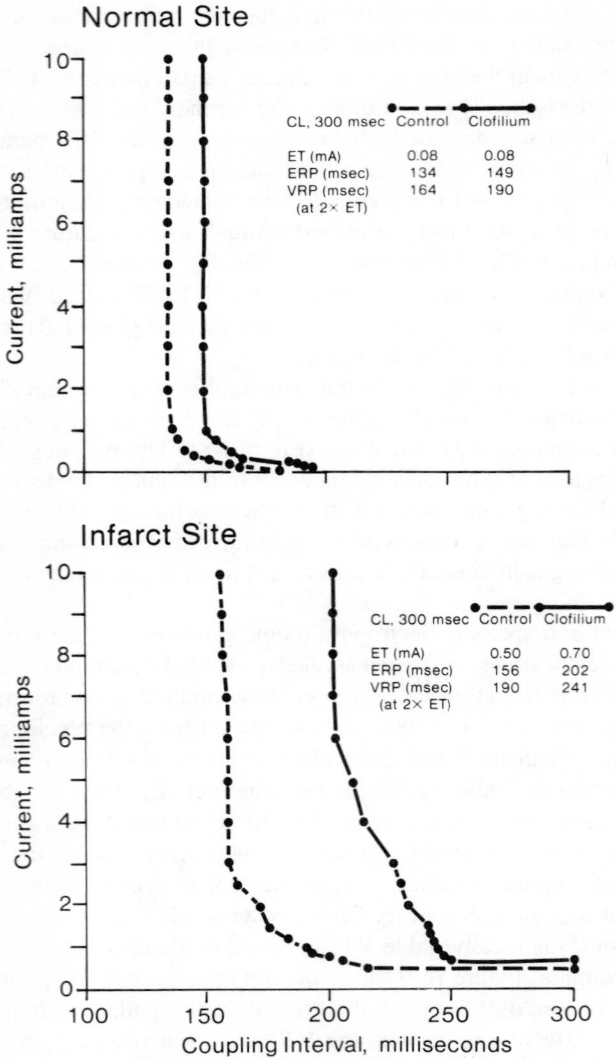

14-7 Typical strength-interval curves before and after clofilium (0.4 mg/kg). The ordinate shows the current in milliamps and the abscissa the longest coupling interval in milliseconds failing to elicit a response. Clofilium increased the effective refractory period (ERP) and refractory period at twice the excitability threshold (ET) in both normal (top) and infarct zones (bottom). However, note that the difference in ERP between normal and infarct zones was 22 ms before the drug, and this difference increased to 53 ms after the drug due to the enhanced sensitivity of the ischemic zone. Only minimal changes were seen in ET in either zone. The left ventricular sites studied were paced at a basic cycle length (CL) of 300 ms.

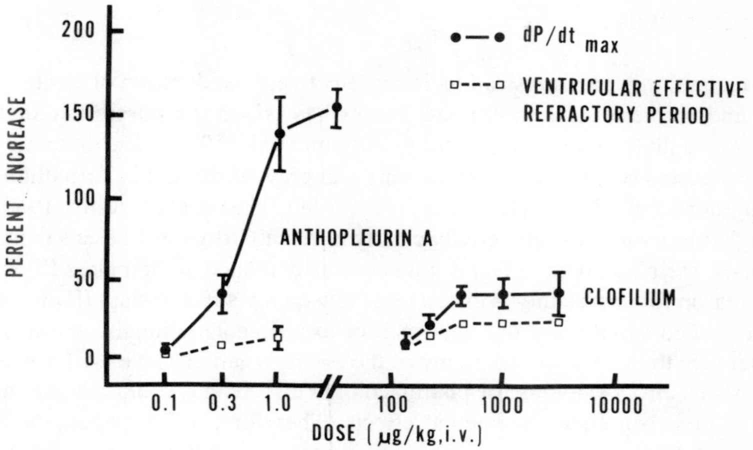

14-8 Effect of anthopleurin A (left) and clofilium (right) on contractility and refractoriness in normal dogs. Ordinate: per cent increase above base-line values (for contractility; 1117 and 1236 mm Hg s^{-1} for anthopleurin, and clofilium, respectively; for VERP; 174 and 176 ms for anthopleurin, and clofilium, respectively). Abscissa: cumulative iv dose. Refractoriness determined as in Figure 14-6. Contractility estimated as the maximum rate of pressure development in the left ventricle (dP/dt_{max}) determined using a fluid-filled polyethylene cannula. All values are the mean ± SE of six experiments.

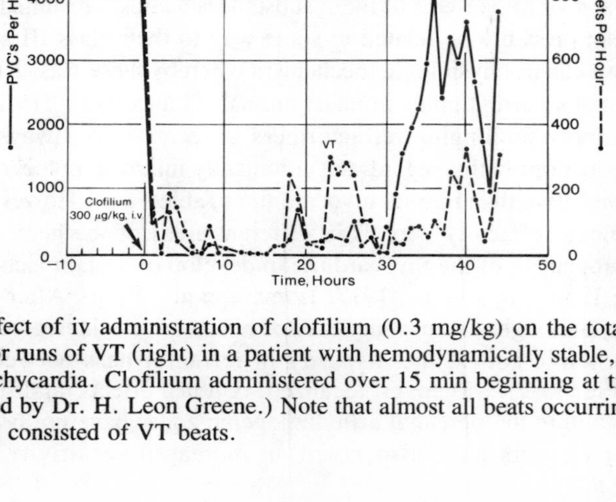

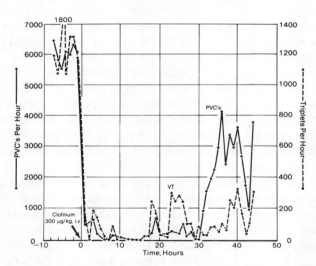

14-9 The effect of iv administration of clofilium (0.3 mg/kg) on the total number of PVC's (left) or runs of VT (right) in a patient with hemodynamically stable, spontaneous ventricular tachycardia. Clofilium administered over 15 min beginning at time 0. (Data kindly supplied by Dr. H. Leon Greene.) Note that almost all beats occurring during the control period consisted of VT beats.

Discussion

The recognition that drugs can increase selectively the duration of electrical systole and refractoriness in cardiac tissues has raised the possibility that such activity might have therapeutic utility (Olsson et al., 1973). The dramatic therapeutic success of amiodarone in treating and preventing cardiac arrhythmias has strengthened this belief (Haffajee et al., 1983; Nademanee et al., 1983). Although drugs with class III activity clearly have antiarrhythmic effects in man and animals, their beneficial effect is not necessarily related to their class III activity. One reason for uncertainty is that, as yet, few highly specific class III agents have been studied extensively in either man or experimental animals. As mentioned earlier (see the introduction), many of the agents listed in Table 14-1 possess additional electrophysiologic or pharmacologic effects that could mediate all or a part of their beneficial therapeutic effects. Therefore, to investigate the advantages and disadvantages of class III activity per se, it is imperative to have available potent and selective agents for experimental and clinical study.

Previous studies with isolated cardiac tissues had revealed a series of drugs (clofilium being one of the more potent members) that prolong the APD without changing the conductance of the membrane for sodium ions or affecting normal automaticity (Sullivan et al., 1978; Steinberg and Molloy, 1979). Automaticity occurring from depolarized potentials in the presence of barium ions (0.3 mM) was also unaffected by high concentrations of clofilium (unpublished data). Moreover, these agents are generally devoid of other noncardiac pharmacologic activity (Steinberg et al., 1983). The results of these studies implied that the specific class III activity demonstrated in single cell studies could also be extended to intact animal models of arrhythmias. As demonstrated in the present study, the lack of effect of clofilium on conduction velocity in normal or infarcted myocardium, at the same time antiarrhythmic effects were evident, supports the concept that the antiarrhythmic effects of these substances against presumed reentrant arrhythmias can probably be related in some way to their class III activity.

The precise electrophysiologic mechanism whereby these class III drugs might prevent or abolish arrhythmias in intact animals is uncertain. The most obvious way is by simply prolonging refractoriness in reentrant pathways but without slowing conduction; in this regard, the chronically infarcted myocardium seemed to be more sensitive than normal myocardium (Table 14-3). However, increased disparity among refractory periods in different areas of the heart may also increase the propensity of the myocardium to develop or sustain tachyarrhythmias (Han et al., 1966; Merx et al., 1977; Isomura et al., 1983). After clofilium administration, although the absolute level of refractoriness increased in both normal and ischemic zones, the disparity in refractoriness between sites also increased (Fig. 14-7). Moreover, localized, regional effects on dispersion of refractoriness within the potential arrhythmogenic zones have not been characterized. Other workers have also noted an increased sensitivity of ischemic myocardium to clofilium in chronically ischemic canine models (G. Kopia, personal communication). In isolated tissue studies, refractoriness and APD were increased both in normal and in ischemic zones but somewhat less in the latter, tending to reduce the disparity of refractoriness between the two zones (Steinberg et al., 1981). Differences between these data obtained in vivo and in vitro might be related to several factors. First, the way a drug is presented to the myocardium can influence its ultimate effect (Zipes et al., 1982); penetration of the drug to ischemic tissues in vitro is obviously different from the situation in vivo. Second, ERP determined in vitro tends to reflect local refractoriness in the immediate vicinity of the stimulating and recording electrodes, while abnormal conduction patterns throughout ischemic tissues, especially in the mottled infarcts present in the chronic canine model (Michelson et al., 1981), might significantly alter refractoriness determined in vivo. Third, the duration of ischemia in the present studies lasted between 4 and 9 days as opposed to only 2 days in the studies in vitro.

The ionic mechanism(s) mediating the cellular effects of specific class III substances is unknown. To date, no experiments under voltage-controlled conditions have been performed with the analogs described in this study. One of us had previously speculated that clofilium, like TEA, might delay the onset or reduce the magnitude of the time-dependent outward current carried by potassium ion in cardiac tissues (Steinberg et al., 1981). The similarities between the structure-activity relationships demonstrated in the present study for quaternary and tertiary amines and those of an analogous group of substances in blocking potassium pores in nerve, lend support to this possibility (Armstrong, 1971; French and Shoukimas, 1981; Swenson, 1981). These voltage clamp studies in squid axon suggested that small quaternary ammonium ions (about 8–10 Å in diameter) can easily fit through the inner mouth of the potassium pore but cannot easily penetrate the narrow outer portion (about 3Å in diameter) in the vicinity of the selectivity filter, thereby blocking the pore. Binding of antagonists within the pore seems to be facilitated by hydrophobic, aliphatic groups positioned on either side of a positively charged nitrogen head (Swenson, 1981). Presumably, the charged amine is required to bind to negative sites along the mouth of the pore. Figure 14-10 represents an attempt to fit this general concept to the structural requirements for potent class III activity found in the present study. Thus, although the N-heptyl, diethyl "head group" is larger than the "best fit" trialkyl-substituted groups studied in squid axon, one could easily envision how the heptyl "head" group might extend into the narrow inner portion of the pore while the "tail" of the molecule (the phenylbutyl portion) remains in the vicinity of the pore mouth. This arrangement could provide more opportunity for hydrophobic binding adjacent to the charged amine site. Somewhat similar concepts have been discussed in regard to the binding of hydrophobic, long chain quaternary ammonium ions to potassium pores in nerve (French and Shoukimas, 1981; Swenson, 1981) and heart (Kass et al., 1982). The fact that long chain trialkyl substitution on the nitro-

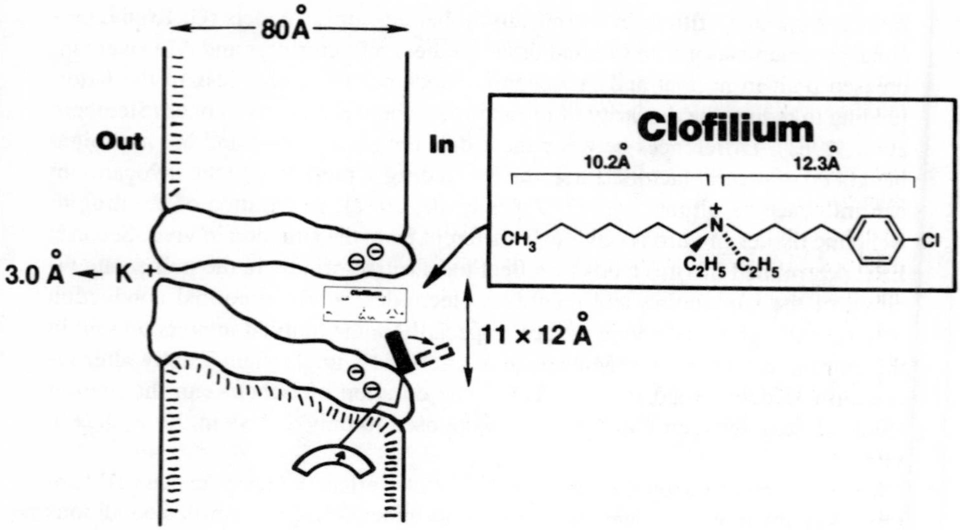

14-10 Hypothetical framework for the interaction of quaternary ammonium ions with potassium pores in myocardial membranes. The entrance to the inner aspect of the pore mouth is voltage- and time-dependent (gate is open for large depolarizations) and is relatively wide, allowing a variety of quaternary ammonium ions with radii of approximately 8–10 Å to enter. Binding within the pore is facilitated by electrostatic interactions between the quaternary nitrogen and anionic sites along the pore wall, as well as by hydrophobic binding of the heptyl and phenylbutyl groups to the pore wall. The selectivity filter (outer end) is wide enough to pass unhydrated or partially hydrated potassium ions, but not the larger quaternary analogs, thus causing the latter to act as potassium antagonists. Bulky, axially directed groups or hydrophilic substitution on the alkyl chains decreases binding affinity. Overall scheme adapted from Armstrong (1971; 1975) and Swenson (1981).

gen and ortho substitution on the phenyl ring markedly decrease potency may indicate that, at least in cardiac Purkinje fibers axially directed, bulky substituents might hinder binding within the pore or access of the molecule to the pore mouth. It is unclear how electronic or steric changes induced by p-phenyl nitro substitution (Fig. 14-4) confer greater class III activity to the tertiary amine molecule than even in the quaternary series. However, the fact that tertiary amines can also be shown to have highly potent and selective class III activity may have importance with regard to their potential improved oral bioavailability over quaternary amines.

Anthopleurin A and a number of other potent naturally occurring polypeptide toxins prolong the activation or delay the inactivation mechanisms of the sodium channel (Honerjäger, 1982; Lazdunski and Renaud, 1982). In general, these substances possess potent class III electrophysiologic properties as well as positive inotropic activity (Ravens 1976; Shibata et al., 1978; Hashimoto et al., 1980). The latter presumably derives from enhanced sodium-calcium exchange facilitated by an increase in intracellular sodium (Honerjäger, 1982). Although clofilium increased dP/dt_{max} during constant ventricular pacing (Fig. 14–8), its inotropic effect for a given increase in refractory period was considerably less than for anthopleurin A. Simply prolonging the APD per se could result in positive inotropic activity (many class III drugs have this activity). Our results suggest that class III activity mediated through increased sodium flux during the upstroke and plateau of the action potential might result in greater inotropic activity than class III activity mediated, for example, by blocking potassium flux as envisioned above.

Whether antiarrhythmic drugs will produce a beneficial effect, no effect or even a proarrhythmic effect depends on numerous complex and interrelated factors (Hoffman and Rosen, 1981). Probably any potent compound capable of altering the critical balance of conduction or refractoriness can be proarrhythmic under appropriate circumstances. Arrhythmogenic effects of class III substances have been seen in both man (Laakso et al., 1981; Sclarovsky et al., 1983) and experimental animals (Dangman and Hoffman, 1981). As indicated earlier, an increased dispersion of refractoriness between normal and ischemic zones could perhaps outweigh any potential benefit of increased local refractoriness within presumed reentrant pathways and predispose to arrhythmias. Arrhythmias could also arise from cells with excessively prolonged APD leading to repetitive early afterdepolarizations during the plateau phase of the action potential (Cranefield, 1977; Dangman and Hoffman, 1981; Ito and Surawicz, 1977). This kind of triggered "automatic" mechanism is consistent with observations made in halothane-anesthetized dogs that clofilium-induced arrhythmias are inversely related to heart rate, suppressed by overdrive pacing, and abolished by sinus arrest (Steinberg et al., 1983; unpublished data). A proarrhythmic potential is, of course, not restricted to class III agents; numerous reports linking the depressant effects of class I agents with arrhythmogenic activity have also appeared (Lui et al., 1982; Patterson et al., 1982; Rinkenberger et al., 1982). On the other hand, any arrhythmogenic potential of these substances must be reconciled with the potent and long-lasting antiarrhythmic activity seen in patients with refractory, spontaneous VT (Fig. 14-9). Important questions that may have a bearing on the ultimate therapeutic utility of specific class III substances include: Should these agents be used in acute or chronic myocardial ischemia? Would the therapeutic index be improved by prolonged oral therapy as opposed to the relatively rapid iv infusions studied so far? Would any benefit be realized by combining a specific class III drug with one of the newer highly specific class I conduction-depressant agents (Roden et al., 1980; Somani, 1980)? Before any firm judgments can be made about the potential role of specific class III substances, these and other problems will have to be answered by careful clinical and experimental studies. These efforts should be aided by the development of newer, specific class III agents with improved pharmacodynamic properties and more favorable therapeutic ratios.

Summary and Conclusion

Class III drugs that possess exceptional specificity and potency can be developed using established intracellular electrophysiologic techniques. Analogous to studies performed using the squid axon, the structure-activity relationships disclosed in the present study suggest, but do not prove, that these compounds act by blocking potassium pores in the cardiac membrane. Potent class III activity can also be demonstrated in vivo by the enhanced ventricular refractoriness in normal and ischemic ventricular myocardium in the absence of conduction changes. Specific class III drugs can possess potent antiarrhythmic action as demonstrated in an ischemic dog model subject to inducible tachycardia and in spontaneous VT in man. Whether pure class III electrophysiologic activity will eventually find therapeutic usefulness for arrhythmia control or whether other electrophysiologic properties alone or in combination with class III activity are preferable, will only be known by continued clinical and experimental studies.

Acknowledgments

We gratefully acknowledge the contributions of our colleagues to the studies cited in the text. These include: Drs. Masahito Naito, Daniel David, E. Neil Moore, Leonard S. Dreifus, Charles Sauermelch, and Mark Sullivan. The expert technical assistance of Mr. Charles Keller and Ms. Sally Wiest are greatly appreciated. Thanks also to Dr. David Robertson for his insight concerning the possible molecular configurations of clofilium in aqueous solution. Finally, it is a pleasure to acknowledge Ms. Denise Wakefield for her secretarial assistance.

This work was supported in part by Clinical Investigator Award 5K08 HL00709 from the National Heart, Lung and Blood Institute, National Institutes of Health, Bethesda, Maryland.

References

Allessie, M.A., Bonke, F.I.M., and Schopman, F.J.G. 1977. Circus movement in rabbit atrial muscle as a mechanism of tachycardia. III. The "leading circle" concept: a new model of circus movement in cardiac tissue without the involvement of an anatomical obstacle. Circ Res 41:9–18.

Armstrong, C.M. 1971. Interaction of tetraethylammonium ion derivatives with the potassium channels of giant axons. J Gen Physiol 58:413–437.

Armstrong, C.M. 1975. Membranes/A Series of Advances. Vol. 3, pp. 325–381. New York and Basel: Marcel Dekker, Inc.

Armstrong, C.M., and Hille, B. 1972. The inner quaternary ammonium ion receptor in potassium channels of the node of Ranvier. J Gen Physiol 59:388–400.

Bexton, R.S., and Camm, A.J. 1982. Drugs with class III antiarrhythmic action. Pharmacol Ther 17:315–355.

Bigger, J.T., and Jaffe, C.C. 1971. The effect of bretylium tosylate on the electrophysiologic properties of ventricular muscle and Purkinje fibers. Am J Cardiol 27:82–92.

Boura, A.L.A., and Green, A.E. 1959. The actions of bretylium: adrenergic neurone blocking and other effects. Br J Pharmacol 14: 536–548.

Brooks, C.McC., Hoffman, B.F., Suckling, E.E., and Orias, O. 1955. Excitability of the Heart. p. 263. New York and London: Grune and Stratton.

Cranefield, P.F. 1977. Action potentials, afterpotentials, and arrhythmias. Circ Res 41: 415–423.

Dangman, K.H., and Hoffman, B.F. 1981. In vivo and in vitro antiarrhythmic and arrhythmogenic effects of N-acetyl procainamide. J Pharmacol Exp Ther 217:851–862.

El-Sherif, N., Mehra, R., Gough, W.B., and Zeiler, R.H. 1982. Ventricular activation patterns of spontaneous and induced ventricular rhythms in canine one-day-old myocardial infarction. Evidence for focal and reentrant mechanisms. Circ Res 51:152–166.

El-Sherif, N., Scherlag, B.J., and Lazzara, R. 1975. Electrode catheter recordings during malignant ventricular arrhythmia following experimental acute myocardial ischemia. Evidence for re-entry due to conduction delay and block in ischemic myocardium. Circulation 51:1003–1014.

French, R.J., and Shoukimas, J.J. 1981. Blockage of squid axon potassium conductance by internal tetra-N-alkylammonium ions of various sizes. Biophys J 34:271–291.

Greene, H.L., Werner, J.A., Gross, B.W., Sears, G.K., Trobaugh, G.B., and Cobb, L.A. 1983. Prolongation of cardiac refractory times in man by clofilium phosphate, a new antiarrhythmic agent. Am Heart J 106:492–501.

Haffajee, C.I., Love, J.C., Canada, A.T., Lesko, L.J., Asdourian, G., and Alpert, J.S. 1983. Clinical pharmacokinetics and efficacy of amiodarone for refractory tachyarrhythmias. Circulation 67:1347–1355.

Haldimann, C. 1963. Effet du tétraéthylammonium sur les potentiels de repos et de'action du ceur de mouton. Arch Int Pharmacodyn Ther 146:1–9.

Hamer, A.W.F., Mandel, W.J., Zaher, C.A., Karagueuzin, H.S., and Peter, T. 1983. The electrophysiologic basis for the use of amiodarone for treatment of cardiac arrhythmias. Pace 6:784–792.

Han, J. 1971. The concepts of reentrant activity responsible for ectopic rhythms. Am J Cardiol 28:253–262.

Han, J., Millet, D., Chizzonitti, B., and Moe, G.K. 1966. Temporal dispersion of recovery of excitability in atrium and ventricle as a function of heart rate. Am Heart J 71:481–487.

Hashimoto, K., Ochi, R., Hashimoto, K., Inui, J., and Miura, Y. 1980. The ionic mechanism of prolongation of action potential duration of cardiac ventricular muscle by anthopleurin-A and its relationship to the inotropic effect. J Pharmacol Exp Ther 215:479–485.

Hauswirth, D., and Singh, B.N. 1979. Ionic mechanisms in heart muscle in relation to the genesis and the pharmacological control of cardiac arrhythmias. Pharmacol Rev 30:5–63.

Hoffman, B.F., and Rosen, M.R. 1981. Cellular mechanisms for cardiac arrhythmias. Circ Res 49:1–15.

Honerjäger, P. 1982. Cardioactive substances that prolong the open state of sodium channels. Physiol Biochem Pharmacol 92:2–80.

Isomura, S., Toyama, J., Kodama, I., and Yamada, K. 1983. Epicardial activation patterns and dispersion of refractoriness initiating ventricular tachycardia in the canine left ventricle during acute ischemia. Jpn Circ J 47: 342–350.

Ito, S., and Surawicz, B. 1977. Transient, "paradoxical" effects of increasing extracellular K^+ concentration on transmembrane potential in canine cardiac Purkinje fibers. Role of the Na^+ pump and K^+ conductance. Circ Res 41:799–807.

Ito, S., and Surawicz, B. 1981. Effect of tetraethylammonium chloride on action potential in cardiac Purkinje fibers. Am J Physiol 241:H139–144.

Josephson, M.E., Horowitz, L.N., and Farshidi, A. 1978a. Continuous local electrical activity. A mechanism of recurrent ventricular tachycardia. Circulation 57:659–665.

Josephson, M.E., Horowitz, L.N., Farshidi, A., and Kastor, J.A. 1978b. Recurrent sustained ventricular tachycardia. Circulation 57:431–447.

Kass, R.S., Scheuer, T., and Malloy, K.J. 1982. Block of outward current in cardiac Purkinje fibers by injection of quaternary ammonium ions. J Gen Physiol 79:1041–1063.

Kaumann, A.J., and Aramendiá, P. 1968. Prevention of ventricular fibrillation induced by coronary ligation. J Pharmacol Exp Ther 164:326–332.

Laakso, M., Pentikainen, P.J., Pyorala, K., and Neuvonen, P.J. 1981. Prolongation of the Q-T interval caused by sotalol—possible association with ventricular tachyarrhythmias. Eur Heart J 2:353–358.

Lazdunski, M., and Renaud, J.F. 1982. The action of cardiotoxins on cardiac plasma membranes. Annu Rev Physiol 44:463–473.

Lui, H.K., Lee, G., Dietrich, P., Low, R.I., and Mason, D.T. 1982. Flecainide-induced QT prolongation and ventricular tachycardia. Am Heart J 103:567–569.

Maruyama, Y., Yamashita, E., and Inomata, H. 1980. Effects of intracellular or extracellular application of tetraethylammonium on the action potential in cultured chick embryonic heart muscle cell. Experientia 36:557–558.

Mason, J.W., Hondeghem, L.M., and Katzung, B.G. 1983. Amiodarone blocks inactivated cardiac sodium channels. Pflügers Arch 396: 79–81.

Merx, W., Yoon, M.S., and Han, J. 1977. The role of local disparity in conduction and recovery time on ventricular vulnerability to fibrillation. Am Heart J 94:603–610.

Mines, G.R. 1914. On circulating excitations in heart muscles and their possible relation to tachycardia and fibrillation. Trans R Soc Can 8:43–52.

Michelson, E.L., Spear, J.F., and Moore, E.N. 1980. Electrophysiologic and anatomic correlates of sustained ventricular tachyarrhythmias in a model of chronic myocardial infarction. Am J Cardiol 45:583–590.

Michelson, E.L., Spear, J.F., and Moore, E.N. 1981. Further electrophysiologic and anatomic correlates in a canine model of chronic myocardial infarction susceptible to the initiation of sustained ventricular tachyarrhythmias. Anat Rec 201:55–65.

Moe, G.K. 1975. Evidence for reentry as a mechanism of cardiac arrhythmias. Physiol Biochem Pharmacol 72:56–81.

Nademanee, K., Singh, B.N., Hendrickson, J., Intarachot, V., Lopez, B., Feld, G., Cannom, D.S., and Weiss, J. 1983. Amiodarone in refractory life-threatening ventricular arrhythmias. Ann Intern Med 98:577–584.

Ochi, R., and Nishiye, H. 1974. Effect of intracellular-tetraethylammonium ion on action potential in the guinea-pig's myocardium. Pflügers Arch 348:305–316.

Olsson, S.B., Brorson, L., and Varnauskas, E. 1973. Class III antiarrhythmic action in man. Observations from monophasic action potential recordings and amiodarone treatment. Br Heart J 35:1255–1259.

Patterson, E., Gibson, J.K., and Lucchesi, B.R. 1982. Electrophysiologic actions of lidocaine in a canine model of chronic myocardial ischemic damage—arrhythmogenic actions of lidocaine. J Cardiovasc Pharmacol 4:925–934.

Platia, E., and Reid, P.R. 1984. Dose ranging studies of clofilium, an antiarrhythmic quarternary ammonium compound. Clin Pharmacol Ther 35:193–202.

Platou, E.S., Refsum, H., Amlie, J.P., and Landmark, K. 1982a. Plasma levels and cardiac electrophysiological effects of melperone in the dog. Eur J Pharmacol 82:1–7.

Platou, E.S., Smiseth, O.A., Refsum, H., Rouleau, J.L., and Chuck, L. 1982b. H. S. Vasodilator and inotropic effects of the antiarrhythmic drug melperone. J Cardiovasc Pharmacol 4:645–651.

Ravens, U. 1976. Electromechanical studies of anemonia sulcata toxin in mammalian cardiac muscle. Naunyn-Schmied Arch Pharmacol 296:73–78.

Rinkenberger, R.L., Prystowsky, E.N., Jackman, W.M., Naccarelli, G.V., Heger, J.J., and Zipes, D.P. 1982. Drug conversion of nonsustained ventricular tachycardia to sustained ventricular tachycardia during serial electrophysiologic studies: identification of drugs that exacerbate tachycardia and potential mechanisms. Am Heart J 103:177–184.

Roden, D.M., Reele, S.B., Higgins, S.B., Mayol, R.F., Gammans, R.E., Oates, J.A., and Woosley, R.L. 1980. Total suppression of ventricular arrhythmias by encainide. Pharmacokinetic and electrocardiographic characteristics. N Engl J Med 302:877–882.

Rosenbaum, M.B., Chiale, P.A., Halpern, M.S., Nau, G.J., Przybylski, J., Levi, R.J., Lazzari, J.O., and Elizari, M.V. 1976. Clinical efficacy of amiodarone as an antiarrhythmic agent. Am J Cardiol 38:934–944.

Scherlag, B.J., Helfant, R.H., and Haft, J.I. 1970. Electrophysiology underlying ventricular arrhythmias due to coronary ligation. Am J Physiol 6:1665–1671.

Sclarovsky, S., Lewin, R.F., Kracoff, O., Strasberg, B., Arditti, A., and Agmon, J. 1983. Amiodarone-induced polymorphous ventricular tachycardia. Am Heart J 105:6–12.

Shibata, S., Izumi, T., Seriguchi, D.G., and Norton, T.R. 1978. Further studies on the positive inotropic effect of the polypeptide anthopleurin-A from a sea anemone. J Pharmacol Exp Ther 205:683–692.

Singer, D.G., Baumgarten, C.M., and Ten Eick, R.E. 1981. Cellular electrophysiology of ventricular and other dysrhythmias: studies on diseased and ischemic heart. Progr Cardiovasc Dis 24:97–156.

Singh, B.N., and Vaughan Williams, E.M. 1970a. The effect of amiodarone, a new antianginal drug, on cardiac muscle. Br J Pharmacol 39:657–667.

Singh, B.N., and Vaughan Williams, E.M. 1970b. A third class of anti-arrhythmic action. Effects on atrial and ventricular intramuscular potentials, and other pharmacological actions on cardiac muscle, of MJ 1999 and AH 3474. Br J Pharmacol 39:675–687.

Singh, B.N., and Vaughan Williams, E.M. 1971. Effects on cardiac muscle of the β-adrenoceptor blocking drugs INPEA and LB46 in relation to their local anaesthetic action on nerve. Br J Pharmacol 43:10–22.

Somani, P. 1980. Antiarrhythmic effects of flecainide. Clin Pharmacol Ther 27:464–470.

Steinberg, M.I., Lindstrom, T.D., and Fasola, A.F. 1984. Clofilium: a class III antiarrhythmic agent. In: A. Scriabine, ed. New Drug Annual. New York: Raven Press. 103–121.

Steinberg, M.I., and Molloy, B.B. 1979. Clofilium—a new antifibrillatory agent that selectively increases cellular refractoriness. Life Sci 25:1397–1406.

Steinberg, M.I., Sullivan, M.E., Wiest, S.A., Rockhold, F.W., and Molloy, B.B. 1981. Cellular electrophysiology of clofilium, a new antifibrillatory agent, in normal and ischemic canine Purkinje fibers. J Cardiovasc Pharmacol 3:881–895.

Strauss, H.C., Bigger, J.T., and Hoffman, B.F. 1970. Electrophysiological and beta-receptor blocking effects of MJ 1999 on dog and rabbit cardiac tissue. Circ Res 26:661–678.

Sullivan, M.E., Steinberg, M.I., and Molloy, B.B. 1978. Selective prolongation of Purkinje fiber action potentials by tetraalkylammonium ions. The Pharmacologist 20:149.

Swenson, R.P., Jr. 1981. Inactivation of potassium current in squid axon by a variety of quaternary ammonium ions. J Gen Physiol 77: 255–271.

Vaughan Williams, E.M. 1974. Electrophysiological basis for a rational approach to antidysrrhythmic drug therapy. In: N.J. Harper and A.B. Simmonds, eds. Advances in Drug Research. pp. 69–101. New York: Academic Press.

Waleffe, A., Bruninx, P., and Kulbertus, H.E. 1978. Effects of amiodarone studied by programmed electrical stimulation of the heart in patients with paroxysmal re-entrant supraventricular tachycardia. J Electrocardiol 11:253–260.

Wit, A.L., and Cranefield, P.F. 1978. Reentrant excitation as a cause of cardiac arrhythmias. Am J Physiol 235:H1–17.

Wit, A.L., Rosen, M.R., and Hoffman, B.F. 1974. Electrophysiology and pharmacology of cardiac arrhythmias. II. Relationships of normal and abnormal electrical activity of cardiac fibers to the genesis of arrhythmias. B. Reentry. Section II. Am Heart J 88:798–806.

Wit, A.L., Steiner, C., and Damato, A.N. 1970. Electrophysiologic effects of bretylium tosylate on single fibers of the canine specialized conducting system and ventricle. J Pharmacol Exp Ther 173:344–356.

Zipes, D.P., Prystowsky, E.N., and Heger, J.J. 1982. Electrophysiologic testing of antiarrhythmic agents. Am Heart J 103:610–615.

Chapter 15

Clinical Effects of Class III Antiarrhythmic Agents

Charles I. Haffajee

Introduction

The development of effective and safe antiarrhythmic agents continues to be very desirable and provides the impetus for basic and clinical research of new agents. The significance of this is highlighted by the fact that sudden arrhythmic cardiac death remains a therapeutic challenge not only in patients experiencing an acute myocardial infarction not reaching a cardiac care unit, but also those who survive an acute myocardial infarction. Significant advances have been made in the understanding of the genesis of many of the clinical cardiac arrhythmias. Progress seemingly has been made in the development and understanding of the modes of action of conventional and newer antiarrhythmic agents. Therein, the classification of antiarrhythmic agents based on their antiarrhythmic mechanism is being accepted and employed in clinical usage. Antiarrhythmic agents that produce a pure prolongation of the action potential duration constitute class III agents. The agents, to date, that have been recognized to belong to this class are amiodarone, bretylium, the oral analog of bretylium, bethanidine, clofilium, N-acetylprocainamide (NAPA), and sotalol. Of these agents, only bretylium in its parenteral form is available for routine use in the United States, whereas the others are still in the investigational stages. However, worldwide, amiodarone has been employed with remarkable efficacy and an expanding body of experience has accrued with this drug in the United States in the past 6 years. This chapter will concentrate on the clinical experience with bretylium and amiodarone.

Bretylium

General Properties and Pharmacokinetics

This agent was first introduced as an antihypertensive. However, its poor tolerance, mainly due to gastrointestinal disturbances and significant orthostatic hypotension, limited its use for hypertension. However, its effects as an antifibrillatory agent, especially in the acute ischemic setting, and its effect against some ventricular tachycardias refractory to other agents led to its resurgence in the last 10 years, predominantly as an antiarrhythmic. It can be given iv, im, and orally. Its preliminary pharmacokinetics have suggested an erratic oral bioavailability, 70–80% excretion unchanged in the urine and a preferential concentration in myocardial cells (50:1 tissue/plasma). Its elimination half-life is 7–8 h. Clinical experience stems from its use as an iv drug in the setting of acute myocardial infarction where it is used for ventricular fibrillation (VF) that is often refractory to lidocaine and defibrillation. Some uncontrolled studies have suggested (Arcidiancono, 1978) that this agent can result in chemical defibrillation.

In normal myocardial and Purkinje tissues, bretylium consistently and homogeneously prolongs the entire duration of the action potential and the effective refractory period, hence classifying it as a class III antiarrhythmic. However, these effects do not occur in atrial muscle and this is consistent with the clinical observation that it has no effect on supraventricular tachyarrhythmias. Furthermore, it has disparate effects on the action potential duration between ischemic and infarcted myocardium which may explain its unique effect in raising the ventricular fibrillation threshold in man during infarction.

Hemodynamics

In the clinical setting, bretylium when given as an iv bolus produces a biphasic response. In the acute myocardial infarction (MI) setting, Chatterjee et al. (1973) demonstrated a rise in heart rate and blood pressure for the initial 10–15 min following the iv bolus. This is presumed to be due to the secondary release of norepinephrine. However, during the second phase which lasts for several hours, there was a fall in blood pressure and heart rate without significant changes in cardiac output or pulmonary capillary wedge pressure. Unlike most antiarrhythmics, however, there does not appear to be any depression of left ventricular (LV) function. Indeed, as there is a decrease in systemic vascular resistance, mainly of the venous capacitance vessels following iv bolus, there may be some decrease in LV work.

Antiarrhythmic Efficacy

Clinical experience in man with bretylium has largely been with the parenteral form in the acute myocardial infarction and in the post-cardiac surgical setting. Reported efficacy for VF in these settings has ranged from 60–90% in the noncontrolled series of Bacaner (1968), Terry et al. (1970), Bernstein and Koch-Weser (1972), Holder et al. (1977), and Dhurandhar et al. (1980) (Table 15-1).

A recent randomized controlled trial by Haynes et al. (1981), comparing bretyl-

Table 15-1 Results of Bretylium in Resistant VT-VF in the Acute MI Setting.

Group	Total No. of Patients	No. of Patients Responding	Success	No. of Patients Experiencing Chemical Defibrillation
			%	
Bacaner and Benditt	31	25	78	—
Bernstein and Koch-Weser	31	18	60	—
Holder et al.	27	20	78	—
Arcidiancono	17	14	84	10
Terry et al.	10	7	70	—
Dhurandhar et al.	18	10	58	—

MI, myocardial infarction; VT-VF, ventricular tachycardia-fibrillation.

ium to lidocaine for the management of VF occurring out of hospital, did not show bretylium to be superior to lidocaine (Table 15-2).

On the other hand, bretylium has been shown by Puddu et al. (1980), to be more effective for VF prophylaxis in the acute MI setting than lidocaine. In this nonrandomized study of 1255 patients, 412 were treated with conventional antiarrhythmic agents, usually lidocaine, whereas 843 patients received bretylium initially. In the lidocaine group, the incidence of primary VF was 5.1% as opposed to a 1.3% incidence in 843 patients treated with bretylium.

Table 15-2 Comparison of Bretylium and Lidocaine in Patients Experiencing an Out-of-Hospital Cardiac Arrest.

	No. of Patients	Percent in Whom an Organized Rhythm Established	Percent in whom a Stable Perfusing Rhythm Established	Cardioversions per Patient	Time (min) to Organized Rhythm	Percent Leaving Hospital
Bretylium	74	89	58	2.8	10.4	34
Lidocaine	72	93	60	2.4	10.6	26

Bretylium is usually administered parenterally either as a 400-mg iv bolus (5 mg/kg) repeated every 6 h, or as an infusion of 1–4 mg/min following the initial bolus. It can also be given im. The poor tolerance, variable absorption, and insufficient evidence regarding the efficacy of the oral form has limited its use and development as an oral agent. To date, there have been no reports of untoward drug interactions with bretylium, in particular with other antiarrhythmics. In fact, it is used for the treatment of torsade de pointes ventricular tachycardia, especially that induced by class IA antiarrhythmics (quinidine, procainamide, disopyramide).

Favorable experience with the oral analog of bretylium, bethanidine, as an antiarrhythmic has been reported recently by Bacaner and Benditt (1982). They found that bethanidine was successful in suppressing and preventing reinduction of VT during programmed ventricular stimulation in 66% of patients. The VT in these patients had been refractory to a wide variety of routine antiarrhythmic agents. This agent also resulted in orthostatic hypotension, which was controlled by the concomitant use of protritryline (Bacaner and Benditt, 1982).

Clofilium

Clofilium is an oral bretylium derivative which to date has not been evaluated extensively in man. Preliminary experience reported by Greene et al. (1981) suggests that this agent has promise in interrupting and preventing reinduction of both ventricular and supraventricular tachycardia.

Amiodarone

General Properties

Although this class III agent is still being investigated in the United States, it has emerged as perhaps the most powerful antiarrhythmic for the chronic prophylaxis of symptomatic and life-threatening ventricular arrhythmias and symptomatic atrial tachyarrhythmias that have proven refractory to most conventional agents. There is a rapid expanding volume of published papers attesting to this agent's efficacy in the world literature and it has been used in France and Argentina since 1969. Although its exact mechanism of action has not been elucidated to date, its effects on the action potential have been discussed in the previous chapter.

Electrophysiologic Effects

In patients undergoing electrophysiologic evaluation before and after receiving high dose oral amiodarone for 4–6 weeks, we have noted a significant prolongation of the atrial and ventricular refractory periods and a shortening of the Wenckebach point. These effects were more marked than those produced by therapeutic quinidine and procainamide administration in the same patients (Table 15-3). It also slows ventriculoatrial conduction and accessory pathway conduction in the orthodromic and antidromic directions. Its effects on H-V conduction and the sinus node are variable.

The ECG of patients taking long term amiodarone reveal slowing of the sinus rate, slight P-R prolongation, no change in QRS width, prolongation of the QT_c interval, and often the appearance of U waves and flattening of the T wave (Table 15-4).

Table 15-3 Comparative Effects of Amiodarone, Quinidine, and Procainamide on Myocardial Refractory Periods in Patients.

Paced CL 600 msec	Amiodarone	Quinidine*	Procainamide*
ARP (msec)	25–45 (m36)	15–35 (m22)	15–30 (m24)
VRP (msec)	20–50 (m38)	15–25 (m20)	20–30 (m24)

*$p < 0.001$.
CL, cycle length of pacing; ARP, right atrial effective refractory period; VRP, right ventricular effective refractory period.

Table 15-4 Electrocardiographic and Electrophysiologic Effects during Chronic Amiodarone in Man.

Electrocardiographic		Electrophysiologic	
H-R	↓	SNF	V
P-R	↓	AH	↑
QRS	↔	CL to Wencke	↓
QT_c	↑	H-V	V
T-U Development		VA	↑
		ARP	↑
		VRP	↑
		ACC P	↑

↑, Increased/Prolonged; ↓, Decreased/Shortened; ↔, No Change; V, Variable; SNF, Sinus Node Function.
ACC P = accessory pathway

Antiarrhythmic Efficacy

Amiodarone and Atrial Fibrillation Refractory to Conventional Agents

The long term efficacy of amiodarone in patients with atrial fibrillation/flutter that has been refractory to conventional agents (digoxin, quinidine, disopyramide, β-blockers) has ranged from 70–95%. In most of the reported series, the daily maintenance dose of amiodarone that was employed ranged from 200–400 mg. The etiology of the atrial fibrillation was similar in the series and patients with Wolff-Parkinson-White Syndrome were included in most of these reports (Table 15-5).

We and others have found that patients with relatively established atrial fibrillation can be primed with oral amiodarone for 4–6 weeks and thereafter subjected to cardioversion with a very high conversion rate to sinus rhythm. If their underlying disease was corrected, such as mitral valve disease, then the majority have continued to remain in sinus rhythm even with residual large left atria. In our own experience, 9 out of 12 such patients have maintained sinus rhythm while on amiodarone during a mean follow-up of greater than 12 months. Only 1 out of 12 patients failed to cardiovert initially into sinus rhythm. These patients had failed to maintain sinus rhythm with a variety of antiarrhythmic agents and repeated cardioversions (Haffajee et al., 1983).

Table 15-5 Results of Amiodarone Therapy.

Recurrent Refractory Atrial Fibrillation.

Group	No. of Patients	Mean Follow-up	Daily Maintenance Dosage	Success	No. of Patients with WPW
		months	mg	%	
Rosenbaum et al.	30	16	200–400	97	7
Moysey et al.	57	42	200–400	75	4
Wheeler et al.	16	11	100–200	60	—
Podrid and Lown	84	27	200–400	76	8
Haffajee et al.	80	11	200–400	73	3

Refractory Supraventricular Tachycardia.

Group	No. of Patients	Mean Follow-up	Daily Maintenance Dosage	Success	No. of Patients with WPW
Rosenbaum et al.	59	16	200–400	97	20
Moysey et al.	17	8.7	200–400	82	—
Leak and Eydt	13	16.8	200–600	100	3
Podrid and Lown	26	27.3	200–400	87	6

Refractory VT-VF.

Group	No. of Patients	Mean Follow-up	Daily Maintenance Dosage	Success	No. of Patients on Additional Antiarrhythmics
		months	mg	%	
Wheeler et al.	7	11	200–400	86	—
Kaski et al.	23	21.5	200–1200	67	—
Podrid and Lown	96	27.3	200–600	78	22
Heger et al.	29	12.7	400–1600	72	—
Waxman et al.	46	8.6	400–800	50–78	9
Nademanee et al.	24	13	200–600	83	—
Haffajee et al.	96	12.4	200–400	81	6

Survivors of Sudden Cardiac Death.

Group	No. of Patients	Mean Follow-up	Daily Maintenance Dosage	Success
		months	mg	%
Peter et al.	27	13	100–600	93
Nademanee et al.	24	10	200–600	83
Morady et al.	23	18	600	91
Haffajee et al.	40	13	200–600	86

WPW, Wolff-Parkinson-White Syndrome; VT, ventricular tachycardia; VF, ventricular fibrillation.

Amiodarone and Supraventricular Tachycardia Refractory to Conventional Agents A review of the published literature reveals a success rate ranging from 65–100% for amiodarone in this group of patients during long term therapy (Table 15-5). Waleffe et al. (1978) and Gomes et al. (1981) have also documented the efficacy of acute iv amiodarone in terminating atrioventricular nodal tachycardia and preventing its reinduction in the vast majority of patients during programmed electrophysiologic studies. Patients with WPW syndrome and atrioventricular tachycardia were included in the series of Waleffe et al. (1978).

Amiodarone and Sick Sinus Syndrome Despite amiodarone's variable effects on the sinus node, the incidence of profound sinus node depression necessitating pacemaker therapy when amiodarone is used long term for control of the atrial tachyarrhythmias of sick sinus syndrome is very low. However, if amiodarone is used in patients with sick sinus syndrome without a pacemaker, careful ECG monitoring and caution has to be exercised.

Amiodarone and Ventricular Tachyarrhythmias Refractory to Conventional Agents In general, amidarone has been used only when conventional agents singly and often in combination have failed to control life-threatening and/or symptomatic ventricular tachyarrhythmias. Its efficacy in these patients has been well documented in Europe, Argentina, and more recently, in the United States. It does require prolonged high dose (0.8–1.6 g/day) oral loading for 3–4 weeks for uniform and reliable effectiveness. Thereafter, low dose maintenance therapy (200–600 mg/day) appears to maintain clinical efficacy in the range of 60–80% for follow-up periods of greater than 12 months in most of the reported series (Table 15-5). The vast majority of patients achieve control with amiodarone alone.

Amiodarone and Survivors of Arrhythmic Sudden Cardiac Death (SCD) Amiodarone's remarkable efficacy has been documented in this high risk group of patients. It has achieved long term efficacy anywhere from 56–90% in the reported series. The effectiveness was similar whether patients were given empiric amiodarone (Kaski et al., 1981; Peter et al., 1981) or in those patients in whom programmed stimulation (EPS)-directed conventional agents had failed (Heger et al., 1981; Nademanee et al., 1982; Haffajee et al., 1983) (Table 15-5). Furthermore, the inducibility of VT-VF during EP testing while on amiodarone (Nademanee et al., 1982; Haffajee et al., 1983) did not preclude long term clinical success of this agent as opposed to the conventional agents (Mason and Winkle, 1980). However, we (Haffajee et al., 1983) and Horowitz et al. (1983) have observed that the patients who experienced a relapse while on chronic amiodarone came from the group who still had VT-VF inducible during EP testing on chronic amiodarone.

It appears that the success of amiodarone can be predicted by long term ECG monitoring once adequate high dose oral loading and probable steady-state with amiodarone (at least 4–6 weeks of high dose loading) is reached. Podrid and Lown (1981), Nademanee et al. (1982), and our group have observed a >85% reduction in ventricular premature beats (VPB) count and elimination of couplets/VT during ECG monitoring in the long term amiodarone responders (Table 15-6).

Table 15-6 The Correlation of VEA Reduction and Clinical Outcome in Patients with Malignant Ventricular Arrhythmias Treated by Long Term Oral Amiodarone.

Group	No. of Patients	>85% Reduction in VEA Counts by Holter Recording	Reduction in Couplets	Long Term Success
		%	%	%
Podrid and Lown	41	70	70	68
Nademanee et al.	13	95	95	100
Waxman et al.	38	29	76	78
Haffajee et al.	40	91	75	85

VEA, ventricular ectopic activity.

Hemodynamic Effects

Virtually all the reported data on the hemodynamic effects of amiodarone in man relate to acute iv administration of this agent. This is not the usual route of administration of this agent for control of cardiac tachyarrhythmias.

Following acute iv administration, Cote et al. (1979), and recently, Schwartz et al. (1983), have demonstrated an initial fall in systemic vascular resistance, decrease in heart rate, and an elevation in pulmonary capillary wedge pressure suggestive of a depression in LV function in patients with coronary or left ventricular disease. However, the net effect of these changes may result in a decrease in LV work and myocardial oxygen demands. This may also be due in part to the decrease in coronary vascular resistance and better myocardial lactate extraction in some patients (Cote et al., 1979).

The only data on the effects of long term oral amiodarone in man relate to LV function as measured by radionuclide ejection. We (Haffajee et al., 1983b) have not noted any change in ejection fraction in 17 patients studied before and during long term oral amiodarone.

Side Effects

This agent has produced a very long list of side effects and drug interactions. However, most of the side effects are relatively minor and can be minimized or rendered tolerable by a reduction in amiodarone dosage. On the other hand, this agent does require careful monitoring for the few but important major side effects (Table 15-7). The side effects in the reported series (Heger et al., 1981; Waxman et al., 1982; Harris et al., 1983) and in our series (Haffajee et al., 1983b), do not appear to respond to dosage reduction and frequently require discontinuation of this agent.

Table 15-7 Side Effects: Amiodarone.

Side Effects	No. of patients	Serum Amiodarone Level
A. Necessitating Discontinuation of Amiodarone (10%)		
		mg/l
1. Worsening or precipitating heart failure	7/173 (4%)	1.1–2.3 (mean 1.6)
2. CNS (parasthesiae, hair loss, nightmares)	4/173 (2%)	1.4–3.6 (mean 2.5)
3. Impotence	3/173 (2%)	1.2–2.5 (mean 1.9)
4. Sun sensitivity	2/173 (1%)	1.4, 1.5
5. Pulmonary fibrosis	1/173 (0.5%)	1.5
6. Generalized weakness, anorexia, and cachexia	1/173 (0.5%)	1.7
B. Symptomatic: Tolerable and/or Controllable (25%)		
1. Sun sensitivity	28/173 (17%)	0.6–4.3 (mean 2.3)
2. CNS	22/173 (13%)	0.8–3.6 (mean 2.2)
3. Skin rash, itchiness	8/173 (5%)	1.2–2.8 (mean 1.9)
4. Visual disturbances	6/173 (5%)	2.1–4.6 (mean 2.8)
5. Sinus node depression	4/173 (2%)	1.7–2.6 (mean 2.3)
6. Clinical hypothyroidism	3/173 (2%)	4.1, 1.8, 1.4
7. Clinical hyperthyroidism	3/173 (2%)	4.3, 1.7, 1.4
8. Drug interactions		
Coumadin	36/45 (80%)	1.2–4.4 (mean 1.8)
Quinidine, Procainamide	3/40 (7%)	—
C. Asymptomatic (19%)		
1. Elevations of liver enzymes (<2× normal)	34/173 (19%)	0.5–3.3 (mean 1.6)
2. Elevated serum T4	31/173 (19%)	0.8–4.3 (mean 1.8)
3. Corneal microdeposits	All	Irrespective

Drug Interactions

Drug interactions are a major concern. Amiodarone potentiates warfarin effects and can result in sudden and unpredictable prolongation of prothrombin time in patients taking this agent with resultant morbidity. The mechanism of this drug interaction has not been unravelled, as yet. Amiodarone displaces digoxin, quinidine, procainamide, and aprindine from protein building in the serum and, hence, results in elevation of the serum levels of these agents and potentiation of their effects.

Amiodarone's Place in Therapy

We feel this agent should be used when conventional first line antiarrhythmic agents have failed. It is attractive because of its dependable efficacy even when used empirically and because of its once-a-day dosing and long elimination half-life. On the other hand, it is an agent that does not lend itself to easy use in the early and often lengthy phase of loading, leaving the patient relatively unprotected, or making continuous hospitalization in patients with life-threatening arrhythmias necessary during this phase. Its pharmacokinetics support a probable three-compartment model and our experience and observations support the concept of a large volume of distribution and tissue uptake of this agent.

Despite the fact that all the published data on this drug have been nonrandomized and noncontrolled, it is fair to emphasize that it has been used mainly when all conventional and some investigational agents have failed in patients with symptomatic and life-threatening arrhythmias. The long term results in this group of patients support the remarkable efficacy of this agent. Often and importantly, the patients' arrhythmias that respond to amiodarone are more malignant than the side effects of this agent.

N-Acetylprocainamide

This major metabolite of procainamide with a longer half-life and lower incidence of lupus induction has class III electrophysiologic actions. Experience in patients is not extensive and has been limited to patients with ventricular arrhythmias. As opposed to procainamide, NAPA does not slow conduction velocity; hence, it does not alter H-V, A-H, P-R, or QRS, nor does it alter sinus cycle length or sinus node recovery times. It does not appear to depress left ventricular function.

Employing long term ambulatory ECG monitoring, Lee et al. (1976) and Kluger et al. (1980), have shown that NAPA significantly suppressed ventricular ectopic activity in 30–40% of patients. However, early data on its ability to prevent reinduction of significant VT during programmed electrical stimulation have not revealed it to be as effective as procainamide or quinidine. Further evaluation is necessary before its place in present day therapy for cardiac dysrhythmias is known.

Sotalol

This promising β-blocker with class III electrophysiologic properties and apparent lack of left ventricular depression has held promise as an antiarrhythmic for the last 10 years. However, very little clinical data on its effectiveness for dysrhythmias in man have been published to date.

References

Arcidiancono, R. 1978. Use of bretylium tosylate in ventricular fibrillation. Clin Therap 84:253–266.

Bacaner, MB. 1968. Treatment of ventricular fibrillation and other acute arrhythmias with bretylium tosylate. Am J Cardiol 21:430–543.

Bacaner, M.B., and Benditt, D.G. 1982. Antiarrhythmic, antifibrillation and hemodynamic actions of bethanidine sulfate: An orally effective analog of bretylium for suppression of ventricular tachyarrhythmias. Am J Cardiol 50:738–734.

Bernstein, J.G., and Koch-Weser, J. 1972. The effectiveness of bretylium tosylate against ventricular arrhythmias. Circulation 45:1024–1034.

Chatterjee, K., Mandel, W.J., Vyden, J.K., Parmley, W.W., and Forrester, J.S. 1973. Cardiovascular effects of bretylium tosylate in acute myocardial infarction. JAMA 223:757–760.

Cote, P., Bourassa, M.G., Delaye, J., Janin, A., Froment, R., and David, P. 1979. Effects of amiodarone on cardiac and coronary hemodynamics and on myocardial metabolism in patients with coronary artery disease. Circulation 59:1165–1172.

Dhurandhar, R.W., Pickron, J., and Goldman, A.M. 1980. Bretylium tosylate in the management of recurrent ventricular fibrillation complicating acute myocardial infarction. Heart Lung 9(2):256–270.

Gomes, J., Kang, P., Behl, A., Lyons, J., and El-Sherif, N. 1981. Intravenous amiodarone: A potent and effective drug for atrioventricular nodal reentrant paroxysmal tachycardia (abstr). Circulation 64(IV):1215.

Greene, H.L., Werner, J.A., Gross, B.W., Kime, G.M., Trobaugh, G.B., and Cobb, L.A. 1981. Selective prolongation of cardiac refractory times in man by clofilium, a new antiarrhythmic agent (abstr). Circulation 64(IV):137.

Haffajee, C.I., Love, J.C., Canada, A.T., Lesko, L.J., Asdourian, G.K., and Alpert, J.S. 1983a. Clinical pharmacokinetics and efficacy of amiodarone for refractory tachyarrhythmias. Circulation 66:1347–1355.

Haffajee, C.I., Love, J.C., Alpert, J.S., and Sloan, K.C. 1983b. Efficacy and safety of long term amiodarone in the treatment of cardiac arrhythmias. Dosage experience. Am Heart J In Press.

Harris, L., McKenna, W.J., Rowland, E., Holt, D.W., Storey, G.C., and Krikler, D.M. 1983. Side effects of long term amiodarone therapy. Circulation 67:45.

Haynes, R.E., Chin, T.L., Copass, M.K., and Cobb, L.A. 1981. A comparison of bretylium tosylate and lidocaine in management of out of hospital ventricular fibrillation: A randomized clinical trial. Am J Cardiol 48: 353–360.

Heger, J.J., Prystowsky, E.N., Jackman, H.M., Naccarelli, G.V., Warfel, K.A., Rinkenberger, R.L., and Zipes, D.P. 1981. Clinical efficacy and electrophysiology during long term therapy for recurrent ventricular tachycardia or ventricular fibrillation. N Engl J Med 305:539.

Holder, D.A., Sniderman, A.D., Fraser, G., and Fallen, E.L. 1977. Experience with bretylium tosylate by a hospital cardiac arrest team. Circulation 55:541–544.

Horowitz, L.N., Spielman, S.R., Greenspan, A.M., Webb, C.R., and Kay, H.R. 1983. Amiodarone—Ventricular Arrhythmia: Use of Electrophysiologic Studies. Amer Heart J 106:881–886.

Kaski, J.C., Girotti, L.A., Messuti, H., Ruzitzky, B., and Rosenbaum, M.B. 1981. Long term management of sustained, recurrent, symptomatic ventricular tachycardia with amiodarone. Circulation 64:273–279.

Kluger, J., Drayer, D., Reidenberg, M., Ellis, G., Lloyd, V., Tyberg, T., and Hayes, J. 1980. The clinical pharmacology and antiarrhythmic efficacy of N-acetylprocainamide in patients with arrhythmias. Am J Cardiol 45:1250–1257.

Leak, D., and Eydt, J.N. 1979. Control of refractory cardiac arrhythmias with amiodarone. Arch Intern Med 139:425.

Lee, W.K., Strong, J.M., Kehoe, R.F., and Dutcher, J.S. 1976. Antiarrhythmic efficacy of N-acetylprocainamide in patients with premature ventricular contractions. Clin Pharmacol Ther 19:508–514.

Mason, J.W., and Winkle, R.A. 1980. Accuracy of the ventricular induction study for predicting long-term efficacy and inefficacy of antiarrhythmic drugs. N Engl J Med 303: 1023–1077.

Moitey, J. 1980. Amiodarone in the management of supraventricular tachycardias. Proceedings of Symposium on Amiodarone in Cardiac Arrhythmias. p. 19. Royal Society of Medicine. London: Academic Press Ltd.

Nademanee, K., Hendrickson, J., Kannan, R., and Singh, B.N. 1982. Antiarrhythmic efficacy and electrophysiologic actions of amiodarone in patients with life threatening ventricular arrhythmias. Potent suppression of spontaneously occurring tachyarrhythmias vs. inconsistent abolition of induced ventricular tachycardia. Am Heart J 103:950–959.

Peter, T., Hamer, A., Weiss, D., and Mandel, W. 1981. Sudden death survivors: Experience with long-term empiric therapy with amiodarone (abstr). Circulation (IV)36:64.

Podrid, P., and Lown, B. 1981. Amiodarone therapy for symptomatic sustained refractory atrial and ventricular tachyarrhythmias. Am Heart J 101:374.

Puddu, P.E., Jouve, R., and Torresani, J. 1980. Bretylium tosylate: A suitable drug in the prevention of primary ventricular fibrillation. 8th European Congress of Cardiology, Paris. June, 1980.

Rosenbaum, M.B., Chiale, P.A., Halpern, M.S., Nau, G.J., Probylski, J., Levi, R.S., Lazzari, L.O., and Elizari, M.V. 1976. Clinical efficacy of amiodarone as an antiarrhythmic agent. Am J Cardiol 38:934.

Rosenbaum, M.B., Chaile, P.A., Ryba, D., and Elizari, M.V. 1974. Control of tachyarrhythmias associated with Wolff-Parkinson-White Syndrome by amiodarone hydrochloride. Am J Cardiol 34:315.

Schwartz, A., Shen, E., Scheinman, M., Morady, F., and Chatterjee, K. 1983. Hemodynamic effects of intravenous amiodarone in patients with recurrent ventricular tachycardia and depressed left ventricular function (abstr). J Am Cardiol 1(2):646.

Terry, G., Vellani, C.W., Higgins, M.R., and Doig, A. 1970. Bretylium tosylate in treatment of refractory ventricular arrhythmias complicating myocardial infarction. Br Heart J 32:21–25.

Waleffe, A., Bruninx, P., and Kulbertus, H.E. 1978. Effects of amiodarone studied by programmed electrical stimulation of the heart in patients with paroxysmal recurrent supraventricular tachycardia. J Electrocardiol 11:253.

Waxman, L.R., Groh, W.C., Marchilinski, F.E., Buxton, A.E., Sadowski, L.V., Horowitz, L.N., Josephson, M.E., and Kastor, J.A. 1982. Amiodarone for control of sustained ventricular tachyarrhythmias. Clinical and electrophysiologic effects in 51 patients. Am J Cardiol 50:1066–1074.

Wheeler, P.J., Puntz, R., Ingram, D.V., and Chamberlain, D.A. 1979. Amiodarone in the treatment of refractory supraventricular and ventricular arrhythmias. Postgrad Med J 55:1.

Chapter 16

Class III Antiarrhythmic Action and the Q-T Interval

E.M. Vaughan Williams

Many of our currently available antiarrhythmic drugs were originally designed for a different role. Verapamil and amiodarone, for example, were introduced as coronary dilators, at a time when it was thought that coronary dilatation was the treatment of choice for angina pectoris. Mexiletine was first intended to be an antiepileptic drug. Dichloroisoprenaline, the first β-blocker, was developed for its agonist activity on bronchial smooth muscle with the objective of controlling asthma. It would be pleasant to believe that such a detailed knowledge of the electrophysiology of cardiac muscle might be acquired that drugs could be designed to eliminate particular pathologies, but in practice, it has been the discovery of the action of such substances as tetrodotoxin, verapamil, and tetraethylammonium which has helped to elucidate the electrophysiology rather than vice versa.

In attempting to provide an explanation for abnormalities of cardiac rhythm, the electrophysiology of the heart can be approached in two ways. The myocardium can be considered simply as an anatomical network of electrically interconnected cells, through which waves of depolarizing and repolarizing current travel from the sinus node in an orderly and appropriate manner to ensure that different parts of the heart contract at the correct time. Disorders of the waves can be deduced from multiple electrocardiographic records, but these tell us nothing of the nature of the ionic currents flowing into and out of individual cells. In this regard, the heart is looked upon merely as a wiring diagram. The other approach is to identify the sources of current in terms of concentration differences of ions inside and outside the cells, and to study the manner in which individual currents are switched on and off. Such studies ignore the anatomy of the heart, and of the vitally important role of the intercellular contacts, the "gap junctions," the number and distribution of which determine the direction in which the depolarizing wave front will travel.

Ideally, one would like to be able to interpret the mode of action of an antiarrhythmic drug in terms of a selective interference with a particular physiologic process, but this can only be done if the nature of that process is already known. Most of our detailed knowledge of excitable tissues has come from large single cellular elements, such as squid axons or snail neurons. In such preparations, reliable voltage clamp studies can be carried out, and both the intracellular and extracellular fluids can be controlled. Complex tissues like cardiac ventricular muscle cannot be studied in the same way. Consequently, it has been assumed that specific ionic membrane channels in cardiac muscle resemble those studied in simpler cells. Recent voltage clamp studies on single rat ventricular muscle cells (Powell et al., 1980) have confirmed previous conclusions from more complex systems that the sodium-selective, voltage- and time-dependent channels carrying fast inward depolarizing current are very similar to those described by Hodgkin and Huxley in the squid axon. The nature of the repolarizing currents in the heart, however, is much more controversial.

Weidmann's early studies (Weidmann, 1955), confirmed by much of the recent work, showed that the fast inward sodium current channels were inactivated rapidly on depolarization, and that the control voltage ranged from −90 mV, at which all channels were available for activation, to −55 mV, at which all channels were inactivated. Thus, the absolute refractory period for the sodium current was determined by the duration of the action potential to −55 mV. As repolarization proceeds to voltages more negative than this, more and more channels recover from inactivation, and stimulation at successive points on the repolarizing limb of the action potential causes a premature response to have faster and faster rates of depolarization. In Purkinje fibers, recovery from inactivation follows repolarization very rapidly (Weidmann, 1955). In atrial and ventricular muscle, however, recovery from inactivation follows repolarization after a delay, and the latter is increased by class I drugs, which "extend the effective refractory period long after the time at which repolarization was already complete" (Szekeres and Vaughan Williams, 1962).

It was obvious that an alternative way of delaying recovery from inactivation would be to prolong the duration of the action potential itself, and for many years a drug with this property was sought. Quinidine itself, in high doses and at low stimulation frequencies, does cause some delay of repolarization, and it was once considered that this could be the main reason for its antiarrhythmic action (West and Amory, 1960). Nevertheless, it was clear that, although prolongation of action duration (APD) could be a contributory factor, quinidine still had a powerful effect in restricting fast inward current in concentrations and at pacing frequencies at which APD was unchanged (Vaughan Williams, 1958), and that several class I drugs, notably lidocaine and mexiletine, actually shortened APD.

In the ventricular conducting pathway, lidocaine and mexiletine shorten APD to a greater extent in the preterminal Purkinje fibers (in which APD is normally longest) than in the bundle of His or in ventricular muscle, thus reducing disparity of APD. Whether or not this property contributes to the antiarrhythmic efficacy of lidocaine is controversial, and has been fully discussed elsewhere (Vaughan Williams, 1980, 1984).

There is much evidence, including human data obtained with monophasic action potential recordings (Olsson et al., 1971), that shortening of APD is an arrhythmogenic factor, which may, at least in part, explain the high incidence of atrial fibrillation in the hyperthyroid state (Freedberg et al., 1970). Conversely, after thyroidectomy, APD is prolonged, and since cardiac arrhythmias are rare in myxedema, this reinforced the theoretical view that a prolongation of APD, provided that APD was uniform and homogeneous, might constitute a "third class" of antiarrhythmic action (i.e., in addition to the two already established, restriction of fast inward current, and antisympathetic effects). There was, however, no drug available at the time with which the hypothesis could be properly tested. Although quinidine and disopyramide (Sekiya and Vaughan Williams, 1963) caused some delay of repolarization, they were primarily class I agents, and in addition, had undesirable anticholinergic effects.

Amiodarone had already been in use for several years as an antianginal drug before it was subjected to detailed electrophysiologic study with microelectrodes. The finding that it caused a large prolongation of APD, but had only a minor antisympathetic action and a negligible class I effect (Singh and Vaughan Williams, 1970a), suggested that it might be the first "class III" antiarrhythmic drug for which we had been looking. We found that amiodarone was a very effective antiarrhythmic drug in guinea pigs, and Charlier and his colleagues (Charlier et al., 1969) observed an antiarrhythmic effect on dogs. The first cardiologist to use it as an antiarrhythmic in man was Ferrero (Ferrero and Abderhamane, 1972), who had already employed the drug for many years in Switzerland as an antianginal agent. During the next couple of years amiodarone was increasingly used in continental Europe (not in England) and South America in patients with arrhythmias, and it was found by Rosenbaum to be exceptionally useful for the control of preexcitation arrhythmias of the Wolff-Parkinson-White type (Rosenbaum et al., 1974).

In spite of this evidence, there was considerable reluctance among cardiologists to accept a drug which prolonged the Q-T interval, having antiarrhythmic properties. Not only was the familial propensity to fainting fits in children with a long Q-T, described independently by Romano (Romano et al., 1963) and Ward (Ward, 1964), associated with ventricular tachycardia or even fibrillation (precipitated by emotion or exercise), but the phenomenon of "R on T" has long been regarded as a harbinger of impending life-threatening arrhythmias, and a long Q-T interval has been proposed as a predictor of sudden death (Schwartz and Wolf, 1978). The long Q-T syndrome will be discussed again later, but meanwhile something must be said about the mode of action of β-blockers, which have been of value in this condition.

β-Blockers have been in use for nearly 20 years as a treatment for hypertension, yet the mechanism by which blood pressure is lowered has still not been fully explained. Long ago, I become interested in the question why the hypotensive action of β-blockers was often delayed in onset, and why weeks or months of therapy might sometimes be required to achieve an optimum result. The mode of action of a drug is customarily analyzed in acute animal experiments, yet patients are treated with β-blockers for years, often for the rest of their lives. It seemed logical to study their effects in animals which also had been treated for prolonged periods, and 10 years ago, I started a program to investigate the long term effects of a number of β-blocking drugs, with and without the subsidiary properties of cardioselectivity, intrinsic sympathomimetic activity, or local anesthetic action. It was first necessary to establish what dosage regime in the animal we used, the rabbit, would be equivalent to therapeutic levels in man. Fortunately the latter were accurately known for propranolol and a few other β-blockers. Coltart and Shand (1970), for example, found that exercise tachycardia was blocked completely by a propranolol plasma concentration of 100 ng ml^{-1}, but only minor blockade was achieved when the concentration had fallen to 10 ng ml^{-1}. They had also measured the relation between propranolol concentration and blockade of the effects of injected isoprenaline, and we found a good correspondence between rabbits and man for blockade and plasma levels (Vaughan Williams et al., 1975; Raine and Vaughan Williams, 1980a,b). The rabbits were injected for several weeks twice daily sc with 4 mg kg^{-1} propranolol, which we knew would provide clinical levels of blockade for at least two-thirds of each day. The treatment was stopped 24 h before the animals were killed, so that when we did experiments on the heart there was no measurable propranolol present in either the plasma or the myocardium.

There was no difference in responses to isoprenaline of hearts isolated from these animals, in comparison with hearts from saline-treated littermates, indicating the absence both of residual blockade and of any hypersensitivity induced by the treatment. In an untreated rabbit, exposure of myocardium to a concentration of propranolol (100 ng ml^{-1}) equivalent to clinical levels has hardly any effect on the action potential. At higher concentrations (200–500 ng ml^{-1}) action potential duration (APD) is shortened slightly and the maximum rate of depolarization (MRD or $\dot{V}_{max}$) is reduced. We found that long term treatment with β-blockers induced a large prolongation of APD, uniformly observed in both atria and ventricles paced at a constant frequency. Since no drug was present at the time, this represented a secondary adaptation to the treatment. A uniform prolongation of ventricular APD should lengthen the Q-T interval, and we found that we were able to follow the rate of onset of the effect noninvasively by measurement of ECG records (Raine and Vaughan Williams, 1980). The effect was not related to intrinsic sympathomimetic activity (ISA), cardioselectivity, or local anesthetic properties.

Several studies have established that a similar prolongation of Q-T interval, persisting for days after cessation of treatment, is induced by long term β-blockade in man (Edvardson and Olsson, 1981; Vaughan Williams et al., 1980b). These observations can explain both the prevalence of arrhythmias in the long

Q-T syndrome, and the efficacy of therapy with β-blockers or by left stellectomy. It must be emphasized that the Q-T interval on the surface electrocardiogram does not measure action potential duration. Oppositely-oriented late repolarization vectors may cancel each other, so that in some leads the end of the T-wave does not signal the end of repolarization. In particular, the septal and apical repolarization vectors cancel in left-right leads. β-adrenergic stimulation shortens (but α-adrenergic stimulation lengthens) APD and absolute refractory period. In the heart, β-adrenoceptors normally predominate. Thus, high sympathetic activity in the left ventricle could shorten a late repolarization vector which normally balanced a similar late repolarization in the right ventricle, so that a T-wave which had previously been "silent," could become apparent. In the long Q-T syndrome, a paucity of right stellate innervation, causing a reduced heart rate response to exercise, is combined with a compensatory excess of left stellate activity. Reduction of right sympathetic activity, as we have seen, would lengthen right ventricular APD and excess left sympathetic stimulation would shorten left ventricular APD, causing great heterogeneity of ventricular APDs, a highly arrhythmogenic factor. Hence the susceptibility of patients with long Q-T syndrome to ventricular arrhythmias. Treatment by β-blockers or by left stellectomy would reduce the imbalance between left and right sympathetic activity, and left ventricular repolarization would be delayed, thus restoring the mutual cancellation of late repolarization vectors and shortening the Q-T interval on the surface electrocardiogram.

One of the exciting developments of the last few years has been the demonstration that prolonged β-blockade protects a significant proportion of postinfarction patients from reinfarction and sudden death (Vaughan William, 1980). The reason for the protection is unknown, but since a uniform prolongation of APD constitutes an antiarrhythmic (class III) action, this could be a contributory factor in reducing the incidence of sudden death.

One of the β-blockers, sotalol, was shown long ago to delay repolarization on acute administration and to have little class I activity (Singh and Vaughan Williams, 1970b), but it was difficult to extrapolate from animal models of arrhythmias any firm conclusion that the prolongation of APD had contributed an antiarrhythmic action in addition to the class II effect.

Amiodarone has proved outstandingly efficacious in the treatment of arrhythmias of the Wolff-Parkinson-White type (W.P.W.), for which class I drugs like lidocaine are less suitable. It is of interest, therefore, to compare the effects of amiodarone and similar agents with those of lidocaine on the ventricular conduction pathway. It was found that amiodarone and L9146, a nonhalogenated analog of amiodarone with a similar pharmacologic profile, lengthened APD in the bundle of His and ventricular muscle much more than in the preterminal Purkinje fibers or "false tendons" (Vaughan Williams et al., 1977). Indeed, if electrophysiologic studies had been confined to such Purkinje fibers, the class III effect of the drug would have been missed. Thus, both in theory and in practice, prolongation of APD does appear to constitute a true class of antiarrhythmic action. In contrast, lidocaine, which is of little value in W.P.W. has the opposite effect on APD in the ventricular pathway, shortening APD throughout.

It would naturally be of interest to know whether amiodarone, sotalol, disopyramide, melperone, bretylium, and long term β-blockade, all of which prolong ventricular APD, achieve this effect in the same way. One can only speculate in terms of the various mechanisms which have been described as responsible for repolarization in cardiac muscle, which are as follows:

1. Activation of two outward currents, designated I_{x_1} and I_{x_2}, described as controlled in the range +20 to −40 mv in accordance with Hodgkin-Huxley type kinetics by Noble and Tsien (Noble and Tsien, 1969a,b) and carried mainly, but not exclusively, by potassium ions.

2. Calcium-activated outward potassium current described by Isenberg (Isenberg, 1975; Isenberg, 1977).

3. Inactivation of slow inward current by a voltage- and time-dependent mechanism (Giebiksch and Weidmann, 1971). "Normal repolarization of sheep ventricle depends on a time-dependent decrease of inward current (Na, Ca) rather than on a time-dependent increase of outward current (K)." In molluscan neurons, it has been observed that calcium conductance is inactivated by raised intracellular calcium (i.e., by direct negative feedback) (Tillotson, 1979), but whether this mechanism is present in cardiac muscle also is uncertain.

4. Return of potassium conductance by reversal of inward-going rectification. Potassium conductance is reduced in the plateau region, but once repolarization has begun, by whatever mechanism, the nearer E_M approaches to E_K the higher the conductance becomes (i.e., there is positive feedback).

Thus, a drug which delays repolarization could act in a variety of ways, since there are so many suggested mechanisms from which to choose. Repolarization could be delayed by an increase in slow inward current, or by a delay of its inactivation; by an interference with channels carrying outward current, normally activated either by a voltage- and time-dependent mechanism or by raised intracellular calcium concentration; also by a restriction of the reversal of inward rectification. Delayed repolarization could even be due to interference with the sodium-calcium exchange mechanism, since it is now believed that this exchange is electrogenic. The plateau may be maintained not only by slow inward current and inward-going rectification, but also by a net inward current provided by the entry of four sodium ions in exchange for a single calcium ion travelling outward (Mullins, 1979; Mullins, 1981).

The "pacemaker potential," i_{k2}, originally said to be a pure outward potassium current activated by depolarization in the range −90 to −55 mv, appears to have been an artifact (DiFrancesco and Noble, 1981). Long-lasting clamp pulses in complex tissues such as cardiac muscle alter the ionic concentrations in the intercellular clefts. What may appear to be a voltage- and time-dependent conductance change could be secondary to a shift of E_K, and it seems possible that I_{x_2}, for example, may have been as artifactual as i_{k2}. Thus, it is not possible to determine the selectivity of drug actions on individual ion channels concerned in the delay of repolarization until valid methods are available for measuring the normal mechanism of repolarization itself.

Meanwhile, returning to consideration of the heart as an electrical network, it is reasonable to conclude that a homogeneous delay of repolarization, however produced, constitutes a distinct class of antiarrhythmic action. New support for this view has recently been provided by evidence that sotalol has a greater antiarrhythmic effect than can be attributed to its β-blocking action alone (Nathan et al., 1982; Bennett, 1982). Bretylium, which prolongs ventricular (Wit et al., 1970), but not atrial, APD, and which has no class I activity (Papp and Vaughan Williams, 1969) can sometimes have dramatic antiarrhythmic effects on ventricular muscle. Another long-established drug which prolongs APD in both atrial and ventricular muscle (Millar and Vaughan Williams, 1982) is the tranquilizer, melperone, but whether it could be useful as an antiarrhythmic drug in man remains to be established, although there are already some promising reports (Mogelvang, et al., 1980). The possible efficacy or danger of combining drugs delaying repolarization with other classes of antiarrhythmic action opens a new field of exploration.

References

Bennett, D.H. 1982. Acute prolongation of myocardial refractoriness by sotalol. Br Heart J 47:521–526.

Charlier, R., Delaunois, G., Bauthier, J., and Deltour, G. 1969. Dans la serie des benzofurannes. XL. Proprieties antiarrhythmiques de l'amiodarone. Cardiologia 54:83–90.

Coltart, D.J., and Shand, D.G. 1970. Plasma propranolol levels in the quantitative assessment of beta-adrenergic blockade in man. Br Med J 3:731–734.

DiFrancesco, D., and Noble, D. 1981. Implications of the re-interpretation of iK_2 for the modelling of the electrical activity of pacemaker tissues in the heart. In: L.N. Bouman and H.J. Jongsma, eds. pp. 95–128. Cardiac Rate and Rhythm. The Hague: Martinus Nijhoff.

Edvardsson, N., and Olsson, S.B. 1981. Effects of acute and chronic beta-receptor blockade on ventricular repolarization in man. Br Heart J 45:628–636.

Ferrero, C., and Ben Abderhamane, M. 1972. Terapia medica del flutter atriale. G Ital Cardiol 2:186.

Freedberg, A.S., Papp, J.Gy., and Vaughan Williams, E.M. 1970. The effect of altered thyroid state on atrial intracellular potentials. J Physiol 207:357–370.

Giebiksch, G., and Weidmann, S. 1971. Membrane currents in mammalian ventricular heart muscle fibers using a voltage clamp technique. J Gen Physiol 57:290–296.

Isenberg, G. 1975. Is potassium conductance of cardiac Purkinje fibres controlled by $[Ca^{2+}]_i$? Nature (Lond) 253:273–274.

Isenberg, G. 1977. Cardiac Purkinje fibres: $[Ca^{2+}]_i$ controls steady state potassium conductance. Pflügers Arch 371:71–76.

Millar, J.S. and Vaughan Williams, E.M. 1982. Differential actions on rabbit nodal, atrial, Purkinje cell and ventricular potentials of melperone, a bradycardic agent delaying repolarization: Effect of hypoxia. Br J Pharmacol 75:109–121.

Mogelvang, J.C., Petersen, E.N., Folke, P.E., and Ovesen, L. 1980. Antiarrhythmic properties of a neuroleptic butyrophenone, melperone, in acute myocardial infarction. Acta Med Scand 208:61–64.

Mullins, L.J. 1979. The generation of electric currents in cardiac fibers by Na/Ca exchange. Am J. Physiol 236:C103–C110.

Mullins, L.J. 1981. Ion Transport in Heart. New York: Raven Press.

Nathan, A.W., Hellestrand, K.J., Bexton, R.S., Ward, D.E., Spurrell, R.A.J., and Camm, A.J. 1982. Electrophysiological effects of sotalol—just another beta-blocker? Br Heart J 47:515–520.

Noble, D., and Tsien, R.W. 1969a. Outward membrane currents activated in the plateau range of potentials in cardiac Purkinje fibres. J Physiol 200:205–232.

Noble, D., and Tsien, R.W. 1969b. Reconstruction of the repolarization process in cardiac Purkinje fibres based on voltage clamp measurements of membrane currents. J Physiol 200:233–254.

Olsson, S.B., Cotoi, S., and Varnauskas, E. 1971. Monophasic action potential and sinus rhythm stability after conversion of atrial fibrillation. Acta Med Scand 190:381–388.

Papp, J.Gy., and Vaughan Williams, E.M. 1969. The effect of bretylium on intracellular cardiac action potentials in relation to its antiarrhythmic and local anesthetic activity. Br J Pharmacol 37:380–390.

Powell, T., Terrar, D.A., and Twist, V.W. 1980. Electrical properties of individual cells isolated from rat ventricular myocardium. J Physiol 302:131–154.

Raine, A.E.G., and Vaughan Williams, E.M. 1980a. Adaptational responses to prolonged beta-adrenoceptor blockade in adult rabbit. Br J Pharmacol 70:205–218.

Raine, A.E.G., and Vaughan Williams, E.M. 1980b. Adaptation to prolonged beta-blockade of rabbit atrial, Purkinje and ventricular potentials, and of papillary muscle contraction. Time-course of development of, and recovery from, adaptation. Circ Res 48:628–636.

Romano, C., Gemme, G., and Pongiglione, R. 1963. Aritmie cardiache rare dell'eta' pediatrica. Clin Pediat 45:656.

Rosenbaum, M.B., Chiale, P.A., Ryba, D., and Elizari, M.W. 1974. Control of tachyarrhythmia associated with Wolff-Parkinson-White syndrome by amiodarone hydrochloride. Am J Cardiol 34:215–223.

Schwartz, P.J., and Wolf, S. 1978. QT Interval prolongation as predictor of sudden death in patients with myocardial infarction. Circulation 42:1074–1077.

Sekiya, A., and Vaughan Williams, E.M. 1963. The effects of pronethalol, dichloroisoprenaline and disopyramide on the toxicity to the heart of ouabain and anesthetics. Br J Pharmacol 21:462–472.

Singh, B.N., and Vaughan Williams, E.M. 1970a. The effect of amiodarone, a new antianginal drug, on cardiac muscle. Br J Pharmacol 39:657–668.

Singh, B.N., and Vaughan Williams, E.M. 1970b. A third class of antiarrhythmic action. Effects on atrial and ventricular intracellular potentials, and other pharmacological actions on cardiac muscle, of MJ1999 and AH3474. Br J Pharmacol 39:675–687.

Szekeres, L., and Vaughan Williams, E.M. 1962. Antifibrillatory action. J Physiol (Lond) 160:470–482.

Tillotson, D. 1979. Inactivation of Ca conductance dependent on entry of Ca ions in molluscan neurons. Proc Natl Acad Sci USA 76: 1497–1500.

Vaughan Williams, E.M. 1958. The mode of action of quinidine on isolated rabbit atria interpreted from intracellular records. Br J Pharmacol 13:276–287.

Vaughan Williams, E.M. 1980. Antiarrhythmic Action. London: Academic Press.

Vaughan Williams, E.M. 1984. Classification of antiarrhythmic actions, reviewed after a decade. In: H.J. Reiser and L.N. Horowitz, eds. Mechanisms and Treatment of Cardiac Arrhythmias: Relevance of Basic Studies to Clinical Management. Baltimore: Urban and Schwarzenberg.

Vaughan Williams, E.M. Hassan M.O., Floras, J.S., Sleight, P., and Jones, J.V. 1980. Adaptation of hypertensives to treatment with cardio-selective and non-selective beta-blockers. Absence of correlation between bradycardia and blood-pressure control, and reduction in slope of the QT/RR relation. Br Heart J 44:473–487.

Vaughan Williams, E.M., Raine, A.E.G., Cabrera, A.A., and Whyte, J.M. 1975. The effects of prolonged beta-adrenoceptor blockade on heart weight and cardiac intracellular potentials. Cardiovasc Res 9:579–592.

Vaughan Williams, E.M., Salako, L., and Wittig, J.H. 1977. The effect on atrial and ventricular intracellular potentials, and other pharmacological actions of L9146, a non-halogenated benzo(b)thiophen related to amiodarone. Cardiovasc Res 11:187–197.

Ward, O.C. 1964. A new familial cardiac syndrome in children. J Ir Med Assoc 54:103–106.

Weidmann, S. 1955. The effect of the cardiac membrane potential on the rapid availability of the sodium-carrying system. J Physiol 127:213–224.

West, T.C., and Amory, D.W. 1960. Single fiber recording of the effects of quinidine at atrial and pacemaker sites in the isolated right atrium of the rabbit. J Pharmacol Exp Ther 130:183–193.

Wit, A.L., Steiner, C., and Damato, A.M. 1970. Electrophysiological effects of bretylium tosylate on single fibers of the canine specialized conduction system and ventricle. J Pharmacol Exp Ther 173:344–356.

Antiarrhythmic Effects of Agents which Selectively Prolong Action Potential Duration (Class III)

Steinberg and Michelson have provided convincing data which shows that a relationship exists between molecular structure and class III antiarrhythmic properties. These data are provocative in suggesting that an organized search for antiarrhythmic drugs with class III activity can be pursued. The antiarrhythmic properties of the presently available class III agents, however, show relatively little structural similarities, providing no obvious explanation for their similarity of electrophysiologic effects. In part the reason for this discrepancy lies in the fact that class III agents were not designed chemically as such, but rather have evolved into this category by their retrospectively discovered class III action. A pertinent example is amiodarone, originally a vasodilator agent.

While the concept of clinical usefulness of the class III agents is unquestioned, to date no agent is a true representative of this drug classification. Each drug designated as a class III type agent has either significant toxicities, additional effects representative of other classifications, or problematic pharmacokinetic parameters (e.g., duration of action or ease of administration). For example, bretylium, often considered the original class III agent, is also a potent adrenergic blocking agent, while melperone, a "newly discovered" class III agent, is also an alpha-antagonist that may produce reflex sympathetic stimulation. Similarily, the more obvious class III agent sotalol has, in addition, beta-receptor-blocking effects. As Dr. Haffajee's chapter emphasized, the greatest experience with a class III agent has been with amiodarone; however, it also has a multitude of cardiovascular effects in addition to its class III antiarrhythmic property. Only clofilium may represent the first, prospectively developed class III agent. However, based upon the overall clinical experience with class III type agents, there appears to be a strong suggestion that this class of agents would be effective in most life-threatening arrhythmias primarily due to reentry. Additional agents with more specific properties exemplified by the class III concept would thus provide an effective therapeutic addition and improvement to the existing antiarrhythmic drug regimen.

Upon considering the mechanism of action of class III antiarrhythmic drugs, some obvious yet confusing considerations become apparent. On one hand it would seem apparent that prolongation of refractoriness prevents the manifestations of reentry, which is the primary mechanism thought to underlie most recurrent, clinical tachyarrhythmias. Since prolongation of action potential duration, a hallmark of the class III type drug, would result in prolongation of refractoriness (presumably the mechanism underlying the antiarrhythmic effect), then one would also expect that prolongation of refractoriness by other drugs should also confer similar antiarrhythmic efficacy. However, a comparison of drugs that increase refractoriness will show that class III agents have much greater efficacy than such class I agents. Furthermore, agents that have virtually no effect on refractoriness may show similar potency to amiodarone in preventing certain arrhythmias thought to result from reentry. This apparent dichotomy no doubt reflects the great complexity of the pathophysiologic system and the diverse effects of drugs; such questions must be seriously considered in analyzing drug effects in the setting of reentry, using refractoriness as a barometer. One additional consideration that has not been fully explored for class III agents relates to their effect on nonventricular arrhythmias. For example, agents that prolong refractoriness, such as the class III agents, should also show significant efficacy against certain atrial arrhythmias. Similarly, arrhythmias originating in the A-V nodal area and related to bypass tracts often are reentrant arrhythmias and also need to be closely evaluated in this regard.

The chapter by Dr. Vaughan Williams on the concept of class III antiarrhythmic action and the Q-T interval addresses a very critical and yet timely topic concerning the potential limitations of class III agents in the clinical setting: the seemingly entrenched reluctance among many cardiologists to accept that a drug that prolongs the Q-T interval could also be an antiarrhythmic agent. While this bias can be appreciated, in part, due to the well described congenital Q-T syndrome as well as the acquired Q-T prolongation in the setting of ischemia, the assumption that such biases carry over to Q-T prolongation in general and to the class III concept in particular, may indeed be false. As Dr. Vaughan Williams points out, one must consider several important facts to fully appreciate that drug-induced prolongation of the Q-T interval may not necessarily be an arrhythmogenic factor. First, it must be emphasized again that the Q-T interval on the surface electrocardiogram does not measure action potential duration per se. Second, the Q-T interval is strongly affected by the balance of right and left stellate sympathetic activity. Thirdly, the Q-T interval incorporates the QRS interval and therefore Q-T prolongation may occur if a drug prolongs QRS duration alone (a more accurate measurement of ventricular repolarization is the J-T interval). An additional point relates to the degree of homogeneity of refractoriness that is imposed upon the atria and ventricles and the various membrane effects inherent in a drug that delays repolarizations. Thus, when considering the concept of Q-T prolongation in relation to a class III antiarrhythmic drug action, one must first separate the congenital and pathophysiologic aspects regarding the Q-T interval. Second, one must appreciate the concept of uniformity and homogenous prolongation of repolarization throughout the myocardium as induced by a drug versus the inhomogeneity of refractoriness associated with ischemia. One must also ask the question of how much Q-T prolongation is therapeutic since, invariably, extreme prolongation of the Q-T interval is likely to be arrhythmogenic. Lastly, much needs to be learned about drug combinations, including class III types of drugs, if any, are desirable or potentially detrimental in the patient with life-threatening arrhythmias.

D. Antiarrhythmic Effects of Calcium Channel-Blocking Drugs (Class IV)

Chapter 17

Cellular Mechanisms of Action of Calcium Channel Antagonists

Frank J. Green and August M. Watanabe

Introduction

The organic calcium antagonist drugs are a group of compounds which are useful as experimental probes in the laboratory and as therapeutic agents in the treatment of a variety of cardiovascular diseases (Henry, 1980). Several recent reviews detail the historical development, structure-activity relationships, vascular effects, and comparative pharmacology of these drugs and related calmodulin antagonists (Triggle, 1981; Fleckenstein, 1977, 1981; Janis and Triggle, 1983; Janis and Scriabine, 1983; Henry, 1982, 1983). The focus of this brief review will be on the mechanisms of action of calcium channel antagonists in the myocardial cell. The term "calcium antagonist" encompasses a large group of compounds with actions vastly different from those originally described by Fleckenstein (Henry, 1980; Nayler, 1983). We will confine our attention to the phenylalkylamines, verapamil and D_{600}; the dihydropyridines, including nifedipine, nimodipine, nisoldipine, and nicardipine; and the benzothiazepine derivative, diltiazem. These are the most powerful and selective calcium channel antagonists, because they inhibit calcium-dependent myocardial contraction by 90% or more before the fast sodium influx is affected (Fleckenstein, 1981). We will begin with a brief review of the properties of calcium channels. Against this background, we will then review the putative mechanisms by which organic calcium channel antagonists alter the function of calcium channels.

The Calcium Channel

The myocardial voltage-dependent calcium channel has attracted considerable attention for the past two decades since the existence of a slow inward current, in addition to the fast sodium current, was first suspected (Coraboeuf and Otsuka, 1956; Cranefield, 1975; Reuter, 1979; McDonald, 1982). Several recent reviews have summarized our current understanding of the calcium channel (Reuter,

1983; Hagiwara and Byerly, 1981; Tsien, 1983). Rises in intracellular calcium effect coupling of excitation of the myocardial membrane to activation of the contractile apparatus. At rest, intracellular calcium concentration, $[Ca^{2+}]_i$, is on the order of 0.05–0.5 μM and rises 1–2 orders of magnitude with depolarization of the cell membrane. It is likely that influx of calcium from outside the cell may not account for the entire amount of calcium necessary to raise intracellular calcium to this level, and a role for calcium-induced release of calcium from sarcoplasmic reticulum has been proposed in cardiac muscle (Fabiato, 1983). The channel is controlled by voltage-dependent gating and is more selective for calcium than is the sodium channel for sodium, although in calcium-depleted conditions sodium also participates in the slow inward current. With depolarization of the membrane, the channel is activated at membrane potentials in the range of −40 to +10 mv, at which inactivation of the sodium channel has already occurred. Inactivation is also voltage-dependent, but occurs more slowly than in the sodium channel (Reuter, 1983). Voltage clamp studies of membrane patches in isolated cells have measured single calcium channel current (Hamill et al., 1981). It is apparent that the calcium channel exists in either an open or closed state and admits a current of uniform amplitude. In response to depolarization of the membrane the probability that an individual channel will open increases (Reuter et al., 1982).

Calcium channel function can be modulated by β-adrenergic agonists, which increase the slow inward current (Reuter, 1967). Single calcium channel studies have shown that in response to isoprenaline, a β-agonist, single channel current amplitude does not change, but the mean duration of channel opening and the frequency of opening increase (Reuter et al., 1982). This increase in calcium influx is mediated by a sequence of intracellular reactions which occur in response to β-adrenergic stimulation. Binding of a β-adrenergic agonist to its receptor on the sarcolemmal membrane activates adenylate cyclase, which catalyzes the formation of adenosine 3′,5′-monophosphate (or cyclic AMP) from ATP. Cyclic AMP, in turn, activates protein kinase by binding with the regulatory subunit of the kinase and this binding leads to release of the catalytic subunit. The free catalytic subunit then leads to phosphorylation of certain proteins, and thereby alteration in the properties of the protein. Evidence for this scheme comes from several different types of studies, including the observation that cyclic AMP itself increases calcium influx. Experimental injection of cyclic AMP into Purkinje fibers mimicked the effects of epinephrine on the action potential (Tsien, 1973). 8-Bromocyclic AMP, a cyclic AMP analog which penetrates cardiac myocytes, also causes an increase in calcium influx (Cachelin et al., 1982). Similarly, injection of catalytic subunit of protein kinase into guinea pig myocytes caused an increase in slow inward current (Osterrieder et al., 1982).

Cyclic AMP-dependent protein kinase has been shown to phosphorylate a number of membrane proteins in vitro (Stull and Mayer, 1979; Wollenberger and Will, 1978; Wray et al., 1973; Jones et al., 1979, 1980; Manalan and Jones,

1982). Studies with intact ventricles provide evidence for phosphorylation of some of these same proteins in response to β-adrenergic stimulation in functioning myocardium (Lindemann et al., 1983). Reuter and Scholz (1977) postulated that catecholamines increased the availability of functional calcium channels through phosphorylation of a site in the channel. This hypothesis has gained wide currency but has not been proven conclusively. Also at issue is the question of whether β-adrenergic stimulation changes the kinetics of individual calcium channels or increases their number. Cachelin et al. (1983) noted an increase in the forward rate constant leading to channel opening. Bean et al. (1984) have presented evidence that isoprenaline increases the number of channels per cell in frog ventricular myocytes and that it slows the time course of activation and inactivation. Thus, it appears that both kinetics of calcium channel function and channel number change in response to β-adrenergic stimulation.

Physiologic Effects of Calcium Channel Antagonists

The mechanism of action of calcium channel antagonist drugs was studied systematically first by Fleckenstein et al. (1967), who likened the effects of verapamil and prenylamine on myocardial contractility to that of calcium withdrawal. In the presence of calcium antagonists, the upstroke and overshoot of the cardiac action potential were unchanged, the action potential plateau slightly abbreviated, and contraction inhibited (Fleckenstein, 1977). This permitted the conclusion that these agents uncoupled excitation and contraction. Numerous subsequent studies have extensively explored the effects of calcium antagonists on the action potential of the myocardial cell. In cells with a fast sodium current such as muscle cells and Purkinje fibers, verapamil, D_{600}, diltiazem, and the dihydropyridines lower the plateau of the action potential and usually shorten its duration (Fleckenstein, 1977; Saikawa et al., 1977; Kohlhardt and Fleckenstein, 1977; Dangman and Hoffman, 1980) without affecting upstroke velocity or overshoot. Occasionally, the action potential duration is prolonged (Cranefield et al., 1974). In sinoatrial and atrioventricular nodal cells, whose action potentials are dependent solely on the slow inward current, nifedipine, verapamil, diltiazem, and D_{600} decrease the rate of impulse formation, increase membrane threshold potential, decrease the amplitude, rate of rise and overshoot of the action potential, and prolong the effective and functional refractory periods (Wit and Cranefield, 1975; Henry, 1982; Kawai et al., 1981; Kohlhardt and Haap, 1981; Zipes and Fischer, 1974).

Calcium-dependent action potentials may be produced in cells which normally have a fast sodium current. If one inactivates the sodium channel by depolarizing the cell with voltage clamping or increasing extracellular potassium, or by treating the cell with tetrodotoxin, the cells become inexcitable. If the cells are stimulated in the presence of elevated extracellular calcium or catecholamines, one produces action potentials which are dependent upon the influx of calcium (Pappano, 1970). These are also known as slow responses, and they are likewise sensitive to calcium antagonists. In preparations exhibiting this slow response, verapamil, D_{600}, and dihydropyridines suppress automaticity, decrease amplitude, upstroke velocity, and action potential duration, and shift the threshold potential for depolarization toward zero (Cranefield et al., 1974; Dangman and Hoffman, 1980; Tung and Morad, 1983; Kohlhardt and Mnich, 1978; Tritthart et al., 1973).

It has been noted that the S(−) enantiomers of verapamil and D_{600} are more potent than the R(+) enantiomers (Bayer et al., 1975c). The implications of this stereoselectivity for binding sites will be described subsequently. In addition, verapamil and D_{600} are well recognized to exhibit frequency or use dependence. Their effects upon the slow response are not evident at slow pacing rates (less than 6/min) but become marked at faster pacing rates (Bayer et al., 1975c; Ehara and Kaufmann, 1978). Dihydropyridines are generally recognized not to exhibit use-dependence; however, Kohlhardt and Haap (1981) noted that the reduction of upstroke velocity produced by nifedipine in rabbit atrioventricular nodal cells was enhanced by repetitive stimulation.

Voltage clamp studies of myocardial tissue have confirmed impressions from studies of the action potential that all of the organic calcium antagonists block the slow inward current (Kohlhardt et al., 1972; Kohlhardt and Fleckenstein, 1977; Kass and Tsien, 1975; Kass, 1982; Tung and Morad, 1983). D_{600}, verapamil, and diltiazem, but not the dihydropyridines, exhibit voltage- and frequency-dependent effects on the slow inward current, such that their effects are more pronounced at less negative holding potentials and increasing rates of stimulation (Ehara and Kaufmann, 1978; Scheuer and Kass, 1982; McDonald et al., 1980; Tung and Morad, 1983). Kanaya et al. (1983) have reported that prolonged single clamp steps also enhance blockade with diltiazem and verapamil. Both verapamil and D_{600} slow the activation and the recovery of the slow inward current (Ehara and Kaufmann, 1978; Nawrath et al., 1977; Henry, 1980), while nifedipine does not (Kohlhardt and Fleckenstein, 1977). This observation may explain the use and voltage-dependent effects of verapamil and D_{600}. In addition D_{600}, diltiazem, nifedipine, and nisoldipine have been noted to decrease the transient outward current. The delayed outward current, I_x, is suppressed by D_{600} and verapamil, not affected by nisoldipine, and accentuated by diltiazem and nifedipine (Tung and Morad, 1982; Kass and Tsien, 1975; Kass, 1982; Henry, 1983).

As a function of concentration, all of the organic calcium antagonists depress contractility of myocardial tissue (Bayer et al., 1975a,b; Fleckenstein, 1977; Kohlhardt and Fleckenstein, 1977; Saikawa, 1977; Tung and Morad, 1983). In response to increasing frequency of stimulation, D_{600}, verapamil and diltiazem depress myocardial contractility to a greater extent, another example of use dependence. This creates an inverse force-frequency relationship which has been referred to as a negative staircase (McCans et al., 1974; Bayer et al., 1975a,b). As in the electrophysiologic effects, the negative inotropic activity resides in the negative isomers of D_{600} and verapamil (Bayer et al., 1975b; Tung and Morad, 1983). Nifedipine reduces the development of tension by the same percentage at each frequency (Bayer et al., 1977; Henry, 1982). Tung and Morad (1983) recently pointed out that D_{600} and diltiazem, but not nisoldipine, each exhibit partial release of this inhibition if the muscle is permitted to rest or is hyperpolarized. Similarly, Linden and Brooker (1980) have shown that verapamil exhibits greater inhibition of developed tension in partially depolarized atria. Thus, the negative inotropic effect of these drugs is voltage-dependent as well. In mammalian myocardium, inhibition of the slow inward current correlates quantitatively with the inhibition of developed tension (Nawrath et al., 1977; Kohlhardt and Fleckenstein, 1977; Fleckenstein, 1981). Because of this, it has been contended that the negative inotropic effect of these drugs is accounted for by the reduction in slow inward current. In frog myocardium treated with diltiazem, however, Morad et al. (1982) have found no quantitative correlation between inhibition of developed tension and slow inward current. Moreover, in some studies the effects of D_{600}, diltiazem, and verapamil on the contractile responses have been noted to be only partially reversible (Ludwig and Nawrath, 1977; McCans et al., 1974; Morad et al., 1982), while the action potential can be restored with washout of the drug.

Several metabolic changes occur in cells in response to the decrease in the slow inward current and reduced tension development. Utilization of high energy phosphate and extra oxygen consumption by the contractile system is reduced to basal levels (Fleckenstein, 1964, 1977). Nayler and Szeto (1972) noted low myocardial oxygen demand in the presence of calcium antagonists. In a variety of experimental models of heart disease, calcium channel antagonists have been observed to have protective effects thought to result from attenuation of the terminal event of calcium overload (Fleckenstein, 1977; Nayler et al., 1976; Henry, 1982).

Effect of Calcium Channel Antagonists on the β-Adrenergic Receptor-Adenylate Cyclase System

Fleckenstein originally recognized that all of the effects of the calcium antagonists resembled those of calcium withdrawal and β-blockade (Fleckenstein et al., 1967; Fleckenstein, 1977). In mammalian heart muscle, verapamil and propranolol are similar in decreasing heart rate, rate and extent of developed tension, and myocardial oxygen demand, as well as increasing the efficiency of contraction (Nayler and Szeto, 1972). It is well recognized that an increase in extracellular calcium concentration or administration of isoproterenol can reverse, at least partially, the effects of calcium antagonists (Fleckenstein, 1977, 1981; Henry, 1983; Kohlhardt and Mnich, 1978; Tritthart et al., 1973). Investigations in our laboratory have examined the possible relationships between the effects of β-blockers and calcium channel antagonists. One preparation we used to study this relationship in intact functioning muscle was the slow response model (see above for general discussion of this model).

Isolated guinea pig hearts were perfused by the Langendorff technique. They were rendered inexcitable by perfusion with 22 mM K^+, which depolarized the hearts to approximately −40 mV as determined by microelectrode study of ventricular muscle strips. Alternatively, tetrodotoxin (TTX) was used to block sodium channels while maintaining a normal resting membrane potential. With these perturbations the hearts were inexcitable even with pacing impulses of 15 v. A slow response action potential and contractions were restored to these depolarized or TTX-inactivated hearts with the addition of isoproterenol ($2–10 \times 10^{-9}$M), or dibutyryl cyclic AMP (3 mM), or increasing extracellular calcium concentrations to 11.5–20 mM. In the presence of isoproterenol, halving extracellular calcium concentration produced approximately a 50% reduction in developed tension, and this reversed with restoration of normal extracellular calcium concentration. These observations supported the hypothesis that these were calcium-dependent responses. The amount of steady-state tension developed rose as a function of the concentration of isoproterenol (Fig. 17-1). Propranolol, 0.3

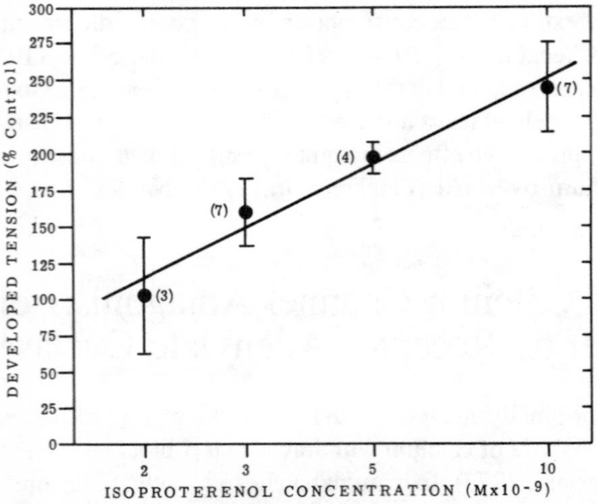

17-1 Developed tension in restored hearts (expressed as a per cent of control) as a function of isoproterenol concentration. Values are means ± SE. Number of hearts studied is given in parentheses. (Reprinted with permission from Watanabe, A.M., and Besch, H.R. 1974. Circ Res 35:316–323.)

μM, reduced the developed tension in response to isoproterenol, but did not inhibit the response to extracellular calcium (Table 17-1). D_{600} and verapamil, however, abolished the response both to isoproterenol and to calcium (Table 17-1). Glucagon and ouabain did not restore excitability or tension.

Identically treated hearts were assayed for tissue cyclic AMP. As a function of concentration, each restoring drug, but not calcium, elevated tissue cyclic AMP levels. Neither ouabain nor glucagon affected tissue cyclic AMP levels (Fig. 17-2). The time course of cyclic AMP generation was examined and is depicted in

Table 17-1 Developed Tension of Hearts Restored with Isoproterenol or Ca^{2+} Alone and in the Presence of Propranolol or D_{600}. (Reprinted with permission from Watanabe, A.M., and Besch, H.R. 1974. Circ Res 35:316–323.)

	Iso (10 nM)	Iso (10 nM) + Prop (0.3 μM)	Iso (10 nM) + D_{600} (1μM)	Ca^{2+} (22 nM)	Ca^{2+} (22 mM) + Prop (0.3 μM)	Ca^{2+} (22 mM) + D_{600} (1 μM)
Tension (% control)	247 ± 27	53 ± 9*	66 ± 15*	213 ± 27	208 ± 13	2 ± 2†
N	7	6	7	3	3	3

Iso, isoproterenol; Prop, propranolol.
*$p < 0.001$ compared with isoproterenol alone.
†$p < 0.01$ compared with Ca^{2+} alone.

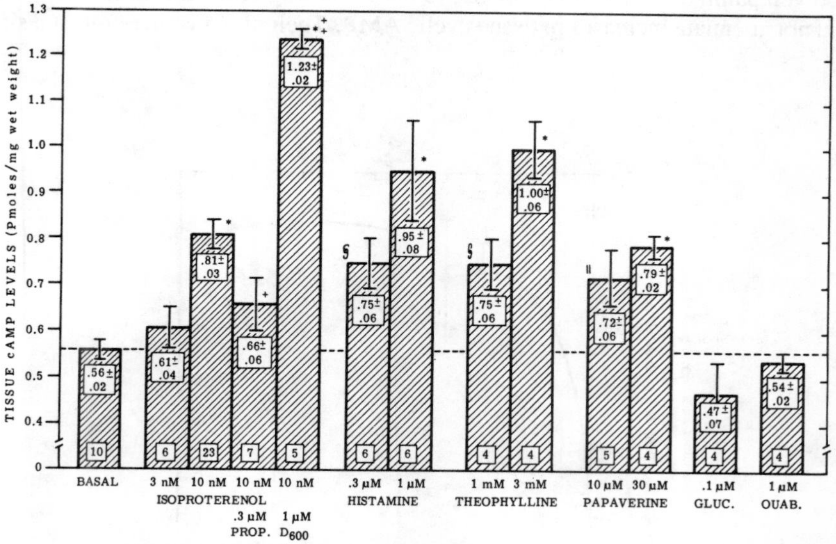

17-2 Tissue cyclic AMP levels in K^+-depolarized hearts after treatment with inotropic agents used to restore excitability and contractions to the hearts. Hearts which were restored were frozen after they reached a steady-state level of contraction. Values are means ± SE. The number of hearts studied is given at the bottom of each bar. PROP = propranolol; GLUC = glucagon; OUAB = ouabain; * $p < 0.0005$ compared with basal; + $p < 0.01$ compared with isoproterenol alone; ‡ $p < 0.0005$ compared with isoproterenol alone; § $p < 0.0025$ compared with basal; ‖ $p < 0.005$ compared with basal. (Reprinted with permission from Watanabe, A.M., and Besch, H.R. 1974. Circ Res 35:316–323.)

Figure 17-3. As early as 45 s after isoproterenol was introduced into the perfusion, cyclic AMP levels were elevated significantly. By 90 s, when contractions began in response to isoproterenol, cyclic AMP levels were approaching their maximum value. The correlation between steady-state-developed tension and tissue cyclic AMP levels was examined, and it is depicted in Figure 17-4. There was a significant correlation ($r = 0.67$, $p < 0.01$) between steady-state-developed tension and the log of tissue cyclic AMP levels.

As depicted in Figure 17-2, cyclic AMP generation in response to isoproterenol, 10 nM, was attenuated by propranolol, 0.3 μM. Propranolol did not attenuate increases in cyclic AMP in response to theophylline and papaverine (not shown). D_{600}, 1 μM, did not attenuate, and in fact, appeared to potentiate cyclic AMP generation.

Thus, restoration of excitability and developed tension in these hearts in which fast sodium channels were inactivated or blocked was related to extracellular calcium concentration and to the generation of intracellular cyclic AMP. Propranolol antagonized the tension response to restoring drugs and attenuated increases in tissue cyclic AMP, but did not alter the response to increased extracellular calcium. This suggests that propranolol's effect was mediated at the β-receptor. D_{600} and verapamil abolished the response to both restoring drugs and to calcium, but did not attenuate increases in tissue cyclic AMP. Their effect is therefore at a site

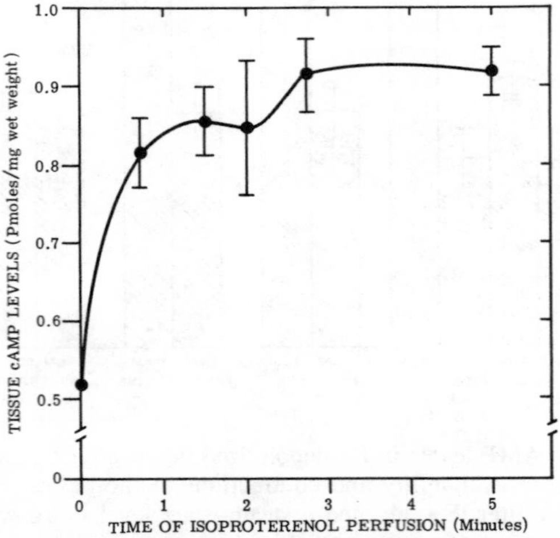

17-3 Time course of tissue cyclic AMP elevation in hearts depolarized with 22 mM K^+ and restored with 1×10^{-8} M isoproterenol. Values are means ± SE for three hearts. (Reprinted with permission from Watanabe, A.M., and Besch, H.R. 1974. Circ Res 35:316–323.)

other than and "distal" to the β-receptor, and a series relationship between increases in cyclic AMP and increases in calcium influx is suggested (Watanabe and Besch, 1974a). This is in agreement with previously described studies documenting the ability of cyclic AMP and its analogs, as well as the catalytic subunit of protein kinase, to increase the slow inward current. In Figure 17-5B, we have summarized the sequence of reactions which we believe occurs in response to β-adrenergic stimulation of the cell. It appears that increases in cyclic AMP and subsequent activation of the catalytic subunit of protein kinase cause an increase in calcium influx. The working hypothesis is that phosphorylation of the calcium channel by protein kinase is the mechanism by which β-adrenergic drugs increase calcium influx (Reuter and Scholz, 1977). This scheme accounts for the observed inhibition of restored contractions by D_{600}, even though increases in cyclic AMP still occur in response to β-adrenergic stimulations. D_{600} blocked the effects of β-agonists at a step "distal" to the β-receptor.

Subsequent in vitro experiments demonstrated that propranolol, but not D_{600}, antagonized epinephrine-induced activation of adenylate cyclase in isolated membrane fractions consistent with the results in intact tissue. In addition, calcium binding by sarcoplasmic reticulum vesicles was examined. Propranolol, 100 and 300 μM, reduced calcium binding by 9 and 18%, respectively. D_{600}, 10 and 100 μM, reduced calcium binding by 11 and 15%, respectively. These

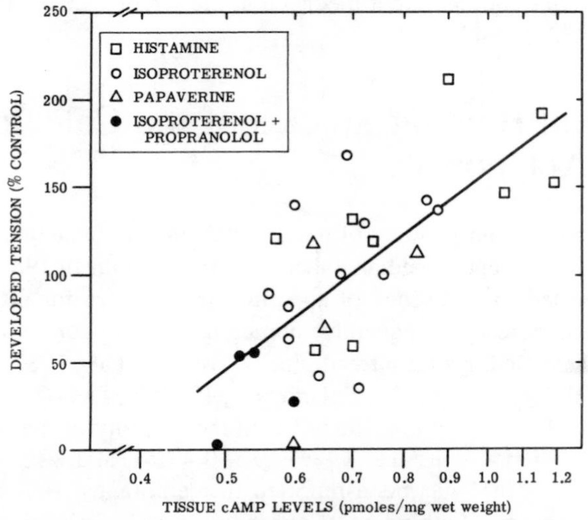

17-4 Correlation between tissue cyclic AMP (cAMP) levels, plotted logarithmically, and steady-state-developed tension of the same hearts. Slope was estimated by least squares method ($r = 0.67$, $p < 0.01$). (Reprinted with permission from Watanabe, A.B., and Besch, H.R. 1974. Circ Res 35:316–323.)

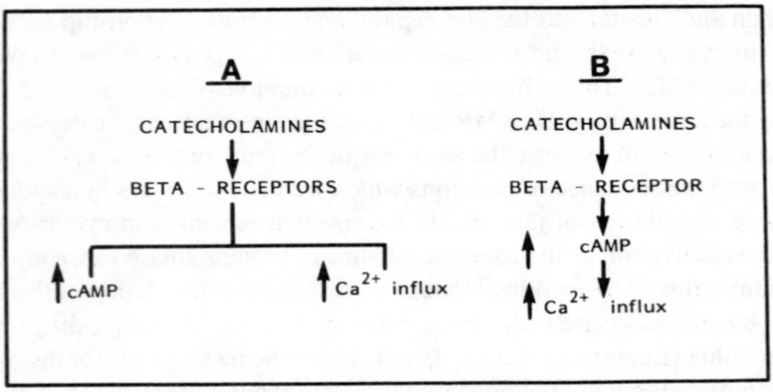

17-5 Two possible relationships between β-adrenergic receptors and slow inward current channels. In A, stimulation of the β-adrenergic receptor causes independent increases in cyclic AMP and calcium influx, a parallel relationship. In B, stimulation of the β-adrenergic receptor causes increases in cyclic AMP which then result in increases in calcium influx, a series relationship. (Reprinted with permission from Lindemann, J.P., Bailey, J.C., and Watanabe, A.M. 1982. Am Heart J 103:746–756.)

concentrations of drug exceeded by 1–3 orders of magnitude the concentrations which were effective in intact hearts and suggested that the effects of these agents on contractility were probably not mediated at the sarcoplasmic reticulum (Watanabe and Besch, 1974b).

Radioligand Binding Studies of the Calcium Channel Antagonists

The stereoselectivity and potency of the organic calcium antagonists suggested the possibility of a receptor-mediated mechanism of action. In 1981, Bellemann et al. first reported the presence of specific binding sites for nitrendipine in myocardial membranes. Subsequently, numerous investigators have confirmed and extended these findings for nitrendipine (Glossman et al., 1982; Murphy and Snyder, 1982; Bolger et al., 1982; Ehlert et al., 1982a,b; DePover et al., 1982), and nimodipine (DePover et al., 1983a,b). In the majority of these reports, the equilibrium dissociation constant, K_D was 0.1–0.4 nM, and a second site with lower affinity of 67 nM has been reported in membranes (Bellemann et al., 1981). In addition, specific binding of nitrendipine and of nimodipine has been described in intact cells (Marsh et al., 1983; DePover et al., 1983a; Green et al., 1983).

The classes of calcium channel antagonists can be contrasted by examining their competition with one another at the dihydropyridine receptor. Dihydropyridines completely inhibited binding of ^{3}H-nitrendipine and ^{3}H-nimodipine to the receptor, and the slope factor of the Hill plot derived was approximately 1, consistent with competitive inhibition at one site (Glossman et al., 1982). In contrast, verapamil and D_{600} only partially inhibited nitrendipine binding, increased the half-time of association and dissociation of the ligand from its receptor, and caused a maximum 4-fold increase in the K_D without changing the maximum number of receptor sites (Ehlert et al., 1982b). This interaction was consistent with negative heterotropic cooperativity.

The interaction of diltiazem with the dihydropyridine receptor is more complex. In membranes, diltiazem inhibited nitrendipine binding partially at 0°C, while at 25°C, some investigators have noted no or partial inhibition. At 37°C, enhancement of nitrendipine binding occurred (Murphy and Snyder, 1982; Ehlert et al., 1982a,b; Ferry and Glossman; 1982; DePover et al., 1982, 1983b). The enhancement of dihydropyridine binding at 37°C has been attributed to an increase in number of dihydropyridine binding sites without a change in receptor affinity (Millard et al., 1983; DePover et al., 1982, 1983b). The pharmacologic significance of this membrane interaction has been suggested by one study in isolated rat hearts in which diltiazem, 250 nM, which by itself produced no effects, potentiated the negative inotropic effects of nimodipine (DePover et al., 1983b). However, Marsh et al. (1983) observed no interaction of diltiazem with nitrendipine in cells.

Dihydropyridine binding has been characterized in subpopulations of membrane vesicles as well. Sarmiento et al. (1983) detected nitrendipine binding in sarcolemmal fractions but found none in fractions of sarcoplasmic reticulum and of mitochondria. Using a different preparation which employed calcium oxalate loading of vesicles followed by fractionation by sucrose density centrifugation, Williams and Jones (1983) had different results. In addition to finding specific nitrendipine binding in the membrane fraction which is enriched in sarcolemmal markers, they also found a high density of sites in those membrane fractions which are enriched in enzymatic markers of sarcoplasmic reticulum, and which demonstrate increased calcium uptake in the presence of ryanodine. DePover et al. (1982a) had similar results using a different preparation to examine nimodipine binding. One of the ryanodine-sensitive membrane fractions, fraction D, contains a 55,000-dalton calcium-binding protein (Jones and Cala, 1981; Campbell et al., 1983). This protein cross-reacts with antiserum to calsequestrin, a skeletal muscle protein localized to terminal cisternae (Jorgensen et al., 1979; Campbell et al., 1983). Circumstantial evidence suggests that this cardiac calsequestrin is also located in junctional sarcoplasmic reticulum (Campbell et al., 1983). It is as yet unclear whether these subfractions contain dyads and triads of junctional sarcoplasmic reticulum and transverse tubules. However, this seems quite possible, and could explain the findings of Williams and Jones. Their observation of substantial ^{3}H-nitrendipine binding to "sarcoplasmic reticulum" may have actually represented binding to the sarcolemmal (T-tubule) portions of dyads and/or triads. As characterization of these membrane fractions progresses, the precise location of dihydropyridine binding sites will be clarified. Recently, using radiation inactivation and target size analysis, Venter et al. (1983) identified a 278,000-dalton protein as the calcium channel in ileal smooth muscle. A nitrendipine analog, which inhibited smooth muscle contraction in response to the muscarinic agonist cis-methyldioxolane, covalently linked to a 41,000-dalton protein which was postulated to be a regulatory subunit of the channel (Venter et al., 1983). Comparable data do not as yet exist for myocardial membranes. The relationship of these sites to the myocardial calcium channel remains to be established.

It is also unclear how the binding of dihydropyridines relates to their pharmacologic effects on myocardium. In isolated atrial and ventricular muscle, the concentration of nifedipine which half-maximally reduced dP/dt, I_{50}, was 0.045 μM. In nonworking Langendorff-perfused guinea pig hearts, the dose of nifedipine which produced half-maximal inhibition of force developed, ID_{50}, was 0.03 μM (Millard et al., 1983). In isolated cells, the concentration of nitrendipine which produced half-maximal block of calcium current was 154 nM (Lee and Tsien, 1983). This contrasts with a binding K_D of 0.1–0.4 nM in membranes and up to 1 nM in isolated myocytes (DePover et al., 1983b; Marsh et al., 1983; Green et al., 1983). Marsh et al. (1983) described a second lower affinity binding site in cultured chick ventricle cells, with a K_D of 19 nM. This corresponded to a concentration of nitrendipine which produced half-maximal inhibition of contraction amplitude, IC_{50}, of 26 nM. Henry (1983) has raised the possibility that discrepancies in binding and pharmacologic effects may be the result of the nature of the coupling of the receptor to the cellular response.

Other Possible Cellular Sites of Action of Calcium Channel Antagonists

As already discussed, a preponderance of studies suggest that the organic calcium channel antagonists are active at the plasma membrane and this is a likely primary site of action of these drugs. The electrophysiologic effects of the calcium channel antagonists are consistent with a sarcolemmal site of action. Recently, Morad et al. (1983) demonstrated in frog ventricles, which are solely dependent upon transsarcolemmal calcium flux for the generation of tension, that photoinactivation of nifedipine and nisoldipine resulted in almost immediate restoration of tension and action potential configurations to pretreatment levels. The effect of the drugs on tension development and action potential was altered by nickel, to which the cell was impermeable. This suggested that the drugs and nickel both acted on the sarcolemma. A quaternary derivative of D_{600}, D_{890}, to which the myocardial cell is impermeable, is ineffective when applied externally to the cell, but suppresses calcium current, tension, and the plateau of the action potential when it is microinjected into the cytosol. This has been interpreted to mean that D_{600} is active at the inner mouth of the calcium channel (Hescheler et al., 1982). The single cell studies of Lee and Tsien (1983) also support a sarcolemmal site of action for calcium antagonists. The drugs block outward as well as inward current through the channel, consistent with the concept of channel blockade.

A number of observations suggest that calcium antagonist drugs may have multiple sites of action on the sarcolemma, particularly at micromolar and higher concentrations. At concentrations of 10^{-5}–10^{-4} M, verapamil has been observed to inhibit competitively ^{3}H-quinuclidinyl benzilate binding to muscarinic receptors and ^{3}H-prazosin binding to α-1 receptors (Karliner et al., 1982). Nayler et al. (1982) observed that D_{600}, (+) and (−) verapamil, diltiazem, and nicardipine inhibited ^{3}H-prazosin and ^{3}H-clonidine binding to α-1 and α-2 receptors, respectively. Micromolar concentrations of verapamil have also been reported to inhibit ATP-dependent calcium transport and activation of calcium-dependent ATPase in sarcolemma (Mas-Oliva and Nayler, 1980). The significance of these observations is that at higher concentrations in experimental preparations the calcium antagonists may have multiple effects, some of which may be unrelated to calcium channel blockade. These concentrations may be attained in myocardium after intravenous administration of verapamil (Keefe and Kates, 1982). Pang and Sperelakis (1983) also demonstrated that nitrendipine is avidly taken up in myocardial cells. Therefore, plasma concentrations of these drugs may not equal myocardial concentrations, nor can we be certain of the effective concentration intracellularly.

Some investigators have questioned whether inhibition of transsarcolemmal calcium influx by calcium channel antagonists accounts entirely for suppression of developed tension. Studying effects of diltiazem in frog ventricular muscle, Morad et al. (1982) found no effects on tension or action potential at concentrations less than 10^{-6} M. A concentration of 2.2×10^{-5} M diltiazem suppressed tension development to a greater extent than the slow inward current and increased the delayed outward current. Diltiazem was demonstrated not to attenuate contractures in response to sodium withdrawal, suggesting no effect on sodium-calcium exchange. Only in sodium-depleted tissues did suppression of contraction and slow inward current correlate. Thus, in this study, diltiazem was felt to exert an effect on a "slowly inactivating" calcium current or an "undefined calcium transport system" (Morad et al. 1982). Whether this reflects the high concentrations of diltiazem used, or a species-specific characteristic is unclear. Morgan et al. (1983) also identified a dissociation between depression of tension development and intracellular calcium concentration as identified by aequorin signal in feline papillary muscle.

Studies of subcellular constituents have demonstrated effects of calcium channel antagonists only when greater than micromolar concentrations of the compounds are used. Early studies by Fleckenstein (1977) demonstrated that in chemically skinned myocardial cells, calcium channel antagonists did not alter myocardial contraction in the presence of ATP and calcium. This suggests that the calcium channel antagonists had no direct effect on myofibrils of the contractile apparatus. As mentioned previously, studies of isolated sarcoplasmic reticulum demonstrated that D_{600} and verapamil had no effect on calcium transport at concentrations which were negatively inotropic (Watanabe and Besch, 1974b; Nayler and Szeto, 1972). Besch et al. (1981) demonstrated that D_{600} had multiple effects on calcium accumulation by sarcoplasmic reticulum vesicles at higher concentrations. In concentrations of 10^{-5} and 10^{-4} M, D_{600} stimulated calcium uptake, but it completely inhibited calcium uptake at 10^{-3} M. All of these responses were attenuated in the presence of potassium. No change occurred in ATP hydrolysis by Ca^{2+}-ATPase at the lower concentrations of D_{600}, but it was inhibited by 10^{-3} M D_{600}.

In normal mitochondria, verapamil and diltiazem had no effect on calcium uptake (Fleckenstein, 1977; Vaghy et al., 1981). Vaghy et al. (1983) demonstrated that calcium channel antagonists in this same concentration range inhibited sodium-induced calcium release from mitochondria as detected by dye indicators. Verapamil (25–200) μM) and diltiazem (50–500 μM) were also demonstrated to inhibit mitochondrial swelling in the presence of elevated concentrations of inorganic phosphate (Vaghy et al., 1981).

Additional in vitro studies have identified other intracellular actions of calcium antagonists at high concentrations. Nimodipine and nicardipine inhibited purified phosphodiesterase activity with an IC_{50} of 3–25 μM. Verapamil more potently inhibited the purified calmodulin-insensitive phosphodiesterase than the calmodulin-sensitive form, with IC_{50} of 9–17 μM and 300 to greater than 1000 μM, respectively (Epstein et al., 1982). The physiologic significance of these observations is not clear. These effects are observed at concentrations greatly exceeding those required to produce negative inotropism, but it is possible that such concentrations of drug are attained inside the cell.

Thayer and Fairhurst (1983) did not detect physiologically important binding of nitrendipine to calmodulin. At concentrations of up to 10 μM, nitrendipine, nicardipine and felodipine did not inhibit the binding of ^{3}H-chlorpromazine or ^{45}Ca to calmodulin, and nicardipine, 10 μM, reduced ^{14}C-pimozide binding to calmodulin by only 26%. Thus, inhibition of calcium binding to calmodulin does not appear to mediate the effects of commonly used calcium channel antagonists.

Determination of the effects of calcium channel antagonists on the uptake of ^{45}calcium is another method of studying the biochemical effect of these drugs.

Thus far, these types of studies have yielded varied results. Nayler and Szeto (1972) observed that verapamil displaced La^{3+}-sensitive calcium. This calcium pool is bound superficially to the cell and can be displaced by lanthanum, to which the cell is impermeable. They suggested that verapamil's mechanism of action might be the result of displacement of calcium from superficial binding sites. Mas-Oliva and Nayler (1980) pointed out that racemic and (−) verapamil were equieffective at displacing this calcium from sarcolemma although only (−) verapamil is negatively inotropic. Thus, it seems unlikely that verapamil's effects are mediated by occupation of superficial calcium binding sites. Church and Zsoter (1980) noted that verapamil did not antagonize lanthanum-resistant ^{45}Ca uptake, an index of cellular calcium. Because verapamil did not appear to affect total cellular calcium content, these authors suggested that verapamil exerted its effect by redistribution of cellular calcium. Pang and Sperelakis (1982) described inhibition of ^{45}Ca binding to sarcolemmal vesicles by verapamil and by nickel but not nifedipine or diltiazem, and thus distinguished these drugs in yet another way. Multiple means of calcium transport exist. ^{45}Ca uptake experiments therefore reflect the net calcium transport process, not merely channel-mediated calcium influx. As noted by Henry (1980), because we lack methods to block selectively the multiple means of calcium transport by cardiac sarcolemma, it is difficult to interpret the effects of calcium antagonists on calcium uptake.

Summary and Conclusions

Our understanding of the calcium channel and of the mechanisms of action of calcium channel antagonists has progressed rapidly in the past decade. The electrophysiologic and contractile response of the myocardial cell to calcium channel antagonists is well established, and it is clear that the negative inotropic effects of these drugs is directly linked to a decrease in the transsarcolemmal influx of calcium. The serial relationship of increases in cyclic AMP and activation of protein kinase to increases in calcium influx is well established. While the existence of receptors for these drugs in myocardium is well documented, it is unclear how the cellular response is coupled to binding of the drug to these "receptors." Differences in the structure of these drugs, corroborated by different effects on kinetics of channel activation and recovery, competition at receptor sites, and possibly different binding sites within the sarcolemmal membrane suggest that these drugs may have different sites of action within the calcium channel. This would be analogous to the variety of ways in which drugs inhibit sodium channel function (Glossman et al., 1982). A sarcolemmal site of action for each of these drugs is well established, but additional intracellular actions remain difficult to disprove (Henry, 1983).

Acknowledgments

Supported in part by the Herman C. Krannert Fund; by grants HL18795, HL06308, HL07182, and HL29208 from the National Heart, Lung, and Blood Institute of the National Institutes of Health; and by the American Heart Association, Indiana Affiliate.

References

Bayer, R., Hennekes, R., Kaufmann, R., and Mannhold, R. 1975a. Inotropic and electrophysiologic actions of verapamil and D_{600} in mammalian myocardium. I. Pattern of inotropic effects of the racemic compounds. Naunyn-Schmied Arch Pharmacol 290:49–68.

Bayer, R., Kaufmann, R., and Mannhold, R. 1975b. Inotropic and electrophysiologic actions of verapamil and D_{600} in mammalian myocardium. II. Pattern of inotropic effects of the optical isomers. Naunyn-Schmied Arch Pharmacol 290:69–80.

Bayer, R., Kalusche, D., Kaufmann, R., and Mannhold, R., 1975c. Inotropic and electrophysiologic actions of verapamil and D_{600} in mammalian myocardium. III. Effects of the optical isomers on transmembrane action potentials. Naunyn-Schmied Arch Pharmacol 290:81–97.

Bayer, R., Rodenkirchen, R., Kaufmann, R., Lee, H.J., and Henneckes, R. 1977. The effects of nifedipine on contraction and monophasic action potential of isolated cat myocardium. Naunyn-Schmied Arch Pharmacol 301:29–37.

Bean, B.P., Nowycky, M.C., and Tsien, R.W. 1984. Beta-adrenergic modulation of calcium channels in frog ventricular heart cells. Nature 307:371–375.

Belleman, P., Ferry, D., Lubbecke, F., and Glossman, H. 1981. ^{3}H-Nitrendipine, a potent calcium antagonist, binds with high affinity to cardiac membranes. Arzneim Forsch 31: 2064–2067.

Besch, H.R., Jr., Jones, L.R., and Maddock, K.A. 1981. Effects of calcium antagonists on sarcoplasmic reticular and sarcolemmal vesicles from canine heart. In: G.B. Weiss, ed. New Prospectives on Calcium Antagonists, pp. 47–57. Bethesda: American Physiological Society. Baltimore: Williams and Wilkins.

Bolger, G.T., Gengo, P.J., Luchowski, E.M., Siegel, H., Triggle, D.J., and Janis, R.A. 1982. High affinity binding of a calcium channel antagonist to smooth and cardiac muscle. Biochem Biophys Res Commun 104:1604–1609.

Cachelin, A.B., dePeyer, J.E., Kokubun, S., and Reuter, H. 1983. Ca^{2+} channel modulation by 8-bromocyclic AMP in cultured heart cells. Nature 304:462–464.

Campbell, K.P., MacLennon, D.H., Jorgensen, A.C., and Mintzer, M.C. 1983. Purification and characterization of calsequestrin from canine cardiac sarcoplasmic reticulum and identification of the 53,000 Dalton glycoprotein. J Biol Chem 258:1197–1204.

Church, J. and Zsoter, T.T. 1980. Calcium antagonistic drugs: Mechanism of action. Can J Physiol Pharmacol 58:254–264.

Coraboeuf, E., and Otsuka, M. 1956. L'action des solutions hyposodiques sur les potentiels cellulaires de tissu cardiaque de mammifires. C R Acad Sci Paris 243:441–444.

Cranefield, P.F. 1975. The Conduction of the Cardiac Impulse: The Slow Response and Cardiac Arrhythmias. p. 76. Mount Kisco, New York: Futura Publishing Company.

Cranefield, P.F., Aronson, R.S., and Wit, A.L. 1974. Effect of verapamil on the normal action potential and on a calcium-dependent slow response of canine cardiac Purkinje fibers. Circ Res 34:204–213.

Dangman, K.H., and Hoffman, B.F. 1980. Effects of nifedipine on electrical activity of cardiac cells. Am J Cardiol 46:1059–1067.

DePover, A., Grupp, I.L., Grupp, G., and Schwartz, A. 1983b. Diltiazem potentiates the negative inotropic action of nimodipine in heart. Biochem Biophys Res Commun 114:922–929.

DePover, A., Lee, S.W., Matlib, M.A., Whitmer, K., Davis, B.A., Powell, T., and Schwartz, A. 1983a. ^{3}H-nimodipine specific binding to cardiac myocytes and subcellular fractions. Biochem Biophys Res Commun 113:185–191.

DePover, A., Matlib, M.A., Lee, S.W., Dube, G.P., Grupp, I.L., Grupp, G., and Schwartz, A. 1982. Specific binding of ^{3}H-nitrendipine to membranes from coronary arteries and heart in relation to pharmacological effects. Paradoxical stimulation by diltiazem. Biochem Biophys Res Commun 108:110–117.

Ehara, T., and Kaufmann, R. 1978. The voltage- and time-dependent effects of (−)-verapamil on the slow inward current in isolated cat ventricular myocardium. J Pharmacol Exp Ther 207:49–55.

Ehlert, F.J., Itoga, E., Roeske, W.R., and Yamamura, H.I. 1982a. The interaction of ^{3}H-nitrendipine with receptors for calcium antagonists in the cerebral cortex and heart of rats. Biochem Biophys Res Commun 104:937–943.

Ehlert, F.J., Roeske, W.R., Itoga, E., and Yamamura, H.I. 1982b. The binding of ^{3}H-nitrendipine to receptors for calcium channel antagonists in the heart, cerebral cortex, and ileum of rats. Life Sci 30:2191–2202.

Epstein, P.M., Fiss, K., Hachisu, R., and Andrenyak, D.M. 1982. Interaction of calcium antagonists with cyclic AMP phosphodiesterases and calmodulin. Biochem Biophys Res Commun 105:1142–1149.

Fabiato, A. 1983. Calcium-induced release of calcium from the cardiac sarcoplasmic reticulum. Am J Physiol 245(Cell Physiol 14):C1–C14.

Ferry, D.R., and Glossman, H. 1982. Evidence for multiple receptor sites within a putative calcium channel. Naunyn-Schmied Arch Pharmacol 321:80–83.

Fleckenstein, A. 1964. Die bedeutung der energiereichen phosphate für kontraktilität und tonus des myokards. Verh Dtsch Ges Inn Med 70:81–99.

Fleckenstein, A. 1977. Specific pharmacology of calcium in myocardium, cardiac pacemakers, and vascular smooth muscle. Annu Rev Pharmacol Toxicol 17:149–166.

Fleckenstein, A. 1981. Fundamental actions of calcium antagonists on myocardial and cardiac pacemaker cell membranes. In: G.B. Weiss, ed. New Perspectives on Calcium Antagonists. Bethesda: American Physiological Society. pp. 59–81. Baltimore:Williams and Wilkins.

Fleckenstein, A., Kammermeier, H., Doring, H., and Freund, H.J. 1967. Zum Wirkungsmechanismus neuartiger Koronardilatatoren mitgleichzeitig Sauerstoff-einsparenden Myokard-Effecten, Prenylamin und Iproveratril. Z Kreislaufforsch 56:716–744, 839–853.

Glossman, H., Ferry, D.R., Lubbecke, F., Mewes, R., and Hofmann, F. 1982. Calcium channels: Direct identification with radioligand binding studies. Trends Pharmacol Sci 431–437.

Green, F.J., Farmer, B.B., Wiseman, G.L., Jose, M.J.L., and Watanabe, A.M. 1983. Effect of membrane potential on binding of ^{3}H-nitrendipine to isolated cardiac myocytes. Circulation 68:III–99 (abstr).

Hagiwara, S., and Byerly, L. 1981. Calcium channel. Annu Rev Neurosci 4:69–125.

Hamill, O.P., Marty, A., Neher, E., Sakmann, B., and Sigworth, F.J. 1981. Improved patch-clamp techniques for high-resolution current recording from cells and cell-free membrane patches. Pflügers Arch 391:85–100.

Henry, P.D. 1980. Comparative pharmacology of calcium antagonists: Nifedipine, verapamil, and diltiazem. Am J Cardiol 46:1047–1058.

Henry, P.D. 1982. Comparative cardiac pharmacology of calcium blockers. In: S.F. Flaim and R. Zelis, eds. Calcium Blockers: Mechanisms of Action and Clinical Applications. pp. 135–153. Baltimore-Munich:Urban and Schwarzenberg.

Henry, P.D. 1983. Mechanisms of action of calcium antagonists in cardiac and smooth muscle. In: P.H. Stone and E.M. Antman, eds. Calcium Channel Blocking Agents in the Treatment of Cardiovascular Disorders. pp. 107–154. Mount Kisco, New York: Futura Publishing Company, Inc.

Hescheler, J., Pelzer, D., Trube, G., and Trautwein, W. 1982. Does the organic calcium channel blocker D_{600} act from inside or outside on the cardiac cell membrane? Pflügers Arch 393:287–291.

Janis, R.A., and Scriabine, A. 1983. Sites of action of Ca^{2+} channel inhibitors. Biochem Pharmacol 32:3499–3507.

Janis, R.A., and Triggle, D.J. 1983. New developments in Ca^{2+} channel antagonists. J Med Chem 26:775–785.

Jones, L.R., Besch, H.R., Jr., Fleming, J.W., McConnaughey, M.M., and Watanabe, A.M. 1979. Separation of vesicles of cardiac sarcolemma from vesicles of sarcoplasmic reticulum. J Biol Chem 254:530–539.

Jones, L.R., and Cala, S. 1981. Biochemical evidence for functional heterogeneity of cardiac sarcoplasmic reticulum vesicles. J Biol Chem 256:11809–11818.

Jones, L.R., Maddock, S.W., and Besch, H.R., Jr. 1980. Unmasking effect of alamethicin on the Na^+, K^+-ATPase, beta-adrenergic receptor-coupled adenylate cyclase, and cAMP-dependent protein kinase activities of cardiac sarcolemmal vesicles. J Biol Chem 255:9971–9980.

Jorgensen, A.O., Falnius, V., and MacLennan, D.H. 1979. Localization of sarcoplasmic reticulum proteins in rat skeletal muscle by immunofluorescence. J Cell Biol 80:372–384.

Kanaya, S., Arlock, P., Katzung, B.G., and Hondeghem, L.M. 1983. Diltiazem and verapamil preferentially block inactivated cardiac calcium channels. J Mol Cell Cardiol 15:145–148.

Karliner, J.S., Motulsky, H.J., Dunlap, J., Brown, J.H., and Insel, P.A. 1982. Verapamil competitively inhibits alpha-1-adrenergic and muscarinic but not beta-adrenergic receptors in rat myocardium. J Cardiovasc Pharmacol 4:515–520.

Kass, R.S. 1982. Nisoldipine: A new, more selective calcium current blocker in cardiac Purkinje fibers. J Pharmacol Exp Ther 223: 446–456.

Kass, R.S., and Tsien, R.W. 1975. Multiple effects of calcium antagonists on plateau currents in cardiac Purkinje fibers. J Gen Physiol 66:169–192.

Kawai, C., Konishi, T., Matsuyama, E., Okazaki, H. 1981. Comparative effects of three calcium antagonists, diltiazem, verapamil, and nifedipine, on the sinoatrial and atrioventricular nodes: Experimental and clinical studies. Circulation 63:1035–1042.

Keefe, D.L., and Kates, R.E. 1982. Myocardial disposition and cardiac pharmacodynamics of verapamil in the dog. J Pharmacol Exp Ther 220:91–96.

Kohlhardt, M., Bauer, B., Krause, H., and Fleckenstein, A. 1972. Differentiation of the transmembrane Na and Ca channels in mammalian cardiac fibers by the use of specific inhibitors. Pflügers Arch 335:309–322.

Kohlhardt, M., and Fleckenstein, A. 1977. Inhibition of the slow inward current by nifedipine in mammalian ventricular myocardium. Naunyn-Schmied Arch Pharmacol 298: 267–272.

Kohlhardt, M., and Haap, K. 1981. The blockade of $\dot{V}_{max}$ of the atrioventricular action potential produced by the slow channel inhibitors verapamil and nifedipine. Naunyn-Schmied Arch Pharmacol 316:178–185.

Kohlhardt, M., and Mnich, Z. 1978. Studies on the inhibitory effect of verapamil on the slow inward current in mammalian ventricular myocardium. J Mol Cell Cardiol 10:1037–1052.

Lee, K.S., and Tsien, R.W. 1983. Mechanism of calcium channel blockade by verapamil, D_{600}, diltiazem and nitrendipine in single dialyzed heart cells. Nature 302:790–794.

Lindemann, J.P., Bailey, J.C., and Watanabe, A.M. 1982. Am Heart J 103:746–756.

Lindemann, J.P., Jones, L.R., Hathaway, D.R., Henry, B.G., and Watanabe, A.M. 1983. Beta-adrenergic stimulation of phospholamban phosphorylation and Ca^{2+}-ATPase activity in guinea pig ventricles. J Biol Chem 258:464–471.

Linden, J., and Brooker, G. 1980. The influence of resting membrane potential on the effect of verapamil on atria. J Mol Cell Cardiol 12:325–331.

Ludwig, C., and Nawrath, H. 1977. Effects of D_{600} and its optical isomers on force of contraction in cat papillary muscles and guinea pig auricles. Br J Pharmacol 59:411–417.

Manalan, A.S., and Jones, L.R. 1982. Characterization of the intrinsic cAMP-dependent protein kinase activity and endogenous substrates in highly purified cardiac sarcolemmal vesicles. J Biol Chem 257:10052–10062.

Marsh, J.D., Loh, E., Lachance, D., Barry, W.H., and Smith, T.W. 1983. Relationship of binding of a calcium channel blocker to inhibition of contraction in intact cultured embryonic chick ventricular cells. Circ Res 53:539–543.

Mas-Oliva, J., and Nayler, W.G. 1980. The effect of verapamil on the Ca^{2+}-transporting and Ca^{2+}-ATPase activity of isolated cardiac sarcolemmal preparations. Br J Pharmacol 70:617–624.

McCans, J.L., Lindenmayer, G.E., Munson, R.G., Evans, R.W., and Schwartz, A. 1974. A dissociation of positive staircase (Bowditch) from ouabain-induced positive inotropism: Use of verapamil. Circ Res 35:439–447.

McDonald, T.F., Pelzer, D., and Trautwein, W. 1980. On the mechanism of slow calcium channel block in heart. Pflügers Arch 385:175–179.

McDonald, T.F. 1982. The slow inward calcium current in the heart. Annu Rev Physiol 44:425–434.

Millard, R.W., Grupp, G., Grupp, I.L., DiSalvo, J., DePover, A., and Schwartz, A. 1983. Chronotropic, inotropic, and vasodilator actions of diltiazem, nifedipine, and verapamil: A comparative study of physiological responses and membrane receptor activity. Circ Res 52:i29–i39.

Morad, M., Goldman, Y.E., and Trentham, D.R. 1983. Rapid photochemical inactivation of Ca^{2+}-antagonists shows that Ca^{2+} entry directly activates contraction in frog heart. Nature 304:635–638.

Morad, M., Tung, L., and Greenspan, A.M. 1982. Effect of diltiazem on calcium transport and development of tension in heart muscle. Am J Cardiol 49:595–601.

Morgan, J.P., Wier, J.G., Hess, P., and Blinks, J.R. 1983. Influence of Ca^{2+}-channel blocking agents on calcium transients and tension development in isolated mammalian heart muscle. Circ Res 52:I47–I52.

Murphy, K.M., and Snyder, S.H. 1982. Calcium antagonist receptor binding sites labelled with ^{3}H-nitrendipine. Eur J Pharmacol 77:201–202.

Nawrath, H., Ten Eick, R.E., McDonald, T.F., and Trautwein, W. 1977. On the mechanism underlying the action of D_{600} on slow inward current and tension in mammalian myocardium. Circ Res 40:408–414.

Nayler, W.G. 1983. The heterogeneity of the slow channel blockers (calcium antagonists). Int J Cardiol 3:391–400.

Nayler, W.G., Grau, A., and Slade, A. 1976. A protective effect of verapamil on hypoxic heart muscle. Cardiovasc Res 10:650–662.

Nayler, W.G., and Szeto, J. 1972. Effect of verapamil on contractility, oxygen utilization, and calcium exchangability in mammalian heart muscle. Cardiovasc Res 6:120–128.

Nayler, W.G., Thompson, J.E., and Jarrot, B. 1982. The interaction of calcium antagonists (slow channel blockers) with myocardial alpha adrenoceptors. J Mol Cell Cardiol 14:185–188.

Osterrieder, W., Brum, G., Hescheler, J., Trautwein, W., Flockerzi, V., and Hofmann, F. 1982. Injection of subunits of cyclic AMP-dependent protein kinase into cardiac myocytes modulates Ca^{2+} current. Nature 298: 576–578.

Pang, D.C., and Sperelakis, N. 1982. Differential actions of calcium antagonists on calcium binding to cardiac sarcolemma. Eur J Pharmacol 81:403–409.

Pang, D.C., and Sperelakis, N. 1983. Uptake of ^{3}H-nitrendipine into cardiac and smooth muscle. Biochem Pharmacol 32:1660–1663.

Pappano, A.J. 1970. Calcium-dependent action potentials produced by catecholamines in guinea pig atrial muscle fibers depolarized by potassium. Circ Res 27:379–390.

Reuter, H. 1967. The dependence of slow inward current in Purkinje fibers on the extracellular calcium concentrations. J Physiol (Lond) 192:479–492.

Reuter, H. 1979. Properties of two inward membrane currents in the heart. Annu Rev Physiol 41:413–424.

Reuter, H. 1983. Calcium channel modulation by neurotransmitters, enzymes, and drugs. Nature 301:569–574.

Reuter, H., and Scholz, H. 1977. The regulation of the Ca conductance of cardiac muscle by adrenaline. J Physiol (Lond) 264:49–62.

Reuter, H., Stevens, C.F., Tsien, R.W., and Yellen, G. 1982. Properties of single calcium channels in cardiac cell culture. Nature 297:501–504.

Saikawa, T., Nagamoto, Y., and Arita, M. 1977. Electrophysiologic effects of diltiazem, a new slow channel inhibitor, on canine cardiac fibers. Jpn Heart J 18:235–245.

Sarmiento, J.G., Jarvis, R.A., Colvin, R.A., Triggle, D.J., and Katz, A.M. 1983. Binding of the calcium channel blocker nitrendipine to its receptor in purified sarcolemma from canine cardiac ventricle. J Mol Cell Cardiol 15:135–137.

Scheuer, T., and Kass, R.S. 1982. Distinction in the modes of action of the calcium current inhibitors D_{600}, diphenylhydantoin, and nisoldipine in cardiac Purkinje fibers. Biophys J 37:341a.

Stull, J.T., and Mayer, S.E. 1979. Biochemical mechanisms of adrenergic and cholinergic regulation of myocardial contractility. In: Handbook of Physiology. Cardiovascular System. Vol. I, Chap. 21, pp. 741–774. Bethesda: American Physiological Society.

Thayer, S.A., and Fairhurst, A.S. 1983. The interaction of dihydropyridine calcium channel blockers with calmodulin and calmodulin inhibitors. Mol Pharmacol 24:6–9.

Triggle, D.J. 1981. Calcium antagonists: Basic chemical and pharmacological aspects. In: G.B. Weiss, ed. New Perspectives on Calcium Antagonists pp. 1–18. Bethesda: American Physiological Society. Baltimore: Williams and Wilkins.

Tritthart, H., Volkmann, R., Weiss, R., and Fleckenstein, A. 1973. Alteration of membrane response as induced by changes of Ca or by promoters and inhibitors of transmembrane Ca inflow. Naunyn-Schmied Arch Pharmacol 280:239–252.

Tsien, R.W. 1973. Adrenaline-like effects of intracellular iontophoresis of cyclic AMP in cardiac Purkinje fibers. Nature New Biol 245:120–122.

Tsien, R.W. 1983. Calcium channels in excitable cell membranes. Annu Rev Physiol 45:341–358.

Tung, L., and Morad, M. 1983. Electrophysiological studies with Ca^{2+} entry blockers. In: G.F. Merrill and H. R. Weiss, eds. Entry Blockers, Adenosine, and Neurohumors. Chap. 2, pp. 19–38. Baltimore:Urban and Schwarzenberg.

Vaghy, P.L., Johnson, J.D., Matlib, M.A., Wang, T., and Schwartz, A. 1982. Selective inhibition of Na^{+}-induced Ca^{2+} release from heart mitochondria by diltiazem and certain other Ca^{2+} antagonist drugs. J Biol Chem 257:6000–6002.

Vaghy, P.L., Matlib, M.A., Szekeres, L., and Schwartz, A. 1981. Protective effects of verapamil and diltiazem against inorganic phosphate induced impairment of oxidative phosphorylation of isolated heart mitochondria. Biochem Pharmacol 30:2603–2610.

Venter, J.C., Fraser, C.M., Schaber, J.S., Jung, C.Y., Bolger, G., and Triggle, D.J. 1983. Molecular properties of the slow inward calcium channel: Molecular weight determinations by radiation inactivation and covalent affinity labeling. J Biol Chem 258: 9344–9348.

Watanabe, A.M., and Besch, H.R., Jr. 1974a. Cyclic adenosine monophosphate modulation of slow calcium influx channels in guinea pig hearts. Circ Res 35:316–323.

Watanabe, A.M., and Besch, H.R., Jr. 1974b. Subcellular myocardial effects of verapamil and D_{600}: Comparison with propranolol. J Pharmacol Exp Ther 191:241–251.

Williams, L.T., and Jones, L.R. 1983. Specific binding of the calcium antagonist, ^{3}H-nitrendipine, to subcellular fractions isolated from canine myocardium: Evidence for high affinity binding to ryanodine-sensitive sarcoplasmic reticulum vesicles. J Biol Chem 258:5344–5347.

Wit, A.L., and Cranefield, P.F. 1975. Effect of verapamil on the sinoatrial and atrioventricular nodes of the rabbit and the mechanism by which it arrests reentrant atrioventricular nodal tachycardia. Circ Res 35:413–425.

Wollenberger, A., and Will, H. 1978. Protein kinase catalysed membrane phosphorylation and its relationship to the role of calcium in the adrenergic regulation of cardiac contraction. Life Sci 22:1159–1176.

Wray, H.L., Gray, R.R., and Olsson, R.A. 1973. Cyclic adenosine 3′, 5′-monophosphate-stimulated protein kinase and a substrate associated with cardiac sarcoplasmic reticulum. J Biol Chem 248:1496–1498.

Zipes, D.P., and Fischer, J.C. 1974. Effects of agents which inhibit the slow channel on sinus node automaticity and atrioventricular conductions in the dog. Circ Res 34:184–192.

Chapter 18

Clinical Antiarrhythmic Effects of Calcium Channel-Blocking Drugs

Leonard N. Horowitz

Introduction

The calcium channel-blocking agents are a unique and new class of antiarrhythmic drugs which block the slow inward current that is carried predominantly by calcium (Singh et al., 1978). Unlike the approved class IA antiarrhythmic drugs whose primary effect is on the fast sodium channel (Fleckenstein, 1971), these drugs have little effect on the sodium channel. The calcium current has many effects and plays an integral role in cardiac electrophysiology and contractility, both of which may contribute to the antiarrhythmic actions of this group of drugs (Singh et al., 1978).

Electrophysiology of Calcium Channel Blockers

The most prominant electrophysiologic effect of the calcium channel-blocking agents is depression of sinoatrial automaticity and atrioventricular nodal depolarization (Cranefield, 1975; Zipes and Fischer, 1974). Depolarization in these tissues is dependent upon the slow calcium inward current which produces a so called "slow action potential." Since the majority of cardiac cells which possess potential automaticity are dependent upon the fast sodium channel for activation, the sodium channel-blocking agents do not have a significant effect on these tissues. The consequences of this slow channel blockade are a slowing of conduction and prolongation of refractoriness within the sinus and atrioventricular nodes. The spontaneous firing rates in these structures are similarly decreased. In usually employed clinical doses, calcium channel-blocking agents have little, if any, significant effect on Purkinje fibers or cardiac muscle cells. In clinical terms, these agents, primarily verapamil and diltiazem, reduce the spontaneous rate of the sinus node and produce sinus bradycardia. Depression of conduction through the A-V node produces prolongation of the P-R interval and a reduction in the ventricular response to atrial tachyarrhythmias (Kawai et al., 1981;

Rowland et al., 1979). These drugs can also interrupt reentrant arrhythmias that depend upon conduction through the A-V node.

In the normal experimental animal, verapamil has been found to have minimal electrophysiologic effects which might have antiarrhythmic significance; however, modest changes in the shape of the action potential and the rate of spontaneous diastolic depolarization have been noted (Rosen et al., 1974). In the abnormal tissue, or in the presence of pathologic states, the marked effects of calcium channel-blocking agents (particularly verapamil) on the His-Purkinje fibers and ventricular electrophysiology have been observed (Cranefield et al., 1974; Tse and Han, 1975). Slow response action potentials in Purkinje fibers have been identified under pathologic conditions that may be involved mechanistically in reentry and ventricular tachyarrhythmias (Wit et al., 1974a,b,c). Verapamil decreases action potential amplitude and abnormal automaticity in Purkinje fibers in which the fast sodium current has been inactivated and replaced by the slow calcium current. Whether these abnormalities identified in vitro actually occur and are responsible for arrhythmias in vivo remains open to question; however, if they do, it is conceivable that the calcium channel-blocking agents will have an antiarrhythmic effect. Furthermore, Purkinje fibers exposed to high concentrations of acetylstrophanthidin or ouabain develop late afterdepolarizations which may be associated with the arrhythmias of digitalis toxicity. Verapamil has been shown to decrease the magnitude of these afterdepolarizations in the setting of digitalis glycoside intoxication and may further indicate verapamil's potential as a ventricular antiarrhythmic in pathologic states (Rosen and Daniel, 1982).

Considerable data suggest that verapamil is an effective agent for suppression of arrhythmias in experimental myocardial infarction (Fondacaro et al., 1978; El-Sherif and Lazarra, 1979; Ribeiro et al., 1981). A variety of postulated mechanisms for its antiarrhythmic action have been described, and as yet, the clinical significance of these remains to be determined. As noted above, the slow current action potential, if present in ventricular tissue or Purkinje fibers, can be suppressed by verapamil. The pathophysiologic alterations produced by acute myocardial infarction (high extracellular potassium concentration, high catecholamine concentrations, and depolarizing currents) may lead to the presence of such verapamil-sensitive slow action potential cells within a myocardial infarction. It might be expected under these conditions that verapamil would be an effective ventricular antiarrhythmic agent. In addition, in the setting of acute myocardial infarction, verapamil has been shown to have effects on ventricular automaticity and conduction (Fondacaro et al., 1978). Several groups have reported that verapamil improves conduction in the ischemic zone during acute myocardial infarction (El-Sherif and Lazarra, 1979; Elharrar et al., 1977). The improvement in conduction within the ischemic zone may suppress establishment of reentrant circuits, and thereby reduce the potential for ventricular tachyarrhythmias. The mechanism by which this improvement in conduction occurs is not clear. It has been postulated that the improvement is not an antiarrhythmic effect, but a reflection of the calcium channel-blocking drug's ability to reduce ischemic injury and thereby allow normal myocardial metabolism to restore normal electrophysiologic function. On the other hand, verapamil may produce an as yet unidentified direct electrophysiologic effect which improves conduction in the ischemic zone (El-Sherif and Lazarra, 1979; Elharrar et al., 1977). In several studies in both acute and subacute myocardial ischemia produced by experimental coronary occlusion, ventricular arrhythmias have been found to be reduced by treatment with verapamil and reduction in arrhythmias correlated with improvement of conduction within the ischemic zone. Similarly, verapamil increases the ventricular fibrillation threshold in the presence of myocardial ischemia (Fondacaro et al., 1978). Increase in the ventricular fibrillation threshold generally correlates with a decrease in the likelihood of ventricular tachyarrhythmias. Again, the mechanism by which the ventricular fibrillation threshold is altered is not known and may reflect a direct antiarrhythmic effect or an effect on improvement of myocardial ischemia. Furthermore, in the presence of myocardial ischemia, the sympathetic activity is augmented significantly and may well be a relevant factor in the production of arrhythmias. In this regard, verapamil has been found to antagonize the effects of adrenergic stimuli in acute infarction and may be an additive factor in verapamil's protection against ventricular arrhythmias in acute myocardial ischemic states (Brooks et al., 1980; Melville et al., 1968).

Clinical Indications

The calcium channel-blocking agents can be used for terminating paroxysmal supraventricular tachycardia, reducing the ventricular response during atrial fibrillation, and chronic prevention of paroxysmal supraventricular tachycardia. Their antiarrhythmic properties in supraventricular arrhythmias are believed to be due to their ability to depress A-V nodal conduction and prolong refractoriness.

Atrial Fibrillation

In most studies, verapamil has significantly reduced the ventricular response in patients with atrial fibrillation (Schamroth, 1971; Heng et al., 1975; Plumb et al., 1982; Waxman et al., 1981). This effect is seen in a majority of, but not all patients. In the study by Waxman et al. (1981), the mean ventricular rate decreased from 146–114/min in 13 of 20 patients. In their study, verapamil was shown to be significantly better than placebo. Similar results have been reported by many groups and there is uniform agreement that verapamil is effective for this arrhythmia. When used for the control of ventricular response in atrial fibrillation, the effect of intravenous verapamil is seen within minutes (Schamroth, 1971). A mild decrease in systemic arterial pressure is common but is rarely clinically significant. Frequently, patients in whom ventricular rate does not fall to acceptable levels are found to have congestive heart failure, explaining their failure to respond.

Detailed comparisons between verapamil and other forms of pharmacologic treatment for atrial fibrillation have not been published. It is obvious that verapamil holds certain advantages over β-blocker therapy in selected patient groups such as those with bronchospastic disorders because of the contraindications to β-blocker therapy. In addition, the rapid onset of action makes it more advantageous than digitalis glycosides.

The effectiveness of oral verapamil in the treatment of both new onset and chronic atrial fibrillation has not been well studied. There are preliminary studies which indicate that the oral administration is effective in controlling the ventricular rate in atrial fibrillation, however (Morganroth et al., 1982; Klein et al., 1979).

Particular caution should be exercised in the administration of verapamil to patients with atrial fibrillation and a preexcitation syndrome (Gulamhussein et al., 1981). The slowing of conduction over the normal A-V pathway may allow an increase in the conduction rate over the accessory pathway and paradoxically increase the ventricular response rate. Although not absolutely contraindicated, it is best to seek other modes of therapy for atrial fibrillation in the setting of the Wolff-Parkinson-White or other preexcitation syndromes.

Verapamil has also been used for the management of atrial fibrillation complicating acute myocardial infarction (Hagemeijer, 1978). Although the drug must be given with greater caution in this setting, generally in 1-mg increments, it can be used safely to control the ventricular response in atrial fibrillation. It has been suggested that the drug be administered in small doses until the arrhythmia is controlled or clinically significant hypotension or increase in pulmonary capillary wedge pressure is noted. The beneficial effects derived from acutely controlling the ventricular rate in atrial fibrillation in this setting are significant and compensate for the potential risk of using the drug in this setting.

Paroxysmal Supraventricular Tachycardia

Most types of paroxysmal supraventricular tachycardia are due to a reentrant mechanism and this reentry usually involves the atrioventricular node. The reentry may be confined wholly within the A-V node or may include parts of the atrium, ventricle, A-V conduction system, as well as an accessory pathway connecting the atrium and the ventricle. Although A-V nodal reentrant paroxysmal supraventricular tachycardia is the most common type of reentrant supraventricular tachycardia, verapamil has been used successfully in all reentrant supraventricular tachycardias for termination of the arrhythmia. In this group of patients, two functionally different electrophysiologic pathways exist. Sustained reentry is dependent upon a fortuitous balancing of conduction and refractoriness, such that the electrical impulse can traverse one path and then the other in sequence and establish a self-perpetuating electrical circuit. Verapamil effectively terminates this reentrant circuit by altering conduction and refractoriness within the A-V nodal segment of the reentrant circuit. This process occurs in any supraventricular tachycardia which involves the A-V node.

The majority of studies investigating the ability of verapamil or diltiazem to terminate supraventricular tachycardia have shown both calcium channel-blocking agents to be highly effective in terminating all types of reentrant paroxysmal supraventricular tachycardia. In a review of the literature, greater than 80% of episodes convert to normal sinus rhythm within minutes of intravenous administration of verapamil. One typical study reported by Sung and co-workers (1980) showed that verapamil converted 15 of 19 episodes of supraventricular tachycardia to sinus rhythm. These patients had supraventricular tachycardia of diverse mechanisms both with and without accessory pathways. In those patients in whom the tachycardia was not terminated, the rate of the tachycardia was usually significantly reduced.

The recommended doses for treatment of paroxysmal supraventricular tachycardia is 0.075–0.15 mg/kg infused over 1–3 min. The usual dose used in adults is 5 or 10 mg intravenously and infused rapidly. The rate of conversion is reduced when lower doses are used or when infusion rates are slower. The effective plasma verapamil concentration at the time of arrhythmia termination generally exceeds 100 ng/ml. It has been suggested that those patients who do not respond to verapamil may have lower verapamil blood levels and further drug administration may terminate the arrhythmia (Sung et al., 1980).

Mild hypotension frequently occurs but is rarely clinically significant. The termination of the arrhythmia and restoration of normal sinus rhythm usually more than compensate for the peripheral effects of the verapamil. It is important to remember that hypotension or bradyarrhythmias may follow the conversion of the arrhythmia.

Studies comparing verapamil to β-blockers for termination of supraventricular tachycardia have not been performed. However, as in the treatment of atrial fibrillation, certain obvious advantages attend the use of verapamil. The rapid onset of action is a distinct advantage. In addition, the ability to use the drug in the presence of bronchospastic disorders or other contraindications for β-blocker use is a significant advantage. Once intravenous calcium channel blockers have been administered, it is dangerous and contraindicated to administer an intravenous β-blocker. At present, intravenous verapamil should be considered the drug of first choice for treatment of paroxysmal supraventricular tachycardia.

The use of oral verapamil in the chronic prophylactic treatment of paroxysmal supraventricular tachycardia has been recently studied. It is reported to be effective in chronic oral use (Wu et al., 1983; Lie et al., 1983; Mauritson et al., 1982).

Diltiazem recently has been reported to be effective for chronic suppressive therapy and may be an effective long term prophylactic agent for this indication (Yeh et al., 1983).

Ventricular Arrhythmias

Although considerable evidence exists in experimental preparation to suggest that calcium channel-blocking drug may be effective against ventricular arrhythmias, little clinical evidence supports this. Verapamil has been found to be of little effect in suppressing sustained ventricular tachycardia (Heng et al., 1975; Wellens et al., 1977). Similarly, in the NAMIS study in which the calcium-blocking agent nifedipine was used in myocardial infarction patients, no beneficial effect was noted in regard to subsequent ventricular arrhythmias (Muller et al., 1983). Conflicting data do, however, exist and further study is necessary.

References

Betriu, A., Chaitman, B.R., Bourassa, M.G., Brevers, G., Scholl, J., Bruneau, P., Gague, P., and Chabot, M. 1983. Beneficial effect of intravenous diltiazem in the acute management of paroxysmal supraventricular tachyarrhythmias. Circulation 67:88–94.

Brooks, W.W., Verrier, R.L., and Lown, B. 1980. Protective effect of verapamil on vulnerability to ventricular fibrillation during myocardial ischemia and reperfusion. Cardiovasc Res 14:295–302.

Cranefield, P.F. 1975. The Conduction of the Cardiac Impulse. Mt. Kisco, New York: Futura Publishing Co.

Cranefield, P.F., Aronson, R.S., and Wit, A.L. 1974. Effect of verapamil on the normal action potential and on a calcium-dependent slow response of canine cardiac Purkinje fibers. Circ Res 34:204–213.

Elharrar, J., Gaum, W.E., and Zipes, D.P. 1977. Effects of drugs on conduction delay and incidence of ventricular arrhythmias induced by acute coronary occlusion in dogs. Am J Cardiol 39:544–549.

El-Sherif, N., and Lazarra, R. 1979. Reentrant ventricular arrhythmias in the late myocardial infarction period. 7. Effect of verapamil and 0-600 and the role of the "slow channel." Circulation 60:605–615.

Fleckenstein, A. 1971. In: P. Harris and L.H. Opie, eds. Specific Inhibitors and Promoters of Calcium Action in the Excitation—Contraction Coupling of Heart Muscle and their Role in the Prevention of Production of Myocardial Lesions, in Calcium and the Heart. pp. 135–188. New York: Academic Press.

Fondacaro, I.D., Han, J., and Yoon, M.S. 1978. Effects of verapamil on ventricular rhythm during acute coronary occlusion. Am Heart J 96:81–86.

Gulamhussein, S., Ko, P., Carruthers, S., and Klein, G.J. 1981. Acceleration of the ventricular responses during atrial fibrillation in the Wolff-Parkinson-White syndrome after verapamil. Circulation 65:348–354.

Hagemeijer, F. 1978. Verapamil in the management of supraventricular tachyarrhythmias occurring after a recent myocardial infarction. Circulation 57:751–755.

Heng, M.K., Singh, B.N., Roche, A.H.G., Norris, R.M., and Mercer, C.J. 1975. Effects of intravenous verapamil on cardiac arrhythmias and on the electrocardiogram. Am Heart J 90:487–498.

Kawai, C., Tomotsuga, K., Matsuyama, E., and Okazaki, H. 1981. Comparative effects of three calcium antagonists, diltiazem, verapamil, and nifedipine on the sinoatrial and atrioventricular nodes. Experimental and clinical studies. Circulation 63:1035–1042.

Klein, H.O., Pauzner, H., and DiSegni, E. 1979. The beneficial effects of verapamil in chronic atrial fibrillation. Ann Intern Med 139:747–749.

Lie, K.I., Duren, D.R., Manger Cats, D., David, G.K., and Durrer, D. 1983. Long-term efficacy of verapamil in the treatment of paroxysmal supraventricular tachycardias. Am Heart J 105:668.

Mauritson, D.R., Winniford, M.D., Walker, S., Rude, R.E., Cary, J.R., and Hillis, L.D. 1982. Oral verapamil for paroxysmal supraventricular tachycardia. Ann Intern Med 96:409–412.

Melville, K.I., Barvey, H.L., and Shister, H.E. 1968. On the cardiac adrenergic blocking action of iproveratril in normal and coronary ligated dogs. Can J Comp Med 27:225–230.

Morganroth, J., Chen, C.C., Sturm, S., and Dreifus, L.S. 1982. Oral verapamil in the treatment of atrial fibrillation/flutter. Am J Cardiol 49:981.

Muller, J., Morrison, J., Stone, P., Rude, R., Rosner, B., Roberts, R., Pearle, D., Turi, Z., Schneider, J., Serfas, D., Hennekens, C., and Braunwald, E. 1983. Nifedipine therapy for threatened and acute myocardial infarction: A randomized double blind comparison. Circulation 68:III–120.

Plumb, V.J., Karp, R.B., Kouchous, N.T., Zorn, G.L., James, T.N., and Waldo, A.L. 1982. Verapamil therapy of atrial fibrillation and atrial flutter following cardiac operation. J Thorac Cardiovasc Surg 83:590–596.

Ribeiro, L.G.T., Brandon, T.A., Debauche, T.L., et al. 1981. Antiarrhythmic and hemodynamic effects of calcium channel blocking agents during coronary arterial reperfusion. Am J Cardiol 48:69–74.

Rosen, M.R., and Daniel, P. 1982. Effects of tetrodotoxin, lidocaine, verapamil and AHR-2666 ouabain induced delayed after depolarization in canine Purkinje fibers. Circ Res 46:117–124.

Rosen, M.R., Ilvento, D.P., Gelband, H., and Merkier, C. 1974. Effects of verapamil on electrophysiologic properties of canine Purkinje fibers. J Pharmacol Exp Ther 189:414–422.

Rowland, E., Evans, T., and Krickler, D. 1979. Effect of nifedipine on atrioventricular conduction as compared with verapamil: Intracardiac electrophysiology study. Br Heart J 42:124–127.

Sakumi, M., Yasuda, H., Kato, N., Nomura, A., Fujita, M., Nishino, T., Fujita, K., Koike, Y., and Saito, H. 1983. Acute and chronic effects of verapamil on patients with paroxysmal supraventricular tachycardia. Am Heart J 105:619–628.

Schamroth, L. 1971. Immediate effects of intravenous verapamil on atrial fibrillation. Cardiovasc Res 5:419–424.

Singh, B.N., Ellrodt, G., and Peter, C.T. 1978. Verapamil: A review of its pharmacological properties and therapeutic use. Drugs 15:169–197.

Singh, B.N., and Nademanie, K. 1983. Calcium Antagonists and Control of Cardiac Arrhythmias, Baylor College of Medicine. Cardiology Series. 6:6.

Sung, R.J., Elser, B., and McAllister, R.G. 1980. Intravenous verapamil for termination of reentrant supraventricular tachycardias. Ann Intern Med 93:682–689.

Tse, W.W., and Han, J. 1975. Effects of manganese chloride and verapamil on automaticity of digitalized Purkinje fibers. Am J Cardiol 36:50–55.

Waxman, H.L., Myerburg, R.J., Appel, R., and Sung, R.J. 1981. Verapamil for control of ventricular rate in paroxysmal supraventricular tachycardia and atrial fibrillation or flutter. Ann Intern Med 94:1–6.

Wellens, H.J.J., Bar, F.W., Lie, K.I., Duren, D.R., and Dohmen, H.J. 1977. Effects of procainamide, propranolol and verapamil on mechanism of tachycardia in patients with chronic recurrent ventricular tachycardia. Am J Cardiol 40:579–585.

Wit, A.L., Rosen, M.R., and Hoffman, B.F. 1974a. Relationship of normal and abnormal electrical activity of cardiac fibers to the genesis of arrhythmias I. Automaticity. Am Heart J 88:515–524.

Wit, A.L., Rosen, M.R., and Hoffman, B.F. 1974b. Relationship of normal and abnormal electrical activity of cardiac fibers to the genesis of arrhythmias II. Reentry section I. Am Heart J 88:664–670.

Wit, A.L., Rosen, M.R., and Hoffman, B.F. 1974c. Relationship of normal and abnormal electrical activity of cardiac fibers to the genesis of arrhythmias. II. Reentry section II. Am Heart J 88:798–807.

Wu, D., Kou, H., Yeh, S., Lin, F., and Hung, J. 1983. Effects of oral verapamil in patients with atrioventricular reentrant tachycardia incorporating an accessory pathway. Circulation 67:426–433.

Yeh, S., Kou, H., Lin, F., Hung, J., and Wu, D. 1983. Effects of oral diltiazem in paroxysmal supraventricular tachycardia. Am J Cardiol 52:271–278.

Zipes, D.P., and Fischer, J.C. 1974. Effects of agents which inhibit the slow channel on sinus node automaticity and atrioventricular conduction in the dog. Circ Res 34:184–192.

EDITOR'S NOTES

Antiarrhythmic Effects of Calcium Channel-Blocking Drugs (Class IV)

In the past decade, the calcium channel-blocking agents have been shown to have a wide therapeutic spectrum in cardiovascular diseases, leading to intense investigations in a variety of pathophysiologic settings. Such investigations have established the clinical utility of calcium channel-blocking drugs in certain settings, but they have also prompted additional research that has significantly advanced our understanding of the cell membrane and subcellular metabolic processes related to calcium regulation. The calcium channel is a complex structure that is expertly reviewed by Green and Watanabe. Interactions of various ions, intracellular enzymes, and drugs such as calcium channel and beta-adrenergic-blocking agents are interrelated and are discussed as such. With respect to arrhythmias, however, a great deal of this information is as yet of only tentative clinical importance. Although many calcium-related abnormal electrophysiologic processes have been identified in isolated tissue, the applicability of these arrhythmic mechanisms to the clinical situation is controversial. Without question, certain calcium channel blockers have profound effects on atrial and A-V nodal electrophysiologic parameters, and this, in turn, has a beneficial effect in the treatment of supraventricular or A-V nodal arrhythmias. More importantly, however, the potential utility of these agents in arrhythmias related specifically to abnormalities of the calcium channel has not been verified in clinical situations, and thus the use of calcium channel blockers for ventricular antiarrhythmic indications and during ischemia remains unsettled. One possible exception regarding ventricular arrhythmias, where calcium-blocking agents may have a certain degree of efficacy, is in the setting of reperfusion arrhythmias. However, these constitute a minor subset of arrhythmias and are not well understood at the clinical level. A major, ultimate impact of calcium blockers may be in the setting of ischemia or infarct size reduction, which could have an indirect influence on the development of arrhythmias since ischemia-related arrhythmias are common.

Part III

Therapeutic Applications of Antiarrhythmic Drugs: Cutting Across Drug Classifications

Chapter 19

Can Antiarrhythmic Drugs Prevent Sudden Death?

Philip J. Podrid

Introduction

Sudden death remains one of the major challenges facing the medical profession, afflicting more than 400,000 Americans each year (Lown, 1979). The magnitude of the problem is enormous not only in the United States but in every industrialized nation. Although the most common underlying cardiac abnormality is coronary heart disease, sudden cardiac death afflicts those with other types of cardiac lesions as well as patients without any definable abnormality (Table 19-1). The

Table 19-1 Causes of Sudden Cardiac Death.

Cardiac
Ischemic
Coronary artery disease with or without myocardial infarction
Coronary artery embolism
Nonatherogenic coronary artery disease
Nonischemic
Cardiomyopathy (obstructive and nonobstructive)
Valvular heart disease (aortic stenosis, mitral valve prolapse)
Congenital heart disease
Prolonged QT syndromes
Preexcitation syndromes
Complete heart block
Arrhythmogenic right ventricular dysplasia
Myocarditis
Acute pericardial tamponade
No structural heart disease (primary electrical disease)
Noncardiac
Sudden infant death syndrome
Drowning
Pickwickian syndrome
Cor pulmonale
Pulmonary embolism
Drug-induced
Airway obstruction

demonstration that sudden cardiac death is the result of ventricular fibrillation (VF) has focused attention on the ventricular premature beat (VPB) (Lown and Ruberman, 1970). It has long been felt that the VPB is the clinical marker for the patient at risk for sudden death. Once VPBs are identified, antiarrhythmic drugs are prescribed for their suppression. However, it is unclear if such therapy will prevent the occurrence of VF. To answer this question, those at risk for sudden death should be treated. Although coronary artery disease is the most frequent cardiac problem associated with sudden death, the annual sudden death mortality in this group of patients is only 2–3% (Stamler, 1962). A randomized study to evaluate the role of antiarrhythmic drugs for preventing sudden death in such patients would require several thousand subjects. Such a study would be limited further by the frequent occurrence of side effects resulting from each of the available antiarrhythmic drugs and the potential for arrhythmia aggravation (Velebit et al., 1982). Patients with a myocardial infarction (MI) represent a subset of those with coronary artery disease who are at an increased risk for sudden death during the first year after the event (Hunt et al., 1977; Moss et al., 1976). There have been a number of studies in this group of patients which have addressed the issue of drug effectiveness for preventing sudden cardiac death.

Randomized Trials

Membrane-Active Drugs

Lidocaine Since the advent of the coronary care unit (CCU), lidocaine has been administered routinely to patients with an acute myocardial infarction to treat as well as prevent ventricular arrhythmia (Lown and Vassaux, 1968). Such therapy has substantially reduced the mortality from VF in the CCU during the immediate post-MI period. However, it has been unclear if the improved survival is a result of lidocaine therapy or the intensive medical care offered.

There have been a number of randomized lidocaine-placebo trials to evaluate the efficacy of lidocaine for preventing VF during the periinfarction period (Table 19-2). Bennet and co-workers (1970) and Chopra and co-workers (1971) showed no difference in the incidence of ventricular arrhythmia or in mortality between lidocaine-treated patients and those receiving placebo. Pitt and co-workers (1970) and Morgensen (1970) also reported that lidocaine did not affect mortality, although they did observe that the incidence of ventricular arrhythmia was significantly reduced. However, in these studies, a low and probably subtherapeutic dose of lidocaine was administered by bolus followed by a constant iv infusion. Valentine and co-workers (1974) and Lie and co-workers (1974) used higher doses of lidocaine (over 1 mg/min) and reported a significant decrease in mortality in those patients who received the drug.

Table 19-2 Results of Randomized Trials with Membrane-Stabilizing Drugs.

Study	Drug	Number of Patients	Duration of Therapy	Mortality or VF Control	Drug	P
				%	%	
Morgensen	Lidocaine	79	Days	11	12	NS
Chopra	Lidocaine	82	Days	—	—	NS
Bennett	Lidocaine	610	Days	7	16	NS
Pitt	Lidocaine	224	Days	—	—	NS
Lie	Lidocaine	212	Days	10	0	<0.05
Valentine	Lidocaine	269	Days	7	2	<0.05
Holmberg	Quinidine	104	15 days	7.2	10.7	NS
Bloomfield	Quinidine	53	5 days	0	0	NS
Jones	Quinidine	103	72 h	12.4	8.9	NS
Jennings	Disopyramide	95	1 yr	10.2	4.3	NS
Zainal	Disopyramide	60	3 wk	26.7	3.3	<0.05
Collaborative	Phenytoin	568	1 yr	11.0	9.4	NS
Peter	Phenytoin	150	2 yr	18	24	NS
Koch Weser	Procainamide	70	2–3 wk	6.1	0	<0.05
Kosowsky	Procainamide	78	1 yr	10.3	3.7	<0.05
Campbell	Mexiletine	97	48 h	3.8	2.3	NS
Chamberlain	Mexiletine	344	1 yr	11.6	13.2	NS
Campbell	Tocainide	68	?	?	?	?
Ryden	Tocainide	112	6 mos	8.9	8.9	NS
Hugenholtz	Aprindine	193	1 yr	9.3	7.3	NS

The results of these studies strongly suggest that lidocaine prophylactically infused at higher doses of 2–3 mg/min after a loading bolus is effective for suppressing ventricular arrhythmia and preventing VF in the setting of an acute MI.

Quinidine Quinidine has long been used for therapy of atrial arrhythmias and has become a first-line agent for ventricular arrhythmia. There have been several studies using oral quinidine in the post MI period (Table 19-2). Holmberg and Bergman (1967) administered quinidine sulfate 600 mg b.i.d. to 49 patients with an acute myocardial infarction while 55 received placebo. Therapy was continued for only 15 days after the infarction. Although quinidine reduced the frequency of ventricular arrhythmia as judged by ausculation, mortality was not affected. Bloomfield and co-workers (1971) utilized a higher dose of quinidine, but therapy was limited to only 5 days. In the group of 53 patients, quinidine substantially reduced the frequency of arrhythmia compared to placebo, but there were no deaths in either group. Jones and co-workers (1974) treated 103 patients for 72 h with quinidine or placebo. Quinidine significantly reduced all ventricular arrhythmias including ventricular tachycardia (VT), as well as uniformed and multiformed VPBs. Total mortality was lower on quinidine compared to placebo (8.9% versus 10.4%), but this was not statistically significant.

As was observed with lidocaine, quinidine was effective for suppressing ventricular arrhythmias, but it was without significant effect on mortality. However, the dose of quinidine used in these studies was low and therapy was for a brief period of time. The effect of quinidine on long-term mortality after an MI is not answered by these studies.

Disopyramide In two studies, disopyramide was administered to patients after an MI (Table 19-2). Jennings and co-workers (1976) gave a dose of 400 mg daily to 40 patients, while 49 received placebo. These investigators observed that there was a significant decrease in the incidence of serious ventricular arrhythmias in patients receiving disopyramide and additional interventions were less often required. There was a reduction in the 1-year mortality among those receiving disopyramide, but the difference was not significant. The authors excluded patients who had complex arrhythmia including salvos of VT, early VPBs, or more than 5 VPBs/min, therefore eliminating from study those patients with more serious arrhythmia who are at greatest risk for a major tachyarrhythmia or sudden death. In a study of 58 patients with an acute MI admitted to an open ward, Zainal and co-workers (1977) found that disopyramide significantly reduced the incidence of VT, VF, and total mortality.

Like quinidine, disopyramide suppresses ventricular arrhythmia in patients postinfarction. The study by Jennings and co-workers demonstrated a small and insignificant reduction in 1-year mortality in the group receiving disopyramide. The lack of significance may reflect the small number of patients studied as well as the exclusion of those patients with complex arrhythmia. Although Zainal and co-workers reported a significant benefit from disopyramide, it is unclear how patients were monitored and arrhythmia detected. Since the endpoint for the study was death, these limitations do not negate the finding that mortality was reduced in the treatment group.

Phenytoin Phenytoin, primarily an anticonvulsive agent, has antiarrhythmic effects although it is not a first-line agent. A long half-life, once-a-day dosing and infrequency of side effects when used long term make it an attractive agent for use in randomized trials in patients postinfarction (Table 19-2). In 1971, a multicenter trial with phenytoin in patients with an acute MI was reported (Collaborative Group, 1971). Phenytoin at a dose of 300–400 mg daily, was administered to 283 patients, while placebo (3–4 mg of phenytoin) was used in 285 patients. Those receiving phenytoin reported a reduction in symptomatic palpitations, while there was a decrease in VPBs observed on the electrocardiogram. After a year's follow-up, there was no difference in mortality.

In a second study, Peter and co-workers (1978) used 400 mg of phenytoin daily in 74 patients, while 76 patients received placebo. Unlike other studies, these authors included patients with congestive heart failure, conduction abnormalities, and atrial and complex ventricular arrhythmias. Mortality after 2 years was not different between the placebo and phenytoin groups. There was no benefit from drug therapy in any subset of patients, which included those with mechanical and electrical abnormalities.

Although patient compliance during long term phenytoin treatment is good, this drug has no beneficial effect on survival in patients after a myocardial infarction. This lack of efficacy is in agreement with the poor results of phenytoin therapy for treatment of chronic ventricular arrhythmia.

Procainamide Two studies used oral procainamide in patients after a MI (Table 19-2). Koch Weser and co-workers (1969) administered procainamide to 37 patients, while 33 received placebo. After a loading dose of 1 g, 250–500 mg were given every 3 h. Treatment was continued for only several days. Compared to placebo, procainamide significantly reduced the frequency and severity of ventricular arrhythmia. There were no episodes of VF in patients receiving procainamide, while two patients receiving placebo had VF. These authors concluded that procainamide was effective for suppressing ventricular arrhythmia and preventing sudden death in the immediate post-MI period. Kosowsky and co-workers (1973) reported on long term use of procainamide in patients following an acute MI. In this study, 39 patients were discharged on drug, while 39 were treated with placebo. However, side effects were frequent and only eight patients continued procainamide for more than 3 months. Nevertheless, the occurrence of major ventricular arrhythmia and sudden death was significantly reduced in the treatment group.

Both studies demonstrate that procainamide is an effective agent for suppression of major ventricular arrhythmias and prevention of sudden death in the immediate postinfarction period. When therapy with procainamide was continued for a year after the MI, there was a significant reduction in the frequency of tachyarrhythmias and sudden death. However, frequent side effects necessitated drug discontinuation in a majority of patients and only a small number could continue therapy for more than 3 months. Its usefulness for long term prophylactic therapy is limited by the need for frequent dosing and the high incidence of side effects.

Mexiletine Mexiletine is an investigational antiarrhythmic agent in the United States, but there have been two European studies using this drug in patients after an MI (Table 19-2). Campbell and co-workers (1979) administered mexiletine to 44 patients while 55 received placebo. A loading dose of 600 mg was followed by 250 mg t.i.d. for 48 h. Mexiletine significantly reduced the incidence of VPBs and VT, but mortality was not affected. Two patients receiving placebo died compared to one on mexiletine. Of importance is that patients were withdrawn if frequent complex ventricular arrhythmia occurred necessitating therapy with lidocaine.

In the second study, Chamberlain and co-workers (1980) administered mexiletine to 181 patients and placebo to 163 patients. Therapy was started 6–14 days after the infarction and continued for 1 year. The investigators observed that the presence of frequent VPBs, couplets, or VT on the entry ambulatory monitor was associated with an increased mortality. Compared to placebo, mexiletine reduced the frequency of VPBs on a repeat monitor, but the occurrence of VT was not affected. Mortality was equivalent in the treated and placebo groups. However, 7 of the 24 patients in the mexiletine group died after the drug was withdrawn because of side effects.

As with quinidine and disopyramide, mexiletine was ineffective for preventing sudden death after infarction. However, in the study by Campbell, therapy was limited to 48 h and patients with significant arrhythmia requiring lidocaine were withdrawn. It is difficult to draw any valid conclusions from this study. Similar to observations of other authors, Chamberlain and co-workers reported that the 1-year mortality was higher in patients who had complex arrhythmia. When mexiletine was administered in a fixed dose the arrhythmias were not suppressed, and importantly mortality was not reduced.

Tocainide Tocainide, an oral form of lidocaine, was reported by Campbell and co-workers (1979) to significantly reduce the incidence of ventricular arrhythmia and prevent VT in patients admitted to the CCU with a suspected or documented MI (Table 19-2). The authors did not specify the duration of therapy and effect on mortality was not commented upon. Ryden and co-workers (1980) administered intravenous tocainide followed by long term oral therapy to 56 patients. Although tocainide reduced the frequency of ventricular arrhythmia during the first 24 h, after 1 month and at 6 months in those receiving tocainide compared to those on placebo, there was no significant reduction in mortality. However, tocainide blood levels were low, suggesting that an inadequate dose was used.

Lidocaine is an effective prophylactic agent for preventing serious ventricular arrhythmia when administered during the early phases of an acute MI. However, it can only be given intravenously, precluding long term use. Tocainide, the oral form of lidocaine, is an effective antiarrhythmic agent for preventing major ventricular arrhythmia and sudden death during the first few days after an infarction, but the long term results are disappointing. However, in the study by Ryden, the blood levels of tocainide were low. It is unclear if a higher dose and blood level of drug would have improved survival, but the results do suggest that individual titration of dose is important.

Aprindine Aprindine is an oral lidocaine congener that has a long half-life and can be given twice per day. There has been one study utilizing this agent in post-MI patients (Table 19-2). The Ghent Rotterdam trial involved 310 patients randomized to aprindine or placebo (Hugenholtz et al., 1978). In a preliminary report, aprindine did not alter the incidence of sudden death in a group of 193 patients who were treated for at least 1 year. There was a reduction in the frequency of complex ventricular arrhythmia on monitoring (Hagemeijer, 1978).

As observed with other membrane-active drugs, aprindine suppresses ventricular arrhythmia for up to 1 year after an MI. However, the preliminary results do not show any protective effect against sudden death.

Summary and Conclusions There have been a number of randomized trials evaluating the efficacy of the membrane-active antiarrhythmic drugs in patients after an MI. Results from these studies have been disappointing and they provide no support for the role of these drugs in the prevention of sudden cardiac death after an MI. However, there are a number of serious problems with these studies, which may account for the lack of benefit:

1. The populations studied were small. The endpoint of the trial, sudden death, is a relatively low frequency event. Larger numbers of patients would be necessary to establish a significant difference from any intervention.
2. The frequency and type of arrhythmia observed in the patients before or during therapy are not reported. Methods for arrhythmia evaluation and duration of observation varied and included ausculation, ECG rhythm strips, observation of a bedside monitor, and rarely ambulatory monitoring. Since monitoring of arrhythmia was inadequate, drug effect is uncertain.
3. Little information is supplied about how the endpoint of each study was documented.
4. Patients were entered into the study and treated in a random double-blind fashion. There was no attention given to entry arrhythmia or the effect of the drug on arrhythmia.
5. There were no criteria provided for what constituted drug efficacy.
6. Only short term therapy was used.in many of the trials and any conclusion about the role of the drug on improving long term survival cannot be determined.
7. There are no data supplied about other therapies that may have been given during the course of the trial. The use of other drugs may have directly affected the outcome or could have resulted in important drug interactions.
8. A fixed dose of drug was used in most of the trials. There was no attempt to adjust or titrate dose to the occurrence of side effects or effect on ventricular arrhythmia. Drug levels could vary widely within the patient group.
9. The occurrence of drug-induced side effects limit their usefulness during long term treatment. A high frequency of "drop outs" could affect the outcome.
10. Patient compliance was not assessed in these trials. Compliance is especially important since multiple doses were used. Moreover, each drug has side effects which limit patient acceptance. Failure to take the drug might have accounted for the lack of effect.
11. Each of the antiarrhythmic drugs can aggravate arrhythmia and provoke serious ectopy (Velebit et al., 1982). This potential complication was not addressed in any of the reported studies (Fig. 19-1).

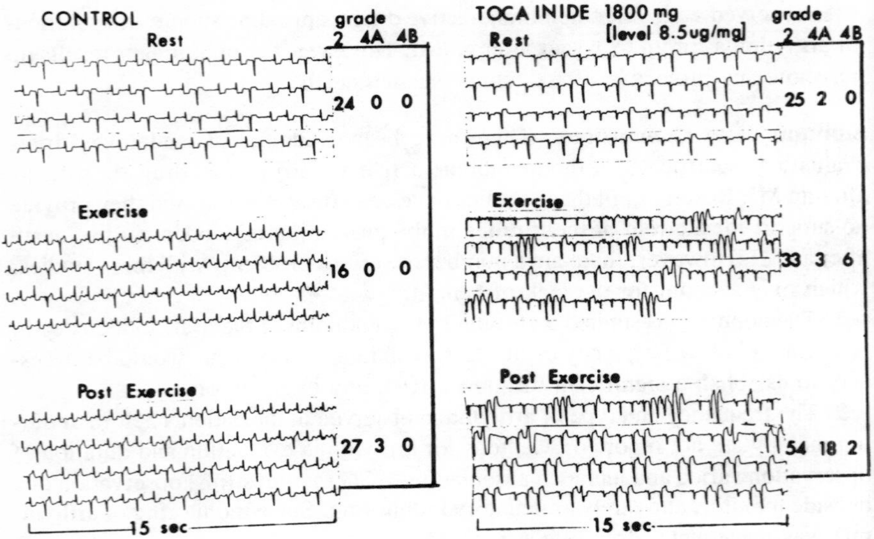

19-1 Aggravation of arrhythmia. During the control period, before drug administration, frequent ventricular premature beats (grade 2) are present at rest and during exercise. During the postexercise recovery period, couplets (grade 4A) are observed. After 3 days of tocainide therapy, the number of couplets has increased and salvos of ventricular tachycardia (grade 4B) are now present.

Although the results of the many trials do not support the role of antiarrhythmic drugs for suppression of sudden death, most studies have serious problems and limitations. The most important is that in none of the studies was therapy directed at arrhythmia suppression. There was no attempt to guide therapy by the elimination of those arrhythmias associated with sudden death.

β-Adrenergic Blocking Agents

The β-adrenergic blocking drugs have also been evaluated in patients after an MI and there are now many such studies (Table 19-3). The first trial was by Snow and Manc (1965) who reported that therapy with propranolol for 1 month significantly reduced the incidence of sudden death. However, a multicenter study in 1966 involving 195 patients failed to confirm these findings. Studies by Balcon and co-workers (1966) and Norris and co-workers (1968) also failed to support the beneficial effect of propranolol on survival after a myocardial infarction. It should be pointed out that therapy with propranolol in these studies was continued for only 28 days, and the doses of drugs used (60–80 mg daily) were low. Similar to the studies with the membrane-active drugs, the number of patients studied was

Table 19-3 Results of Randomized Trials with β-Blocking Drugs.

Study	Drug	Number of Patients	Duration of Therapy	Sudden Death Control %	Sudden Death Drug %	Sudden Death P
Snow, Manc	Propranolol	101	28 days	12.0	6.0	<0.03
Multicenter	Propranolol	195	28 days	9.3	7.1	NS
Balcon	Propranolol	114	28 days	10.5	12.3	NS
Norris	Propranolol	454	3 wk	7.5	8.8	NS
BHAT	Propranolol	3,857	3 yr	4.6	3.3	<0.01
Norwegian	Propranolol	560	1 yr	8.2	4.0	0.038
Wilhelmsson	Alprenolol	230	2 yr	9.6	2.6	<0.05
Ahlmack	Alprenolol	162	1 yr	11.1	1.2	<0.05
Anderson	Alprenolol	282	1 yr	20.6	9.2	<0.01*
Multicenter	Practolol	3,038	1 yr	3.6	2.0	<0.01
Hjarlmarsen	Metoprolol	1,395	90 days	8.9	5.7	<0.03*
Norwegian	Timolol	1,884	33 mos	13.9	7.7	<0.001
Julian	Sotalol	1,456	1 yr	8.9	7.3	NS
Taylor	Oxprenolol	1,103	6 yr	9.3	8.2	NS*

*Total cardiac mortality

small and there are no data about the type and frequency of arrhythmia present before and during therapy. Treatment was not directed against arrhythmia, but was random.

In 1982, the results of the Beta Blocking Heart Attack Trial (BHAT) were reported (BHAT Research Group, 1982). This multicenter trial involved 3857 patients randomized to placebo or propranolol therapy at a dose of 120 or 240 mg daily as guided by blood levels. After an average follow-up of 25 months, there was a 26% reduction in both total cardiac mortality and sudden cardiac death in the propranolol-treated group. These findings were supported by results from a multicenter Norwegian trial involving 560 patients treated with 160 mg of propranolol or placebo for 1 year (Hansteen et al., 1982).

Other β-adrenergic blocking agents have been used in randomized trials and the results support the beneficial effect of those drugs. Wilhelmsson and co-workers (1974) and Ahlmack and co-workers (1974) independently reported that alprenolol significantly reduced the incidence of sudden cardiac death after an MI, although in a study by Anderson and co-workers (1974), the reduction of the incidence of sudden death was observed only in patients less than 65 years of age. A multicenter practolol trial involving 3,038 patients reported a significant reduction in the incidence of sudden death during a one year follow-up (Multicenter Study, 1977). However, this reduction in mortality was primarily in patients with an anterior wall infarction. In a 90-day trial with metoprolol, the incidence of sudden death was decreased in all patient subgroups (Hjalmarsen et al., 1981). A timolol study involving 1884 patients showed a 44% reduction in mortality from sudden death after a 3-year follow-up (Norwegian Study Group, 1981). Although many different β-adrenergic blocking agents may partially protect against sudden death post MI, this effect does not appear to be a class effect as not all of the β-adrenergic blocking agents are of benefit. A trial with sotalol failed to show a reduction in mortality (Julian et al., 1982). This observation is interesting since this drug also prolongs action potential duration and has direct antiarrhythmic effects independent of its β-blocking activity. In a study by Taylor and co-workers (1982), oxyprenolol was without any effect when the entire population was analyzed. However, when the patients were subdivided into three groups, differences were observed. In the first group, oxyprenolol therapy was initiated within the first 4 months after an infarction. The 6-year survival rate was 95% in those receiving oxyprenolol compared with 77% for those on placebo. However, when oxyprenolol therapy was begun 5–12 months after infarction (group 2) survival was not affected. In group 3, in which oxyprenolol therapy was initiated more than 12 months after an infarction, survival was reduced compared to placebo (79% versus 92%). It can be concluded that the protective effect of oxyprenolol occurs during the first 4–6 months after a myocardial infarction while initiation of drug therapy after this period is without benefit. It is of interest that in the BHAT study with propranolol and in the Norwegian timolol trial, the improvement in survival primarily occurs during the first 6 months with the curves becoming parallel thereafter. This finding is important since epidemiologic studies report that the risk of sudden death is greatest during the first 6 months after an MI.

Overall, the results of the β-blocking drug trials are very encouraging. However (like the studies with membrane drugs), there are a number of methodologic problems which urge caution in interpretation. Although the β-blocker trials involved large numbers of patients, the majority of patients (admitted to hospital with an MI) who could have entered were excluded. In the BHAT and Norwegian propranolol studies 77% of patients were excluded because of contraindications to β-blocker therapy (CHF, conduction abnormalities, bradycardia, lung disease) or the need for β-blockers to treat other conditions (angina, hypertension, or arrhythmia). Patients already receiving β-blockers or those who might require surgical intervention were also excluded. Additionally, the Norwegian propranolol study eliminated patients who were "low risk" (a term not defined), patients under 35 or over 70 and those needing antiarrhythmic drugs. These trials therefore excluded those patients at highest risk and only patients expected to do well were entered. This is apparent from the low mortality in patients receiving placebo. A major problem is the absence of any data regarding presence of ventricular arrhythmia prior to therapy or effect of the β-blocker on the arrhythmia in survivors and those who died. These studies do not address the mechanism of the protective effect nor do they provide guidelines about duration of therapy or required dose.

It can be concluded that in certain subsets of patients, the β-adrenergic blocking agents may protect against sudden death after an MI. This beneficial effect is especially apparent during the first 6 months postinfarction, although the mechanism is not known. Many of the agents of this class are effective suggesting that interference with catecholamine activity on the heart may be important. The effect of these drugs on ventricular arrhythmia is unknown since such data during long term therapy were not reported in any of the studies.

There are many randomized trials with membrane-active drugs and β-adrenergic blocking agents, but the results are not decisive. It remains unclear if antiarrhythmic drugs will prevent sudden death in high risk patients after an infarction, in survivors of out-of-hospital sudden cardiac death, or in the much larger group of patients with coronary artery disease who are at risk. What emerges from these studies is that drug therapy cannot be administered in a uniform and nondirected way. It is clear that no one drug or dose will be effective for every patient but that therapy must be "tailored" to the individual. Since VPBs are the clinical manifestation of underlying electrical instability of the myocardium, therapy must be directed at their suppression. Thus, there is need for a systematic approach to drug therapy.

Ventricular Premature Beats: Their Role in Sudden Cardiac Death

The ventricular premature beat (VPB) has long been felt to be the harbinger of more serious arrhythmia. An important issue that should be addressed is the relationship between the VPB and sudden cardiac death. There is mounting epidemiologic evidence that there exists a close causal association. Hinkle and co-workers (1969) utilized 6-h monitoring in 665 asymptomatic men and categorized the frequency of arrhythmia as the number of VPBs per 1000 complexes. After a $2^1/_2$ year follow-up these investigators observed a direct relationship between the frequency of VPBs and yearly cardiac mortality. Other studies have also associated the presence of VPBs with cardiac death. However, VPBs themselves are ubiquitous and can be demonstrated in 88–90% of those with coronary artery disease (Lown et al., 1975; Calvert et al., 1977). Since VPBs are present in almost all patients with coronary artery disease, their very presence cannot be a risk factor for sudden cardiac death.

In the early days of the coronary care unit, Lown and Wolf (1971) observed an association between certain types of ventricular ectopy and the occurrence of sustained malignant ventricular arrhythmia. On the basis of these observations, they developed a grading system for ventricular premature beats (Table 19-4). It was implicit in this system that the higher grades or complex forms of arrhythmia were more serious and imparted enhanced risk. Although this grading system was empiric, based only on observation, subsequent studies have confirmed that the higher grades of ventricular arrhythmia, primarily repetitive forms, are associated with an increased risk of sudden death.

Table 19-4 Lown Grading System of Ventricular Premature Beats (VPBs).

Grade	
0	No VPBs
1A	<30 VPBs/h and <1/min
1B	<30 VPBs/h and occasionally >1/min
2	>30 VPBs/h
3	Multiform VPB
4A	Repetitive VPBs-couplets
4B	Repetitive VPBs-ventricular tachycardia (>3 sequential)
5	Early R on T VPBs

Vismara and co-workers (1975) reported that complex arrhythmia was twice as frequent in those who died post-MI compared with survivors. Moss and co-workers (1979) reported that, in a population of 978 subjects with a definite or suspected MI, annual mortality was significantly greater in those patients with complex VPBs compared to those without these forms. One of the most persuasive studies was reported by Ruberman and co-workers of the Health Insurance Plan (HIP) of New York (1981). After a 5-year follow-up of 1,739 men with at least one MI, they observed that complex arrhythmia significantly increased the risk of sudden death. The 5-year mortality in those without VPBs was 5%, but it was 25% in those with repetitive or early VPBs. The presence of any other VPB was associated with a 12% mortality. The risk of sudden death was constant during each year after the base-line observation. Bigger and co-workers (1981) reached similar conclusions and reported that the presence of VT increased the mortality to 38% during the 1st year after a myocardial infarction, while mortality was only 12% when VT was absent. The conclusion of both these studies is that the presence of repetitive arrhythmia, especially VT, or Lown grade 4B, is an independent risk factor for sudden cardiac death.

Systematic Approach to Drug Therapy

It may be concluded that the risk of sudden death has a strong association with the presence of repetitive ventricular activity and not simple VPBs. It seems logical, therefore, to target antiarrhythmic drug therapy at suppression of these forms of arrhythmia, if those at risk are to be protected against a fatal arrhythmia. Empiric therapy is doomed to failure, as is evident from the negative results of the many randomized antiarrhythmic drug trials in post-MI patients. This concept is also confirmed by data from the Seattle Heart Watch Program (Schaffer and Cobb, 1975). In this program, over 75% of patients who had a second episode out-of-hospital sudden death were receiving antiarrhythmic drugs at the time of recurrence. If the patient is to be protected, an effective and well tolerated drug must be selected, mandating individualization of therapy. Unfortunately, drug selection is a tedious task and there are no clinical or electrophysiologic guidelines that permit

Table 19-5 Systematic Approach to Arrhythmia Management.

Phase 0	Control period: data collection.
Phase 1	Acute drug testing: rapid screening for drug efficacy.
Phase 2	Short term maintenance: evaluate drug efficacy and patient tolerance.
Phase 3	Long term therapy: outpatient management.

the easy identification of a drug that will suppress arrhythmia in an individual patient. Therefore, a systematic approach to drug therapy is essential. We have developed such an approach for drug selection which includes four phases of study (Lown et al., 1980) (Table 19-5).

A. Phase 0

Phase 0 represents a control period during which base-line data about type and frequency of arrhythmia are obtained. Studies include 48 h of ambulatory monitoring and exercise testing on a motorized treadmill adhering to a Bruce protocol. Once the type, density, and reproducibility of the ventricular arrhythmia are established, a decision is made to pursue either a noninvasive or invasive method for drug evaluation. If frequent and reproducible arrhythmia is present, repeat monitoring and exercise testing are utilized for assessment of drug effect. If arrhythmia is either infrequent or nonreproducible, invasive electrophsyiologic testing is employed to provoke repetitive activity.

B. Phase 1

Phase 1 acute drug testing (Gaughan et al., 1976; Podrid and Lown, 1977) is a rapid screening technique to identify drugs that are effective for arrhythmia suppression. This involves the oral administration of a large dose of drug, generally one-half of the standard daily dose. In our experience, this will establish a ''therapeutic'' blood level within 1–2 h. The patient is continuously monitored for 3 h, permitting observation of the drug effect (Fig. 19-2). Low level activity is performed with bicycle ergometry prior to drug administration and each hour thereafter as an additional means of evaluating drug effect. If the patient is undergoing electrophysiologic testing (Fig. 19-3), this is repeated 2 h after drug administration. Blood samples are obtained for drug concentration and ECG rhythm strips are recorded for measurement of intervals.

C. Phase 2

Phase 2, short term maintenance, involves the use of the drug or combination of drugs which was effective and well tolerated during phase 1 acute drug testing.

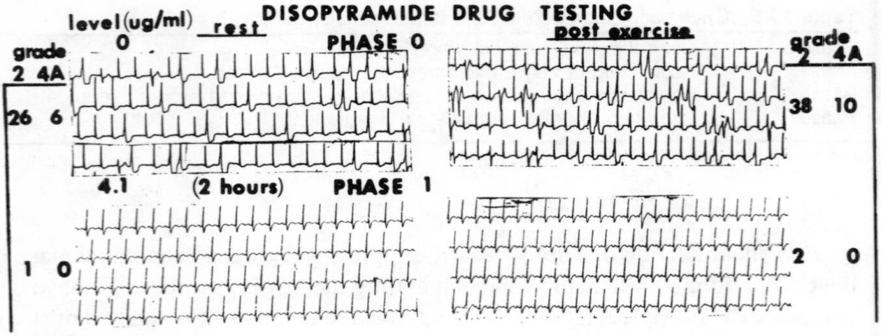

19-2 Acute drug test with disopyramide. During phase 0 control studies, frequent ventricular premature beats (grade 2) and couplets are present at rest and after exercise on a bicycle. Two hours after administration of disopyramide (300 mg), arrhythmia is virtually eliminated.

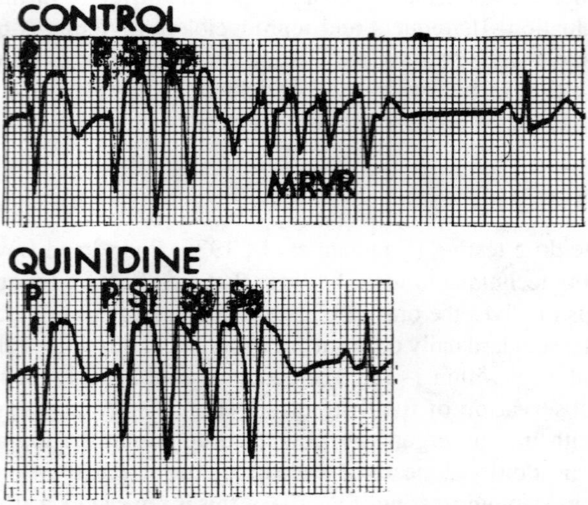

19-3 Drug testing utilizing electrophysiologic testing. During control, three extrastimuli (S_1, S_2, S_3) during a paced (P) rhythm provoke nonsustained ventricular tachycardia (five multiple repetitive responses). After a single dose of quinidine (600 mg), three extrastimuli fail to provoke arrhythmia.

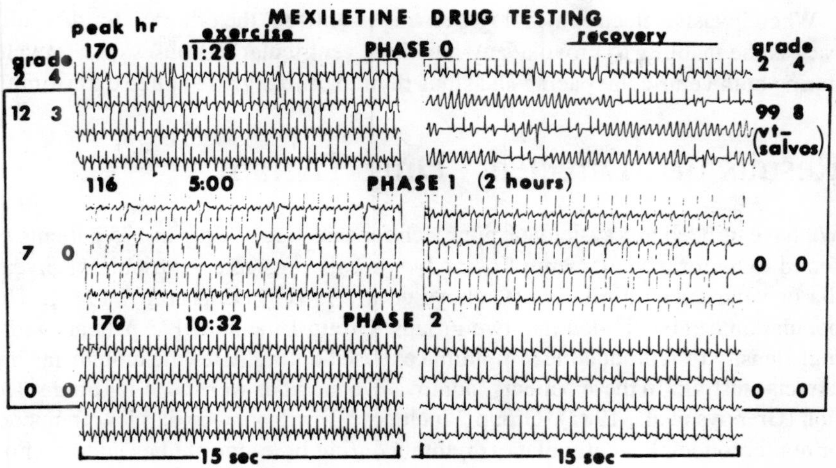

19-4 Response to mexiletine. During control studies, exercise on a treadmill provokes frequent ventricular premature beats (grade 2) and repetitive forms (grade 4). Salvos of ventricular tachycardia (VT) occur in recovery. During phase 1 acute drug testing with mexiletine (400 mg), including 5 min of bicycle ergometry, there is a marked reduction in ventricular arrhythmias and abolition of VT. After 3 days of therapy (phase 2), arrhythmia continues to be suppressed at rest and during a repeat exercise on a treadmill.

Evaluation of efficacy is with repeated monitoring and exercise testing or electrophysiologic study (Fig. 19-4). Blood is obtained for determination of drug concentration.

D. Phase 3

Phase 3 involves long term maintenance with the one or more agents judged to be effective during phase 2. Patients are seen every 3–6 months with monitoring and exercise testing repeated on a regular basis.

One of the major controversies involves criteria for drug efficacy. It has been our philosophy and practice to eliminate repetitive early forms while being less concerned about the frequency of simple VPBs. The criteria we have established reflect this point of view.

When noninvasive methods are employed, the drug is judged effective if the following criteria are met during both ambulatory monitoring and exercise testing.

1. Elimination of salvos of VT.
2. $\geq$90% reduction in couplets.
3. $\geq$50% decrease in VPB frequency.

When invasive electrophysiologic testing is utilized, the criterion for drug efficacy is the inability to provoke any repetitive ventricular responses of >2 cycles during both ventricular pacing and sinus rhythm utilizing up to three extrastimuli.

Results of "Directed" Drug Therapy

We have utilized this systematic approach for selection of drug in 175 patients referred to us for management of hemodynamically unstable ventricular tachycardia or ventricular fibrillation (Graboys et al., 1982; Podrid et al., 1983). This population can be divided into two groups. Group 1 includes 123 patients with a high density of reproducible arrhythmia exposed during base-line monitoring and exercise testing. In these patients, noninvasive methods were used for drug selection (Graboys et al., 1982). Group 2 includes 52 patients who had low frequency or nonreproducible ventricular arrhythmia during base-line studies and in whom electrophysiologic testing was employed (Podrid et al., 1983). Except for the presence of frequent and reproducible arrhythmia, there were no differences between these two groups in age, sex, underlying heart disease, left ventricular dysfunction, extent of disease, presenting arrhythmia, or previous drug therapy.

Repetitive forms of ventricular arrhythmia (primarily salvos of VT, or Lown grade 4B) were suppressed by antiarrhythmic drugs in 98 of 123 group 1 patients (79.7%), while in 25 patients, VT was still present despite therapy with an antiarrhythmic agent felt to be the most effective. In the whole group, there were 23 sudden deaths during a 29.6-month follow-up or an 8.2% annual mortality.

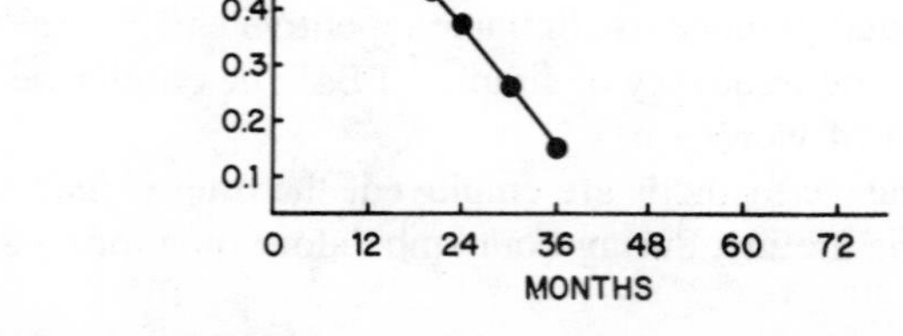

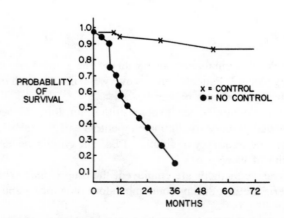

19-5 Sudden cardiac death among 123 patients treated with antiarrhythmic drugs selected noninvasively. In the patients deemed controlled (X), annual sudden death mortality was 2.3% compared to 43.6% among those not deemed controlled (•).

Among the 98 patients deemed controlled, only six died suddenly during a follow-up period of 31.5 months, yielding a 2.3% yearly sudden death mortality. There were 17 sudden deaths among the 25 not deemed controlled, representing a 43.6% annual sudden death mortality (Fig. 19-5). There were no differences in type or extent of heart disease or presence of left ventricular dysfunction between those controlled and not controlled. The only difference was in the presence or absence of salvos of VT while receiving antiarrhythmic drugs.

The results of therapy in the group 2 patients are similar. Seven of the 52 patients did not have inducible arrhythmia and were discharged without antiarrhythmic drugs. All are still alive. Of the remaining 45 patients, 36 (80%) were controlled with antiarrhythmic drugs. Only one patient (2.8%) has had a recurrence after an average follow-up of 22 months. In contrast, five of the nine patients (56%) not controlled have had a recurrence during the follow-up period. It can be concluded from these studies that a careful and systematic evaluation of antiarrhythmic drugs is essential for selection of an effective agent which suppresses spontaneously occurring or electrophysiologically induced repetitive ventricular arrhythmia. If repetitive ventricular arrhythmia is eliminated, survival is improved. Nondirected or empiric therapy is ineffective, but a medical program established as outlined is successful.

There are several other reports that support these findings, although drug selection in these was guided with electrophysiologic testing. Ruskin and co-workers (1980) reported on 31 sudden death survivors, 25 of whom had inducible arrhythmia during electrophysiologic testing. As with our studies, the criterion for drug efficacy was the inability to provoke >2 repetitive responses. In 19 patients, an effective therapeutic program was established; none of these patients died suddenly during an average follow-up of 15 months. Three of the six patients who still had inducible arrhythmia died suddenly. Similar results were reported by Horowitz and co-workers (1978). Nine patients were discharged on an effective drug; only one had a recurrence after 12 months. In contrast, 8 of 11 discharged on a drug that was partially effective or ineffective had recurrence of arrhythmia. Mason and Winkle (1978) reported similar results in a group of 21 patients. Although protocols for electrophysiologic study vary among different centers, the concept unifying these reports is the prevention of inducible repetitive activity. If nonsustained or sustained VT can not be induced while the patient is receiving an antiarrhythmic drug, arrhythmia does not recur. It should be emphasized that all the patients in these studies have survived an episode of serious arrhythmia documented to be VT or VF. Such patients have therefore identified themselves as being at high risk for a recurrence. It is not yet established that these results can be applied to the much larger group of patients with coronary artery disease who have not had sudden death. The prevention of serious tachyarrhythmia requires simple and noninvasive screening techniques to identify those at risk so that antiarrhythmic therapy can be appropriately instituted.

Conclusion

When a patient has had a serious and sustained ventricular tachyarrhythmia, recurrence can be prevented by antiarrhythmic drugs which have been judged effective after a careful and systematic evaluation. It has not been established if these agents will prevent the occurrence of these arrhythmias in patients after an MI or in those patients with coronary artery disease but no MI. Studies using antiarrhythmic drugs in patients after an MI have been uniformly disappointing. However, these trials did not attempt to identify those patients with complex or repetitive arrhythmia who have an enhanced risk of sudden death. Treatment was empiric using a single agent and fixed dose. There was no attempt to guide therapy by the suppression of ventricular ectopy. There is now substantial evidence that if complex or repetitive arrhythmia can be suppressed, survival is improved. It is likely that suppression of these arrhythmias in those with underlying heart disease will prevent the occurrence of sudden death. The major challenge, therefore, is the identification of the patient at risk for VT or VF before this occurs so that therapy can be initiated. There is a pressing need to develop a noninvasive strategy that can be employed widely to screen large numbers of patients and expose those requiring therapy.

Acknowledgment

Supported in part by grant HL-07776 from the National Heart, Lung and Blood Institute, National Institutes of Health, United States Public Health Service, Bethesda, Maryland.

References

Ahlmack, G., Saltre, H., and Korsgren, M. 1974. Reduction of sudden death after myocardial infarction. Lancet 2:1563.

Andersen, M.P., Frederikson, J., Jurgensen, H.G., Pedersen, F., Becksgaard, P., Hansen, D.A., Nielsen, B., Pederson-Bjergaard, and Rasmussen, J.L. 1974. Effect of alprenolol on mortality among patients with a definite or suspected acute myocardial infarction. Lancet 2:865–867.

Balcon, R., Jewitt, D.E., Davies, J.P.H., and Oran, S. 1966. A controlled trial of propranolol on acute myocardial infarction. Lancet 2:917–920.

Bennett, M.A., Wilner, J.M., and Pentecoste, B.C. 1970. Controlled trial of lignocaine in prophylaxis of ventricular arrhythmias complicating myocardial infarction. Lancet 2:909–911.

Beta Blocker Heart Attack Trial Research Group. 1982. A randomized trial of propranolol in patients with acute myocardial infarction. I. Mortality results. JAMA 247: 1707–1714.

Bigger, J.T., Weld, F.M., and Rolmitzky, L.M. 1981. Prevalence, characteristics and significance of ventricular tachycardia (three or more complexes) detected with ambulatory electrocardiographic recording in the late hospital phase of acute myocardial infarction. Am J Cardiol 48:815–823.

Bloomfield, S.S. Rombilt, D.W., Chou, T.L., and Fowler, N.O. 1971. Quinidine for prophylaxis of arrhythmia in acute myocardial infarction. N Engl J Med 285:967–986.

Calvert, A., Lown, B., and Gorlin, R. 1977. Ventricular premature beats and anatomically defined coronary heart disease. Am J Cardiol 39:627.

Campbell, R.W.F., Achuff, S.C., Pottage, A., Murray, A., Prescott, L.F., and Julian, D.G. 1979. Mexiletine in the prophylaxis of ventricular arrhythmias during acute myocardial infarction. J Cardiovasc Pharmacol 1:43–52.

Campbell, R.W.F., Bryson, L.G., Bailey, B.J., Murray, A., and Julian, D.G. 1979. Circulation 59 (suppl II) (abstr):70.

Chamberlain, D.R., Julian, D.G., Boyle, D.M., Jewitt, D.E., Campbell, R.W.F., and Shank, R.G. 1980. Oral mexiletine in high risk patients after myocardial infarction. Lancet 2:1324–1272.

Chopra, M.D., Thadane, U., Portal, R.W., and Abu, C.P. 1971. Lignocaine therapy for ventricular ectopic activity after acute myocardial infarction. A double blind trial. Br Med J 3:668–670.

Collaborative Group. 1971. Phenytoin after recovery from myocardial infarction. Controlled trial in 568 patients. Lancet 2:1055.

Gaughan, C.E., Lown, B., Lanigan, J., Voukydis, J., and Besser, W. 1976. Acute oral testing for determining antiarrhythmias drug efficacy. I. Quinidine. Am J Cardiol 38:677–684.

Graboys, T.B., Lown, B., Podrid, P.J., and DeSilva, R. 1982. Long term survival of patients with malignant ventricular arrhythmias treated with antiarrhythmic drugs. Am J Cardiol 50:437–443.

Hagemeijer, F., Van Durme, J.P., Bogaert, M., Lubsen, J., Grazer, B., and Hugenholz, P.G. 1978. Antiarrhythmic effectiveness of aprindine in patients with ventricular arrhythmias after an acute myocardial infarction. Circulation 57 (suppl II) (abstr):176.

Hansteen, V., Moinichin, E., Lorenstsen, E., Anderson, A., Stromo, L., Soiland, K., Dyrbekh, D., Refsum, A.M., Trumsdaal, A., Knudsen, K., Eika, C., Bakken, J., Smith, P., and Hoff, P.I. 1982. One year's treatment with propranolol after myocardial infarction. Preliminary report of the Norwegian Multicenter Trial. Br Med J 284:155–160.

Hinkle, L.E., Carver, S.T., and Stevens, M. 1969. The frequency of asymptomatic disturbances of cardiac rhythm and conduction in middle aged men. Am J Cardiol 24:629–650.

Hjalmarsen, P., Herlitz, J., Malek, I., Rydén, L., Vedin, A., Waldenstrom, A., Wedel, H., Elmfeldt, D., Holmberg, S., Nyberg, G., Swedberg, K., Waagstein, F., Waldenstrom, J., Wilhelmsen, L., and Wilhelmsson, C. 1981. Effect on mortality of metoprolol in acute myocardial infarction. Lancet 2:823–826.

Holmberg, S., and Bergman, H. 1967. Prophylactic quinidine treatment in myocardial infarction. Acta Med Scand 181:297–304.

Horowitz, L.N., Josephson, M.E., Farshidi, A., Spielman, S., Michelson, E.L., and Greenspan, A.M. 1978. Recurrent sustained ventricular tachycardia. III. Role of the electrophysiologic study in the selection of antiarrhythmic regimens. Circulation 58:986–997.

Hugenholtz, P.G., Hagemeijer, F., Lubsen, J., Glazer, B., VanDurmer, J.P., and Bogaert, M.G. 1978. One year follow-up in patients with persistant ventricular dysrhythmias after myocardial infarction treated with aprindine or placebo. In: E. Sandoe, D.G. Julian, and J.W. Bell, eds. Management of Ventricular Tachycardia Role of Mexiletine. pp. 572–604. Excerpta Medica.

Hunt, D., Sloman, G., Christie, D., and Pennington, C. 1977. Changing patterns and mortality of acute myocardial infarction in a coronary care unit. Br Med J 1:795.

Jennings, G., Jones, M.B.A., Besterman, E.M.M., Model, D.G., Turner, P.P., and Kidner, P.H. 1976. Oral disopyramide in prophylaxis of arrhythmias following myocardial infarction. Lancet 1:51–54.

Jones, D.T., Kostuk, W.J., and Gunton, R.W. 1974. Prophylactic quinidine for the prevention of arrhythmias after acute myocardial infarction. Am J Cardiol 33:655–666.

Julian, D.G., Jackson, F.S., Prescott, R.J., and Szekeley, P. 1982. Controlled trial of sotalol of one year after myocardial infarction. Lancet 1:1142–1147.

Koch Weser, J., Klein, S.W., Foo-Canto, L.L., Kastor, J.A., and DeSanctis, R.W. 1969. Antiarrhythmic prophylaxis with procainamide on acute myocardial infarction. N Engl J Med 281:1253–1260.

Kosowsky, B.D., Taylor, J., Lown, B., and Ritchie, R.F. 1973. Long term use of procainamide following acute myocardial infarction. Circulation 47:1204–1210.

Lie, K.J., Wellens, H.J., VanChampell, F.S., and Durrer, D. 1974. Lidocaine in the prevention of primary ventricular fibrillation. A double blind randomized study of 212 consecutive patients. N Engl J Med 291:1324–1326.

Lown, B. 1979. Sudden cardiac death. The major challenge confronting contemporary cardiology. Am J Cardiol 43:313–328.

Lown, B., Calvert, A.C., Armington, R., and Ryan, M. 1975. Monitoring for serious arrhythmias and high risk of sudden death. Circulation 51 (suppl III):189–198.

Lown, B., Podrid, P.J., DeSilva, R.A., and Graboys, T.B. 1980. Sudden cardiac death. Management of the patient at risk. Curr Prob Cardiol 4 (no. 12):1–62.

Lown, B., and Ruberman, W. 1970. The concept of precoronary care. Mod Concepts Cardiovasc Dis 39:97–102.

Lown, B., and Vassaux, C. 1968. Lidocaine in acute myocardial infarction. Am Heart J 76:586.

Lown, B., and Wolf, M. 1971. Approaches to sudden death from coronary heart disease. Circulation 44:130–142.

Mason, J., and Winkle, R. 1978. Electrode catheter arrhythmia induction in the selection and assessment of antiarrhythmic drug therapy on recurrent ventricular tachycardia. Circulation 58:971–985.

Morgensen, L. 1970. Ventricular tachyarrhythmias and lignocaine prophylaxis in acute myocardial infarction. Acta Med Scand (suppl 513):1–80.

Moss, A.J., Davis, H.T., DeCamilla, J., and Bayer, L.W. 1979. Ventricular ectopic beats and their relation to sudden and nonsudden cardiac death after myocardial infarction. Circulation 60:998–1003.

Moss, A.J., DeCamilla, J., Davis, H., and Bayer, L. 1976. The early posthospital phase of myocardial infarction. Circulation 54: 58–64.

Multicenter International Study. 1977. Reduction in mortality after myocardial infarction with long term beta adrenoceptor blockade. Br Med J 2:419–421.

Multicenter Trial. 1966. Propranolol in acute myocardial infarction. Lancet 2:1435–1437.

Norris, R.M., Laughey, D.E., and Scott, P.J. 1968. Trial of propranolol in acute myocardial infarction. Br Med J 2:398–400.

Norwegian Multicenter Study Group. 1981. Timolol induced reduction in mortality and reinfarction in patients surviving acute myocardial infarction. N Engl J Med 304: 801–807.

Peter, T., Ross, D., Duffield, A., Luxton, M., Harper, R., Hunt, D., and Sloman, G. 1978. Effect on survival after myocardial infarction of long term treatment with phenytoin. Br Heart J 42:1356–1360.

Pitt, A., Lipp, H., and Anderson, S.T. 1970. Lignocaine given prophylactically to patients with acute myocardial infarction. Lancet 1:612–616.

Podrid, P.J., and Lown, B. 1978. Selection of an antiarrhythmic drug to protect against ventricular fibrillation. In: Proceedings of the First US-USSR Symposium on Sudden Death. Yalta, October 3–5, 1977. p. 259. DHEW Publication No. (NIH) 78–1470.

Podrid, P.H., Schoeneberger, A., Lown, B., Lampert, S., Matos, J., Porterfield, J., Raeder, E., and Corrigan, E. 1983. Use of nonsustained ventricular tachycardia as a guide to antiarrhythmic drug therapy in patients with malignant ventricular arrhythmia. Am Heart J 105:181–188.

Ruberman, W., Weinblatt, E., Goldberg, J.D., Frank, L.W., Chaudhary, B.S., and Shapiro, S. 1981. Ventricular premature complexes and sudden death after myocardial infarction. Circulation 64:297–305.

Ruskin, J.N., DiMarco, J., and Garan, H. 1980. Out of hospital cardiac arrest. Electrophysiologic observations and selection of long term antiarrhythmic therapy. N Engl J. Med 303:607–613.

Rydén, L., Arnman, D., Conradson, T.B., Hofvendahl, S., Mortensen, O., and Sondegard, P. 1980. Prophylaxis of ventricular tachyarrhythmias with intravenous and oral tocainide in patients with and recovering from acute myocardial infarction. Am Heart J 100:1006–1012.

Schaffer, W.A., and Cobb, L.A. 1975. Recurrent ventricular fibrillation and modes of death in survivors of out of hospital ventricular fibrillation. N Engl J Med 293:259–262.

Snow, P.J.D., and Manc, M.D., 1965. Effect of propranolol in myocardial infarction. Lancet 2:551–555.

Stamler, J. 1962. Cardiovascular diseases in the United States. Am J Cardiol 10:319–326.

Taylor, S.H., Silke, B., Ebbutt, A., Sutton, G.C., Prout, B.J., and Burley, D.M. 1982. A long term prevention study with oxyprenolol in coronary heart disease. N Engl J Med 307:1293–1301.

Valentine, P.A., Freur, J.L., Mashford, M.L., and Sloman, J.G. 1974. Lidocaine in the prevention of sudden death in the pre-hospital phase of acute infarction. A double blind study. N Engl J Med 291:1327–1331.

Velebit, V., Podrid, P.J., Cohen, B., Lown, B., and Graboys, T.B. 1982. Aggravation and provocation of ventricular arrhythmias by antiarrhythmic drugs. Circulation 65:886–894.

Vismara, L.A., Amsterdam, E.A., and Mason, D.T. 1975. Relation of ventricular arrhythmias in the late phase of acute myocardial infarction to sudden death after hospital discharge. Am J Med 59:6–12.

Wilhelmsson, C., Wilhelmsen, L., Vedin, J.A., Tibblin, G., and Werko, L. 1974. Reduction of sudden death after myocardial infarction by treatment with alprenolol. Lancet 2:1157–1160.

Zainal, N., Griffiths, J.W., Carmichael, D.J.S., Besterman, E.M.M., Kidner, P.H., Gillham, A.D., and Scimmers. G.D. 1977. Oral disopyramide for the prevention of arrhythmias in patients with acute myocardial infarction admitted to open wards. Lancet 2:887–889.

EDITOR'S NOTES

Therapeutic Applications of Antiarrhythmic Drugs: Cutting Across Drug Classifications

Can antiarrhythmic drugs prevent sudden death? That is the question posed by Dr. Podrid in the concluding chapter of this monograph. While this question is not new, unfortunately the answer can still not be definitive for most clinical situations. Most studies using antiarrhythmic drugs in patients who are at risk of sudden death have shown either equivocal or negative results. In fact, in several of such studies, up to 70% of patients were on existing antiarrhythmic drug therapy at the time of sudden death. However, many of these studies were also considered to be flawed either by design or patient characteristics. The more recent beta-blocker trials have shown conclusive evidence that sudden cardiac death can be prevented in the postinfarction population; however, whether this is an antiarrhythmic effect or anti-ischemic effect remains to be resolved. The most encouraging results have been reported in the evaluation of patients with recurrent life-threatening arrhythmias. Using a systemic approach to drug therapy, either with Dr. Podrid's techniques, which are outlined in his chapter, or electrophysiologic techniques previously described, the reduction in sudden death among patients at highest risk for this complication of organic heart disease is excellent. At least two approaches to selection of drug therapy in this population of patients have been advocated and supported by positive clinical results. The appropriate treatment modality for individual patients remains to be determined, but it is clear that in patients at highest risk of sudden death, antiarrhythmic drug intervention can successfully alter this prognosis.

An additional question concerns patients with ventricular arrhythmias and organic heart disease who are not at high risk of sudden death (i.e., greater than 20% of patients with organic heart disease per year). These patients have not been studied to determine whether antiarrhythmic drugs can prevent sudden death. The bulk of clinical data would suggest that these drugs are not effective in this group; however, as we have previously mentioned, adequate trials are really not available. Since the number of patients with potentially life-threatening arrhythmias is so large, the impact of such a study would be tremendous. With the advent of newer agents, this question assumes even greater priority. In this regard, issues raised by Dr. Podrid beyond efficacy, such as proarrhythmic effects and drug-related toxicity, must be prospectively considered.

Without question, the issue of preventing sudden death remains as a major challenge, both to the clinician and the drug industry, to develop effective therapeutic agents. As potentially useful agents are proposed for clinical research, a major task will also be to develop discriminating and meaningful clinical trials to evaluate such agents. Considering the staggering statistics of lives claimed on a minute-to-minute basis by electrophysiologic abnormalities leading to sudden death, research in both the basic and clinical setting must continue at a high intensity.

Index

Italics indicate figures and tables